Thieme

Ultrasound of Abdominal Transplantation

Paul S. Sidhu, B.Sc., M.B.B.S., M.R.C.P., F.R.C.R., D.T.M.&H.
Consultant Radiologist
Department of Radiology
Kings College Hospital
Denmark Hill
London, UK

Grant M. Baxter, M.B.Ch.B., F.R.C.R.
Department of Radiology
Western Infirmary NHS Trust
Dumbarton Road
Glasgow, UK

With contributions by

Syed Babar
Richard C. Beese
Matthew Bowles
Richard Edwards
David Hamilton
Bryon C. Jaques
Rahul M. Jindal
Ajai Khanna
Heather Maxwell
Jon G. Moss
Suzanne Norris
N.H. Patel
Mohamed Rela
R. Stuart C. Rodger
Suzanne M. Ryan
Ashley Shaw
Z. Song
Jonathan Tibballs

257 Illustrations

Thieme
Stuttgart · New York

Library of Congress Cataloging-in-Publication Data
is available from the publisher.

Sponsored by

acuson
A Siemens Company

All clinical images acquired with
The Acuson Sequoia® Ultrasound Platform

Important Note: Medicine is an ever-changing science undergoing continual development. Research and clinical experience are continually expanding our knowledge, in particular our knowledge of proper treatment and drug therapy. Insofar as this book mentions any dosage or application, readers may rest assured that the authors, editors, and publishers have made every effort to ensure that such references are in accordance with **the state of knowledge at the time of production of the book.**
Nevertheless, this does not involve, imply, or express any guarantee or responsibility on the part of the publishers in respect of any dosage instructions and forms of application stated in the book. Every user is requested to examine carefully the manufacturers' leaflets accompanying each drug and to check, if necessary in consultation with a physician or specialist, whether the dosage schedules mentioned therein or the contraindications stated by the manufacturers differ from the statements made in the present book. Such examination is particularly important with drugs that are either rarely used or have been newly released on the market. Every dosage schedule or every form of application used is entirely at the user's own risk and responsibility. The authors and publishers request every user to report to the publishers any discrepancies or inaccuracies noticed.

Cover drawing by Martina Berge, Erbach

Typesetting by primustype R. Hurler GmbH,
D-73274 Notzingen, Typeset on Textline

Printed in Germany by Staudigl, Donauwörth

ISBN 3-13-131081-2 (GTV)
ISBN 1-58890-101-7 (TNY) 1 2 3 4 5

Preface

Over the last two decades, renal and liver transplantation have become an almost routine aspect of medicine, allowing the replacement of an organ to be part of the treatment option for a number of previously fatal diseases. This has come about through advances in immunosuppressive therapy, better surgical techniques, improved medical and nursing care, and technical advances associated with anesthetic equipment. In this overall scene of advancement, imaging has allowed assessment of disease processes that were but a figment of the imagination 20 years ago. However, it has not been due (as perceived mainly by nonradiologists) to advances in CT and MRI. Rather, ultrasound has led the way, particularly color Doppler ultrasound. Ultrasound, especially in the postoperative period, allows complications to be detected early, often at the bedside, directing further imaging or altering medical management. Ultrasound is nearly always the preliminary investigation prior to radiological intervention and is often used to direct the interventional procedure itself, bypassing the need for CT and MRI.

To this effect, we have compiled a textbook that specifically deals with the role of ultrasound in imaging of abdominal transplantation. We have included chapters on intervention in liver and renal transplantation, as an ultrasound examination invariably leads directly to intervention, often by the same radiologist. It is important that the radiologist has an overview of transplantation and works as a "team member" with physicians, surgeons, and nursing staff. To this end, we have included an overview of the medical work-up to transplantation, medical diseases that result in the need for transplantation, and the surgical technique itself. An understanding of the surgical technique is of paramount importance to a successful ultrasound examination. We have also included chapters on pancreatic and small bowel transplantation, currently in its infancy but likely to become more important in the future.

Our aim was to produce a textbook with high-quality images that allows the practicing radiologist, sonographer, or physician insight into techniques of transplant ultrasound and that gives, as well, an overview of medical and surgical management of transplantation.

Paul S. Sidhu and Grant M. Baxter

Acknowledgments

To publish a book requires a lot of effort, enthusiasm, and dedication across many fronts. Our thanks go to the many unnamed heroes involved in the successful completion of our project, i.e. in illustrating, typesetting, designing, and printing this book. Although we cannot thank them all individually in print, we do wish to thank them collectively for their cooperation and tireless effort.

In addition, the editors are aware of the time and effort invested by each of the contributors and would like to thank them for this. We apologize for pushing (encouraging) them on occasion but we are proud to say that this is the only book we have worked upon that has truly run to schedule.

Finally we would like to acknowledge the support of our families during this project and the work and guidance of our secretaries, Mrs. R. McQueen and Mrs. P. Warren, who essentially manage our working lives as efficiently as we will let them, take the strain of many of the organizational aspects of our job, and still manage to smile. Last but not least, we would like to thank our wives, Nuala and Monica, together with our children (Matthew, Joshua, Jamie, Francesca, and Gianluca), all of whom have been reluctantly understanding!

Contributors

Syed Babar, D.M.R.D., F.R.C.R.
Specialist Radiology Registrar
Department of Radiology
Royal Free Hospital
London, United Kingdom

Richard C. Beese, B.Sc., M.B.B.S., M.R.C.P., F.R.C.R.
Consultant Radiologist
Department of Radiology
Kings College Hospital
Denmark Hill
London, United Kingdom

Matthew Bowles, M.S., F.R.C.S. (Gen)
Consultant Transplant Surgeon
Institute of Liver Studies
Kings College Hospital
Denmark Hill
London, United Kingdom

Richard Edwards, M.R.C.P., F.R.C.R.
Consultant Interventional Radiologist
Gartnavel General Hospital
Glasgow, United Kingdom

David Hamilton, Ph.D., F.R.C.S.
Consultant Surgeon
Transplant Unit
Western Infirmary
Glasgow, United Kingdom

Bryon C. Jaques, F.R.C.S., Ph.D.
Consultant Transplant and Hepatobiliary Surgeon
Freeman Hospital
Newcastle upon Tyne, United Kingdom

Rahul M. Jindal, M.D., F.R.C.S., M.Sc.
Director of Transplantation
Department of Surgery
University of Glasgow
Glasgow, United Kingdom

Ajai Khanna, M.D., Ph.D., F.R.C.S. (Eng. & Glasg.)
Director Pediatric Abdominal Transplantation
and Transplantation Research
Department of Surgery
University of California San Diego
and Childrens Hospital and Health Center of San Diego
San Diego, California, USA

Heather Maxwell, M.D.
Consultant Paediatric Nephrologist
Renal Day Unit
Royal Hospital for Sick Children
Yorkhill NHS Trust
Yorkhill
Glasgow, United Kingdom

Jon G. Moss, F.R.C.S., F.R.C.R.
Consultant Interventional Radiologist
Gartnavel General Hospital
Glasgow, United Kingdom

Suzanne Norris, M.R.C.P.I., Ph.D.
Consultant Hepatologist
Institute of Liver Studies
Kings College Hospital
Denmark Hill
London, United Kingdom

N.H. Patel, M.D.
Associate Professor of Radiology
Department of Radiology
Indiana University
Indianapolis, Indiana, USA

Mohamed Rela, M.S., F.R.C.S.
Consultant Transplant Surgeon
Institute of Liver Studies
Kings College Hospital
Denmark Hill
London, United Kingdom

R. Stuart C. Rodger, M.B.Ch.B., F.R.C.P.
Consultant Physician/Honorary Clinical
Senior Lecturer
Renal Unit
Western Infirmary
Glasgow, United Kingdom

Suzanne M. Ryan,
M.B.B.Ch.B.A.O., M.R.C.P.I., F.R.C.R.
Specialist Radiology Registrar
Department of Radiology
Kings College Hospital
Denmark Hill
London, United Kingdom

Ashley Shaw, M.B.Ch.B., M.R.C.P.
Specialist Radiology Registrar
Department of Radiology
Kings College Hospital
Denmark Hill, London
United Kingdom

Z. Song, M.D.
Research Assistant
Department of Surgery
University of Glasgow
Glasgow, United Kingdom

Jonathan Tibballs, M.R.C.P., F.R.C.R., F.R.A.N.Z.C.R.
Consultant Radiologist
Department of Radiology
Royal Free Hospital
London, United Kingdom

Contents

Section 1: Introduction

Section 2: Renal Transplantation

Section 3: Liver Transplantation

Section 4: Multivisceral Transplantation

Historical Introduction: The Impact of Imaging on Organ Transplantation

D. Hamilton

Only within our generation has rapid progress been made towards the ancient goal of replacement of human tissue with that from other persons or animals. In the early part of the twentieth century the first step was taken when the old myth that allografts (i.e., grafts from other persons, then called homografts) could succeed by chance was replaced by a realization that there was a consistent barrier to transplantation. Until that time many skin and organ fragment transplants had been attempted in the absence of any objective measurement of outcome, and the large and contradictory literature on such early grafting used subjective, fallible outcome criteria. When improved understanding of immunology emerged and biochemical and radiological assessments appeared in the 1930s, the approach to transplantation had a more rigorous basis. These aids were not, however, exploited until the modern continuous period of organ transplantation in the 1950s, when management became increasingly dependent not only on laboratory medicine, but also on a growing variety of imaging techniques and radiological interventions. There is debate on the importance of immunology in day-to-day transplantation. There is no doubting the value of modern imaging in transplant management.
The long road to the initial successes of the 1960s will be reviewed in this chapter.

Ancient Times

The tales of ancient civilizations record stories of magical repair and replacement of lost parts of the human body. Since it was believed that the inflicting of disease and illness and even the outcomes after injury were in the hands of the gods, it was also assumed that supernatural forces could replace lost tissue, and folklore in all parts of the world has remarkably similar tales of magical transplantation.[1] Helpful attributes in the recipient—notably a state of grace or personal worth—were also thought to enable the treatment to succeed. In the Christian tradition, for example, there were numerous such incidents, and at the medieval shrines in Britain, notably Canterbury, miraculous restoration of lost tissues was often reported. The best-known legend was the miracle involving the posthumous intervention by the twins St. Cosmas and St. Damian, who replaced a cancerous leg with that of a recently dead donor.

Skin Grafting: Flaps and Other Methods

A limited amount of conventional plastic surgery had been carried out in India in ancient times, as recorded in the Hindu text *Susruta* of the third century BCE. It described sensible, practical, reconstruction procedures for cosmetic defects, particularly following the mutilating punishments of the time. But thereafter, the ancient texts are silent on such matters, and the illustrious Greek medical writers in particular accorded little place to surgery in general, and even less to plastic surgical operations.[2]

The Middle Ages

Belief in divine healing declined and conventional surgery improved in the Middle Ages. The first known revival of the ancient Indian restorative surgery came in Italy in the fourteenth century, when it was discovered in use by skilled surgical empirics in Sicily, and through them the methods came to the notice of the talented trained surgeons of the northern Italian towns and universities. Gaspare Tagliacozzi (1545–1599) is remembered for accepting these techniques into the academic canon, and in his great text on plastic surgery of the face he usually employed an upper arm flap to replace nose or lip defects.[3] He taught that success with allografts was prevented by the "power and force of individuality." But it was a method ahead of its time, and the first of the early English surgical texts, James Cooke's *The Marrow of Surgery*, largely ignored the subject of replacement of tissue. There was a remarkable discontinuity in the practice of plastic surgery, and European surgical texts ignored the earlier sensible plastic surgery of Tagliacozzi until 1800, although enthusiastic surgeons made occasional claims for successful reimplantation of large detached bits of skin or parts of the nose or fingers.
Some nonclinical interest in tissue grafting was kept up by the protobiologists of the day, and the new pragmatic Royal Society in mid-seventeenth century London took some interest in transplantation of skin, teeth, and blood, but their experiments and results were inconclusive, leaving them to concentrate, with success, on the physical sciences instead. In Holland, shortly after, Trembley worked with the tiny pond pol-

yps and showed their remarkable powers of fusion from divided parts of each other. This success encouraged uncritical allografting later.

John Hunter made a number of valuable observations in tissue transfer in the later 1700s.[4] He judged graft success by successful adhesion of donor tissue and noted importantly that donor tissue must be grafted quickly after removal, otherwise the "life principle" in the graft, as he called it, would be lost. His grafts, notably of testis, deceptively appeared vascularized and viable, but he wisely claimed only tissue survival rather than functional replacement. He also taught that separated tissues would unite by the host and donor blood vessels rejoining in continuity, rather than ingrowth of new vessels from the host rescuing the graft. This faulty theoretical background, as seen in Hunter's writings, came from a familiar source, horticulture, where the trunks of one species then and now are routinely merged with desirable roots from another to give an improved hybrid. He noted that "as the transplanting of teeth is very similar to the ingrafting of trees, I thought the term 'scion' for the graft might be transferred from gardening to surgery." He also coined the word "transplant" for his procedure.

But he misled surgery for a while with his claims for successful human tooth transplantation. Using human donor teeth, Hunter obtained a reputation for tooth transplants, but the practice revealed for the first time the danger of introducing disease from a graft, when he found that syphilis had been transferred along with a tooth grafted from an apparently normal donor. The first ethical concerns with transplantation also arose at this time, since paid tooth donation was in use, and Joseph Fox complained for the first time that this "involved a defect of the moral principle."

Plastic Surgery Revives

In London, in 1812, closely following the ancient Indian methods, Carpue treated two patients whose noses were damaged by syphilis or trauma. It was an ancient treatment, observed by some colonists, that had mysteriously returned to favor.[5] Surgical repair by plastic surgery was rapidly being taken up in the increasingly specialized clinics of Germany and France, though Britain lagged behind. Modern methods of plastic surgery were further encouraged in the mid-nineteenth century when Jacques-Louis Reverdin in Paris, aided by the teachings of Paul Bert and others in Claude Bernard's circle at the Collège de France, finally put free skin grafting on a sound basis and into regular use. Reverdin used multiple, thin, small "lambeaux cutanes"[6] rather than single full-thickness grafts—and his grafts succeeded because new vessels grew in quickly. Bert also noted that that animal donor tissue vitality is temperature-dependent. He made the first demonstration that grafts would survive better if cooled, and explained this as retention of Hunter's "life principle."

This new simple method of split skin grafting spread rapidly from Paris, and enthusiasts in London and Boston adapted it and published on the method. These new "pinch" grafts met a need for covering the many unhealed ulcers, burns, and open wounds of the time. Ironically, the success with thin skin autografts seemed to encourage the uncritical use of skin grafts from unrelated human donors and even the use of xenografts, and a confused scientific literature emerged in the late 1800s describing the treatment of many human ills by the use of fragments of spleen, pancreas, nerve, thyroid, and ovary taken from other humans or animals.[7]

Vascular Surgery

Attempts at organ grafting progressed when the first attempts at human and experimental vascular surgery started in 1900. Crude suturing with the stitching materials then available without the support of anticoagulation gave dismal results, but Payr's intravascular metal stents allowed occasional restoration of vessel flow, and successful experimental organ transplants were reported by a number of distinguished surgical scientists in Vienna.

The modern era of vascular surgery commenced when members of the Department of Surgery in Lyon, headed by Mathieu Jaboulay, devised better methods and materials for vascular anastomosis. Jaboulay carried out the first ever attempt at a human kidney transplant in 1906, but the xenografts placed in the arm of patients in chronic renal failure never functioned.[8]

Attached to Jaboulay's department in Lyon was the young Alexis Carrel, and he improved the departmental vascular surgical methods by adding triangulation and the use of finer nonpenetrating stitches. Carrel, out of favor in France, emigrated to Chicago and with Charles Guthrie published a remarkable series of technical papers on organ transplantation and preservation. He later moved to the Rockefeller Institute and established routine success with autografting of the dog kidney, but showed a consistent barrier to kidney allografting with this model. For this work he become America's first Nobel Prize winner in 1912.[9] He had realized that an immunological response might be involved in graft loss. Noticing that his Rockefeller Institute colleague, James B. Murphy, had shown that the allograft reaction was mediated by the lymphocyte and that this reaction was delayed by radiation or the drug benzol,[10] Carrel suggested that this might be the way forward; but, remarkably, the matter was not taken any further for about 40 years.

The Hesitant 1920s and 1930s

These empirical approaches to successful transplantation by Carrel were forgotten. The famous European surgical and scientific centers such as Vienna never recovered after the war, and in British surgery little in the way of experimental or research studies emerged. The scattered transplant events in this period included the repetition of Carrel's work confirming the success of kidney autografts and the failure of allografts by Mann's group at the Mayo Clinic. The fruitful suggestions made earlier regarding immunosuppression were ignored. In the Soviet Union, Yu Yu Voronoy, a Ukrainian surgeon, built on his laboratory experience by performing the first human cadaveric allograft kidney transplant in 1933. The organ, which was removed 6 h after the donor's death, was transplanted into an anuric victim of mercury poisoning. Because of a blood group incompatibility, and donor damage, little function was obtained.[11]

Not only was the interwar period a time of clinical stagnation, but the existence of allograft rejection was often denied and surgeons, ignoring Carrel's documented ground rules, uncritically returned to the use of allograft skin once more. The American surgeon Holman deplored the publicity given to such surgery, saying "grafting is frequently employed to the wondering delight of the credulous laity. That such grafting is most often a failure seems little known." Matters became even less creditable when gland grafters such as Thorek and Lydston in Chicago and Voronoff in Paris used human and animal testis grafts to treat the ills of old age and escaped immediate ridicule.[12]

Sense Returns

One man took a patient long-term interest in allografting at this time, and built quietly on Carrel and Murphy's sound analysis. Leo Loeb, the St. Louis pathologist, reaffirmed the ubiquity of allograft reaction in all species, and emphasized that the graft response was not in place simply to outwit surgeons, but suggested other roles for this mysterious mechanism.[13] Loeb's other influence was on the local St. Louis surgeons Barrett Brown and Earl Padgett, and these men convinced the surgical world yet again that allografts, particularly of the skin, invariably rejected. The work by C.C. Little at Bar Harbor, Maine, and others at Cold Spring Harbor, New York, gave the subject greater precision when they developed the use of inbred mice for transplantation studies. Reluctantly, these pioneer breeders accepted Loeb's dictum that the only test of final inbreeding is graft acceptance. In London, Peter Gorer was encouraged by his mentor J.B.S. Haldane to study tissue transplantation using these new mouse strains, and he not only detected a powerful controlling antigen in mouse tumor rejection, but also demonstrated that an antibody arose after such tumor loss. His work was carried forward with precision by Snell at Bar Harbor, who introduced the term "histocompatibility genes" to explain this phenomenon. When Snell and Gorer finally met in 1946, they found themselves in broad agreement on their views of transplantation immunology.[14]

ROENTGEN RAYS.

PHOTOGRAPHY OF RENAL CALCULUS; DESCRIPTION OF AN ADJUSTABLE MODIFICATION IN THE FOCUS TUBE.

BY JOHN MACINTYRE, M.B., C.M. GLASG., F.R.S. EDIN.

DURING the past four months I have, at the request of several physicians and surgeons, tried to photograph some cases in which the presence of renal calculus was suggested by the symptoms present. A control experiment was first undertaken at the request of Dr. Finlayson, who gave me a

Fig. 1.**1** The first report of imaging of kidney pathology came from Macintyre's pioneering *Lancet* 1896 paper from Glasgow, which described detection of (but did not illustrate) a renal calculus by the new Roentgen rays

Organ Assessment and Imaging Commence

During this lull in transplantation matters, methods of assessing kidney function—radiological and biochemical—emerged in the 1930s. Imaging of the kidney may be said to have started earlier in Glasgow, when Lord Kelvin told John Macintyre, a physician and hospital "electrician" at Glasgow's Royal Infirmary, of Roentgen's work, and in 1896, one year after this discovery, Macintyre managed for the first time to obtain a faint image of a human renal calculus in the body[15] (Fig. 1.**1**). This image, never published, involved a 12-minute exposure. A faint renal outline could also be seen. Soon after, in 1897, aided by the new cystoscopes, Tuffier passed a radiopaque catheter up the ureter and plain films showed its outline and hence the course of the ureter. The first human genitourinary contrast studies were performed by Wülff in 1904 when he used a bismuth mixture to outline the bladder. In the following year Voelcker and von Lichtenberg injected collargol—a silver colloid—through a ureteric catheter to obtain the first retrograde pyelograms, and for the first time were able to display obstructive and neoplastic changes. These silver preparations were fairly toxic and were soon replaced by iodine compounds. Kelling reported at this time that accidental retroperitoneal insufflations of air could be used deliberately to outline the kidneys and adjacent structures. The method had its uses, but eventually was restricted to study of the adrenal glands.

The birth of nephrography involved an episode of classical serendipity.[16] In 1923, Rowntree at the Mayo Clinic learned from a colleague working in the syphilis clinic that when intravenous sodium iodide was used in therapy it gave a faint outline of the kidney and ureter. In Hamburg at this time, systematic production of new chemicals based on salvarsan was carried out by the chemist Binz, and these compounds were tested for their value in kidney infections by Moses Swick, then a visiting research worker from New York. Like the Mayo group, he noted good visualization of the uri-

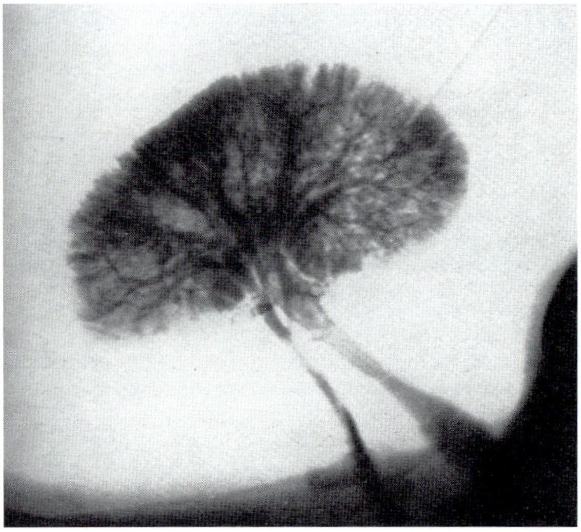

Fig. 1.**2** The first imaging of a transplanted kidney came in 1950 during Dempster's experimental dog kidney transplants. The organ was placed in the neck and for imaging was exteriorized prior to intra-arterial contrast injection. (From Dempster,[19] by courtesy of the *British Journal of Surgery*)

nary tract, and this eventually resulted in the use of Uroselectan and related compounds for kidney studies. Imaging of the kidney had by now become crucial in clinical medicine. However, there was a delay before transplantation emerged and was able to employ this assistance.

Understanding the Rejection Mechanism

A paper from Glasgow in 1942, by Gibson and Medawar, is considered to mark the beginning of our modern continuous interest in tissue transplantation. The war in Europe prompted the Medical Research Council in Britain to study burns sustained by aviators, and the Council gave support to young Peter Medawar at Oxford to pursue this work, including a visit to the busy Burns Unit at Glasgow's Royal Infirmary, where he joined plastic surgeon Tom Gibson in making a series of classic observations firmly concluding that there was an immunological basis for transplant failure. Medawar and Gibson's study showed that a "second set" of skin grafts was more quickly lost than the first, and they proposed that antibody rather than a cellular mechanism was at work.
Medawar's later painstaking animal studies further highlighted the serious challenge of tissue rejection. Neither matching by blood group, the use of young or cultured skin, nor superior surgical skill affected graft survival. Nor were the interesting "privileged sites" of the brain and anterior chamber of the eye of much practical use. In Britain, surgeons were generally uninterested, but American plastic surgeons posted to Britain during the war, like John Converse and Barrett Brown, did pursue transplantation interests on their return home, and later organized the first international conferences on the subject.[17]

Experimental Kidney Transplants

In the early 1950s, Morten Simonsen of Denmark[18] and William Dempster in London[19] revived interest in experimental dog kidney transplantation, neglected since Carrel's era. For the first time, combined radiological, biochemical, and histological studies were made. These two investigators confirmed that loss of the organ was an immunological event, but noted the absence of any antibody appearing in response to the rejection. Simonsen, impressed with the lymphocytes in the rejecting graft, went on thereafter to study the graft-versus-host reaction in simpler systems. Dempster tried immunosuppression in his dog kidney model with both radiation and the new biological agent cortisone, but was unlucky since this animal's immune system is insensitive to the first and the second is toxic to dogs. Simonsen did not image the transplanted kidney directly, but Dempster did, swinging the whole functioning organ on its pedicle out of the neck to obtain the first transplant arteriogram after direct intra-arterial injection of contrast (Fig. 1.**2**).
Medawar, previously alone in his interest in transplantation immunology, extended his group at this time in the late 1940s. The work of Avrion Mitchison, Medawar's pupil, revealed that the powerful allograft rejection mechanism was, after all, a lymphocyte-mediated one, making it unnecessary to find the transplantation antibody.

Boston and Paris

Though it was generally thought that the powerful innate rejection mechanism could not be surmounted, a series of human cadaveric kidney transplants were carried out in the early 1950s in Paris and Boston.[20] These attempts were encouraged by the availability of the pioneering artificial kidneys, which were then mainly used to treat acute renal failure, but could treat patients with hopeless established failure for a short time.[21] The growing use of such dialysis was made possible by the revolution in clinical biochemistry at the time, which gave a steadily increasing range of rapid estimations, particularly of electrolytes. These kidney transplants without immunosuppression, though controversial, did serve to show that the human operation was technically possible, and that thrombosis of the graft was surprisingly uncommon. Occasional kidney survival in both centers in this series gave hope for the future. No kidney allograft urograms were published from this era, although one retrograde pyelogram was carried out on a briefly functioning graft in the Boston series, the kidney being, as usual, placed in the thigh (Fig. 1.**3**).

Back to the Laboratory

This series ended with no immediate hope for successful long-term kidney transplant function, and the mood was to wait for a solution from the scientists. Medawar meantime was reluctantly diverted from his small-animal work into looking at the veterinarian's old problem of distinguishing at birth between identical and nonidentical cattle twins. He was puzzled to find that skin grafts between nonidentical pairs did not reject. He proposed that the animals were "tolerant" of each other's skin as a result of the prenatal exchange of blood.[22] This hypothesis was supported by similar suggestions from Ray Owen of Wisconsin and Macfarlane Burnet of Australia. Experimental work by Brent in Medawar's team followed, and was rewarded by a Nobel Prize for Medawar and Burnet in 1960. This discovery gave renewed hope for allografting in general, and, in particular, hopes for the practical use of this powerful, specific method of attaining graft survival.

The mysterious indolent-looking lymphocyte was now the center of attention and gave up many of its secrets. Its life span was found to be long rather than short, and Gowans showed that it recirculated and was thus suited to a role in systemic sensitization and memory. This cell soon could be induced to perform remarkably in vitro.[23] The apparently functionless thymus gained a central role as producer of the T-cell lymphocyte, now distinguished neatly from the bone marrow-derived B lymphocyte.

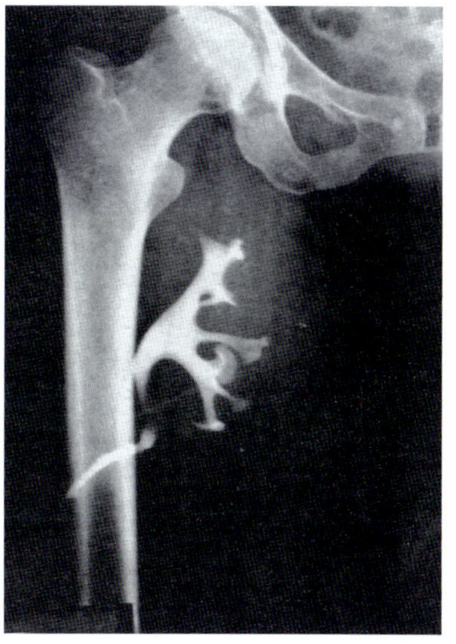

Fig. 1.**3** The first imaging of a human kidney allograft came in 1953 in one of the nonimmunosuppressed Boston cadaver transplant series. The graft was placed in the thigh, and during brief function a retrograde pyelogram showed normal appearances in the ureter and pelvis. (By courtesy of *Annals of Surgery*)

The Twins

The Boston team ceased attempts at unmodified human kidney allografts in 1954, but shortly after, a patient in chronic renal failure appeared together with a healthy twin and was transplanted with success. The team then carried out a series of kidney grafts from identical twin donors to sick twin sibs with remarkable results from 1954 to 1958.[24] Not all these cases went smoothly, and about 25% had ureteric problems. These complications were diagnosed clinically without radiological assistance and managed with a policy of early reexploration when malfunction occurred. With this sustained function in a kidney graft for the first time, radiology was used occasionally, and the first intravenous urogram (IVU) in a successful well-established transplant was published from Boston (Fig. 1.**4**) A number of fears regarding the function of the transplant proved groundless, and even the denervated ureter performed well on "cine-fluorography" studies. During this series the Boston team encountered multiple arteries in the donor twin, but, after debate, decided against arteriography of the donor kidneys. However, from about 1963, led by Starzl's policy, the pioneer units increasingly felt that the risks of angiography were less than the problems posed by multiple arteries, and aortography was used to anticipate such variants and to choose which kidney to take in any donor. Occasionally, when the vasculature was simple, the imaging would pick up debatable abnormalities in one kidney and the less favorable organ could then be taken. If several willing donors were available, the offer from those with arterial abnormalities on angiography could be turned down. From the late 1960s, all living donor kidney vasculature was assessed radiologically in this way, with the addition in the 1970s of selective arterial catheterization as a finer check on the anatomy, until magnetic resonance (MR) angiography replaced it in the 1990s.

The operations involving the twins were invaluable in providing nonimmunological lessons. The noninnervated kidney and ureter functioned better than predicted by skeptics, chronic sepsis and fibrosis were absent, and even one kidney could return all biochemical and hematological values to normal. The donors showed no long-term harm, but the original disease could return quickly in the transplant. New levels of informed consent were required. Above all, the twin transplants sustained researchers' hopes for ultimate success.

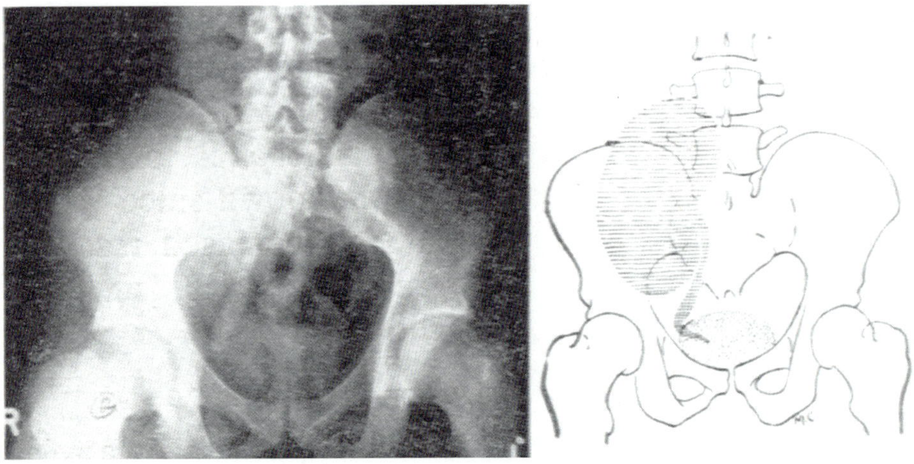

Fig. 1.**4** The first renogram showing a functioning human transplanted kidney, reported in 1955. The kidney was transplanted from one twin to another and placed for the first time in the pelvic position. (By courtesy of the *Journal of the American Medical Association*)

Radiation and Immunosuppression

Study of the biological effects of radiation revived during the Cold War in the 1940s and 1950s and means of protection against lethal exposure were developed, notably by bone marrow infusion from allogeneic sources. The surviving animals were thus chimeric and could accept grafts from the marrow donors.[25] This offered a method, albeit using a blunt weapon, akin to neonatal tolerance induction, which could be applied to adult human grafting.

John Merrill, the Boston nephrologist, had been involved in all the Brigham transplants and considered that the radiation/marrow rescue regimen might be useful in transplantation; after studying the experimental methods at Harwell and elsewhere, he began to use a similar protocol in human patients. Lethal radiation and bone marrow were used only for the first two of the new Boston transplant series, since it was found that radiation was an unexpectedly powerful human immunosuppressive agent when used alone. This unpredictable and uncontrollable approach required special isolation facilities and was used in Boston, Paris, and Edinburgh from 1958 to 1962. In each center there were one or two long-term survivals of kidneys after irradiation, but otherwise kidney loss and mortality were high.

Chemical Immunosuppression

The effects of the poison nitrogen mustard had been identified in World War I and included a capacity to destroy white cells and reduce antibody production. This agent and its interesting effects had largely been forgotten until it emerged again as a reserve defense weapon in World War II, when accidents in Europe, and experimental studies in America, confirmed its destructive effect on bone marrow. The crude drug was used in the therapy of leukemia, and in 1953 a better derivative was produced, the purine analogue 6-mercaptopurine (6-MP). In 1958, Schwartz and Dameshek showed the immunosuppressive potential of the drug. This was noticed by Roy Calne in London, who had been working on dog kidney grafting and had confirmed Dempster's failure to prolong kidney survival with steroids and radiation. Calne now obtained modest dog kidney survival with the new agent,[26] as did Zukoski in Richmond.[27] Calne continued this work during a Boston visit, where he studied variants on the drug 6-MP prepared by George Hitchings and Gertrude Elion of Burroughs Wellcome, who were to share a Nobel Prize in 1988 with James Black. Calne found with Joseph Murray that among the variants, BW57–322, later known as azathioprine (Imuran), was less toxic and more effective in dog kidney transplantation, although mortality was high and the surviving kidneys few. Murray, who had also been the activist in the Boston twin transplants, was awarded a Nobel Prize in 1992. Using azathioprine, human kidney transplants were attempted in London, Boston, Paris, and elsewhere. The results were poor, with high mortality, but were an improvement on radiation. The mood changed in 1963 when Starzl in Denver noted that the neglected steroids, when added to azathioprine, could reverse human kidney rejection episodes when all else had failed.[28] Starzl then was the first to use steroids as "prophylaxis," i.e., from the time of transplant, together with azathioprine, with remarkable results.

Initially huge doses of steroids were used in the immediate post-transplantation period, on the "more is better" approach, but the dose could be reduced in the weeks following grafting, as the mysterious "adaptation" emerged and rejection became less active. Good renal function in a few cases allowed imaging of the allograft kidney for the first time, and the cases of lower ureteric obstruction or leakage encountered were diagnosed with urography. The first detailed report of imaging showing the now-familiar lower ureteric obstruction came in Starzl's pioneering series, in patient LD 39 in 1964. This historic case was dealt with by surgical reimplantation, and this became normal practice until the rise of interventional radiological methods in the 1980s (Fig. 1.5). Nonfunction in cadaveric organs was a common puzzle at this time and was investigated with angiography, eventually differentiating between thrombosis, rejection, and acute tubular necrosis. It was soon realized that blood group incompatibility could destroy a kidney, as could preformed antibodies from an earlier blood transfusion. The radiological appearances of such hyperacute rejection before and after removal were characteristic (Fig. 1.6). Optimism was the mood of the times; Reemstma, Hume, and Starzl even attempted monkey kidney transplants in humans and these achieved short-term function. Starzl started, stopped, and restarted liver transplantation in Denver,[29] and was joined in this effort by Roy Calne in Cambridge in the 1970s, with jointly increasing confidence in the technique. Second kidney transplants after failure of a first graft were also found to do surprisingly well.

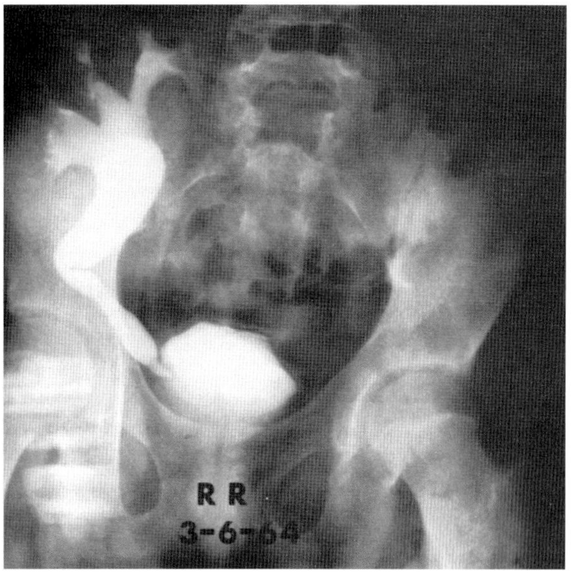

Fig. 1.5 The first reported urogram image showing hydronephrosis in a cadaveric kidney transplant. (From Starzl[28])

Dialysis Back-Up

Belding Scribner's invention of the simple plastic arteriovenous shunt in 1960 (the same year as the introduction of azathioprine) resulted in increased availability of the artificial kidney and regular dialysis, and in keeping such access open, a little niche use of "shuntograms" emerged to explain any technical malfunction.[30] Regular availability of dialysis had a revolutionary impact and made patients fitter than before for transplant surgery. Hemodialysis was available immediately after transplantation but not after loss of the kidney, making heroic and prolonged antirejection efforts necessary. For new patients, both treatments, dialysis and transplantation, were available in the mid-1960s, and each modality had its advocates. The choice was a difficult one for patients and their advisors, and only when regular dialysis became available in the late 1960s after transplant rejection did the two modalities become an integrated renal replacement service.

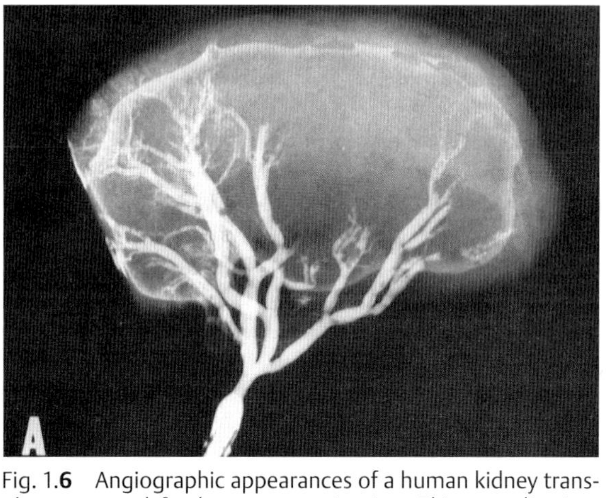

Fig. 1.6 Angiographic appearances of a human kidney transplant removed for hyperacute rejection. This complication, found in the early 1960s, was later prevented by pretransplant serological testing. (From Starzl[28])

Tissue Typing

Another product of the optimistic 1960s was the emergence of tissue typing methods for human organ allografting. Previously, Gorer and Snell had shown the presence of histocompatibility genes in laboratory animals, but in 1958, Jean Dausset (later to be awarded a Nobel Prize with George Snell) started to unravel the hugely complex human system. This work had immediate use in pointing to the best donor in a family of willing living related donors, but in spite of massive investment and development, it was to fail in the main aim of ensuring routine success with cadaveric organs.[31]

The Heart Transplants and After

The short-term success of Christiaan Barnard's first case in 1967[32] liberated others immediately from any constraints, and many heart transplant operations were quickly reported from other centers. Few of the grafts showed long-term survival. This initial period of heart transplantation lasted for a little over a year, ceasing in the spring of 1969, occasioned by poor results and serious complications. Adverse public reaction to some aspects of these transplants was added to by the controversial use of the first prototype artificial heart. Calls from both outside and inside the profession for a moratorium in heart transplantation fol-

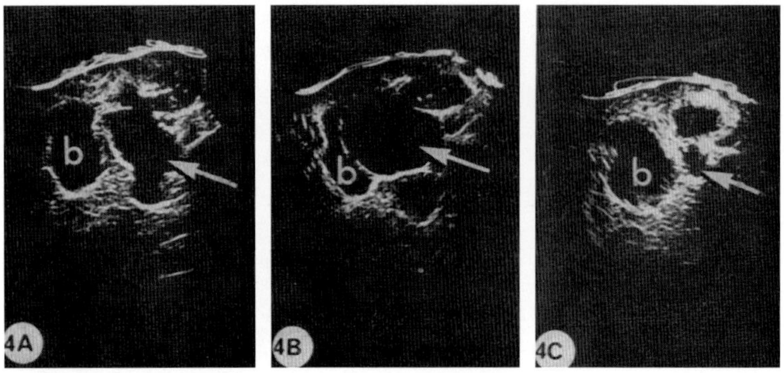

Fig. 1.**7** Early use of ultrasound in 1975 to detect lymphoceles adjacent to transplanted kidneys. (From Morley et al.[28])

lowed, and had to be heeded. The call was yet again for basic immunological studies rather than clinical experimentation—a view welcomed by immunologists but also by many clinicians, concerned if only about the cost of such surgery compared with providing for more obvious, simple needs. The study of the ethics of transplantation and of the day-to-day allocation of scarce resources emerged as serious growth areas in academia at this time.[33]

Formal acknowledgment of "brain death" started in 1968 with a set of suggestions from Harvard University for judging when to terminate pointless ventilatory support of irrecoverable patients.[34] Whilst primarily a matter for intensive care policy, the changes helped the service of transplantation, and by the mid-1970s these or similar guidelines were widely used to allow the use of organs from "heart-beating donors." Cautious governments followed medical opinion, not by new laws on the diagnosis of death, but simply by encouraging national clinical guidelines for brain death diagnosis and, separately, standardizing the procedures for brain-death donation.[35] This innovation was crucial in improving the quality of organs and ensuring the necessary immediate function of liver and heart grafts—a feature not required for kidneys. A low-key program of human heart transplantation was allowed in Shumway's unit in California, and by 1972 his results had reached a 50% one-year survival, aided by regular intracardiac biopsy guided by radiology.[36] In the United Kingdom and elsewhere, heart transplant operations were nervously resumed in 1980, 12 years after the first attempts, such was the sensitivity of the times.

The 1970s

The two-drug regimen of steroids and azathioprine was the mainstay of therapy for almost 20 years, with temporary enthusiasm for other drugs and modalities. Cytotoxic drugs such as cyclophosphamide, biological agents such as antilymphocyte serum, and interventions such as thoracic duct drainage, macrophage blockade, and targeted radiation all had brief vogues. It was a time of clinical refinements, including improved quality of donor kidneys and the use of better preservation methods.[37] This period was a time of consolidation and steadily improving results largely based on clinical experience and a major input from radiology and the laboratories.

Isotope scanning with technetium (^{99m}Tc-DTPA) was being increasingly used in the postoperative period and gave reassurance that blood flow was normal during the period of nonfunction due to acute tubular necrosis, common at this time before the general acceptance of brain death and heart-beating donation. The scans gave characteristic patterns of isotope accumulation inside or outside the transplant when the ureter was blocked or leaking. Total thrombosis was easily diagnosed, and intermediate appearances were seen in rejection.

However, the 1970s also brought the rise of ultrasonography—simple, economical, safe and repeatable—which was to emerge in a key role and partly displace isotope scanning.[38] The centers with experience in interpreting the difficult early abdominal scans were first to report regular imaging of kidney grafts and, although the hope was to detect early swelling and hence rejection of the graft, one surprise was the incidence of large, unsuspected lymphoceles accumulating adjacent to transplanted kidneys[39] (Fig. 1.**7**). Angiography still had an important role once it was realized that the transplant kidney could develop a form of renal artery stenosis. This appeared a short distance from the suture line at about six months after the operation, and was suspected from the clinical findings of deteriorating function plus hypertension which was difficult to control. The first report of this complication came in 1971, and posed an unpleasant surgical challenge,[40] for the donor renal artery is encased in fibrous tissue, yet, when reached, has a friable wall, and the tricky surgery requires interruption of blood flow to the kidney.

Prolonged use of modest doses of steroids was found to give rise to many problems, notably infections, common and uncommon, all giving a radiological challenge.[41] A new form of bone disease appeared—avascular necrosis—which could be detected at an asymptomatic stage by regular skeletal surveys (Fig. 1.**8**) and which proved less of a problem when steroid dosage was reduced in the mid-1970s.[42] The appearance also

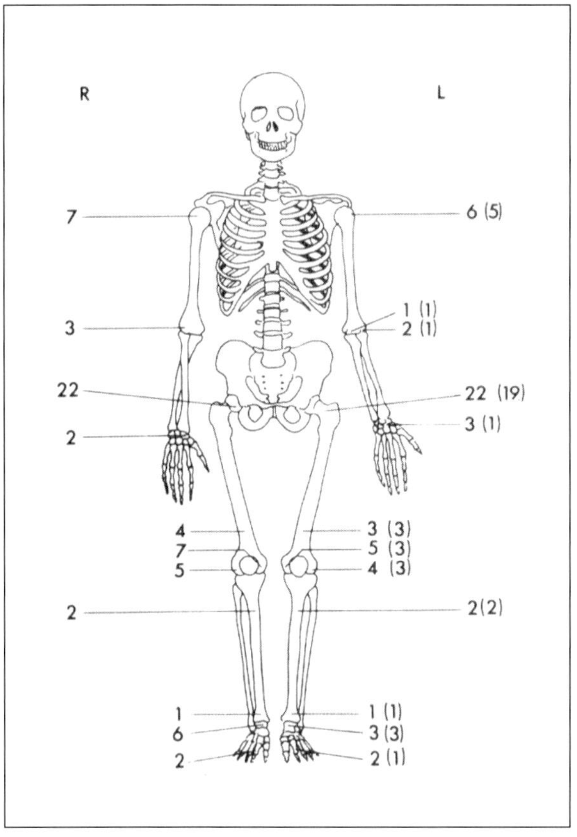

Fig. 1.**8** Detailed regular skeletal surveys detected widespread presymptomatic bone necrosis in kidney transplant patients in the high-dose steroid era of the 1970s. (From Davidson et al.[42])

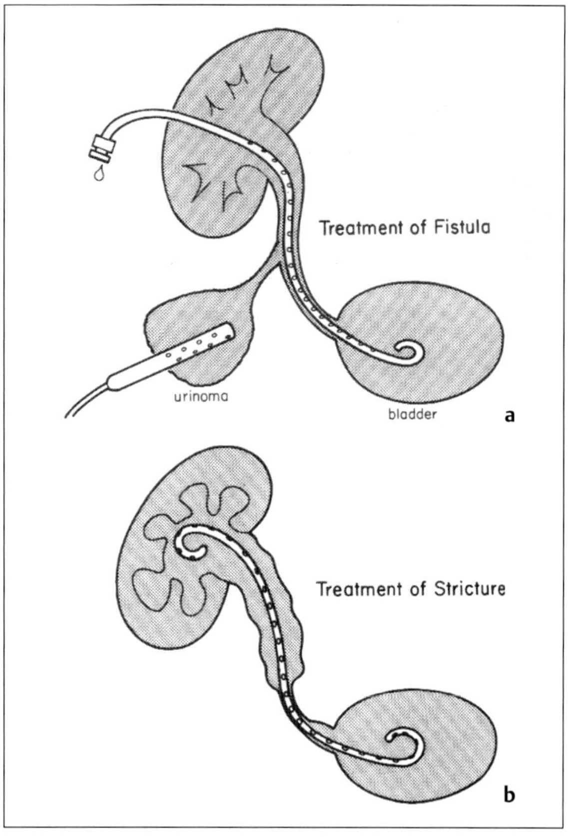

Fig. 1.**9** Interventional radiological methods from the 1980s enabled placement of an external nephrostomy or internal stents in kidney transplants with lower ureteric obstruction or leakage. (From Lieberman et al.[45])

of tumors in allograft recipients raised fundamental questions about tumor origin and surveillance by the immune system, and these de novo malignancies were studied from the first by the Denver Tumor Registry.

Cyclosporine

In the late 1970s, cyclosporine (known then as cyclosporine A, CsA) emerged during routine testing of fungal extracts for biological activity and was the first drug to challenge and replace the traditional core regimen of azathioprine and steroids.[43] It was a difficult drug to use, but with experience results improved, rejection episodes became less frequent and less abrupt, and it partly negated the effects of adverse tissue typing and prior blood transfusion. The search for methods for early diagnosis of rejection was put aside. As CsA was nephrotoxic, ultrasound-guided needle biopsy was increasingly required as a diagnostic method in graft dysfunction. CsA helped greatly to improve the results of heart, liver, and pancreas transplantation, elevating them into routine clinical services. As always, improved management skills, including use of each new imaging method, played a continuing role in the 1980s in the improving results of transplantation, in both graft and patient survival.

In the CsA era, ultrasound also came to have a dominant role in clinical organ transplant management. Regular surveillance of transplant kidneys by ultrasound, rather than occasional scans, was increasingly routine and valuable, and, importantly, picked up the early and late ureteric obstructions. Ultrasound also demonstrated urine leaks in the postoperative period at the new entry into the bladder or from ureteric necrosis. In this complication, cystograms were surprisingly unhelpful, and the anterior position of the new ureteric orifice made retrograde studies almost impossible.[44] Hematomas around kidneys and lymphoceles (which became commoner later with the third-generation immunosuppressants) were still routinely detected. Confidence with scanning led to the helpful diagnosis of hydronephrosis in transplanted organs, and accurate percutaneous nephrostomy placement soon followed in the 1980s (Fig. 1.**9**). Soon after, methods evolved in which double

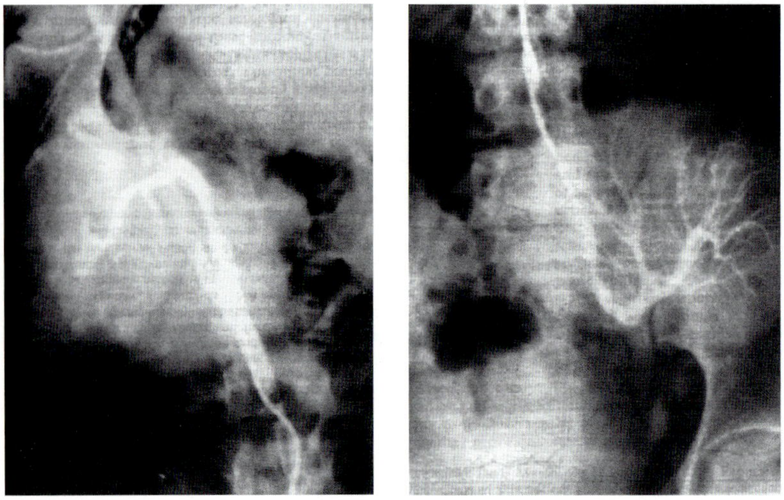

Fig. 1.**10** An early report from Glasgow in 1980 of the use of balloon dilatation for donor renal artery stenosis. (From Quin et al.,[51] by courtesy of the *British Medical Journal*)

pigtail stents could be passed into the transplant and left in situ from pelvis to bladder. These dealt with some early lower-end ureter blockages, with the stent being removed via the bladder later.[45]

The remarkable rise of interventional radiology in the 1990s added balloon dilatation to the management of lower ureteric strictures.[46] This simple noninvasive procedure importantly obviated the need for open reimplantation, a procedure associated with further complications and one notorious for consequent sepsis and mortality. The success of these methods of dealing with ureteric obstruction meant it was no longer necessary to leave the donor ureter long at the time of transplant in case it was required for reimplantation. Confident use of a short length of ureter from the start meant avoiding the use of the ischemia-prone lower end. Postoperative donor arterial suture line aneurysms were also detected by scanning before catastrophic rupture. The puzzle of the natural history of the little aneurysm on the donor renal artery (often associated with fatal cerebral berry aneurysms in the donor) was solved by demonstrating on serial ultrasound examinations that they neither enlarged nor ruptured. Also proving largely innocuous were the iatrogenic arteriovenous fistulae within the kidney following biopsy, detected by ultrasound. If they were suspected of bleeding, radiological embolization could be carried out, based on the knowledge that the intrarenal arteries are end arteries.[47] These therapeutic choices shifted the professional boundaries in transplant patient care.

Ultrasound also aided the study of native kidneys in patients with acute or chronic renal failure, notably revealing any immediately treatable lesion such as obstruction. Biopsy success increased when ultrasound guidance became feasible. From the 1970s onwards, scanning could make the important diagnosis of polycystic kidneys, a disease previously remarkably underdiagnosed, and if desired detect the presence of early cystic disease in the family. Ultrasound of kidneys in prospective living donors occasionally revealed unsuspected renal pathology. Lastly, ultrasound made possible prenatal diagnosis of some diseases requiring future transplantation, notably biliary atresia.

Isotope scanning of nonfunctioning kidneys was supplanted in the early 1980s by duplex Doppler ultrasonography,[48] to which was added color scanning in the 1990s,[49] and which easily detected thrombosis in the transplant vasculature. It could display variations in arterial and venous flow,[50] and this was particularly timely as renal vein thrombosis was becoming slightly commoner in the CsA era. This was not necessarily an effect of the new agent, but was perhaps related to other changes, including the higher viscosity resulting from erythropoietin use. With prompt surgery, venous blockage can be reversed, unlike the immediate graft loss with arterial occlusion. In addition, Doppler flow studies gave a pulsatility index, which when used sequentially gave an indication of overall graft dysfunction.

Donor artery stenosis was still an unpleasant surgical challenge. The early cumbersome dilatation equipment for peripheral vascular stenosis was soon used to avoid surgical intervention, and the first cases of balloon angioplasty of transplant renal arteries appeared in 1980[51] (Fig. 1.**10**). Noninvasive diagnosis by Doppler studies or MR angiography emerged and advances in interventional radiology meant that the lesions could be first imaged angiographically and then treated by balloon dilatation.[52] Recurrent stenoses were soon found to affect about 15 % of cases thus treated, and these could benefit from endoprosthesis stenting methods rather than repeated dilatation.

The 1990s

Further new immunosuppressant drugs emerged, and mycophenolate, tacrolimus, and sirolimus have found favor. With one-year graft survival reaching over 90 %, attention has moved from short-term survival figures to the longer-term influences of chronic rejection and the side effects of these agents, notably on cholesterol metabolism and diabetes provocation. Some agents have been found to have a niche use in special cases such as pancreatic islet transplantation.

From the 1980s, CT scanning added little to the routine management of intra-abdominal transplantation, but was invaluable in a range of miscellaneous postoperative diagnostic problems. The advent of routine MR angiography in the 1990s, on the other hand, gave the important capability to assess living related donor kidney vasculature noninvasively. In the widening range of patients considered for transplantation, whether as recipients or donors, co-morbidity was an increasing concern, and cardiac thallium scanning proved valuable in showing latent problems in those with obesity and diabetes.

Organ Supply

As the service of organ transplantation has become successful, the need has outstripped the supply of organs. In spite of publicity campaigns and donor drives initiated by governments and other agencies, in many countries in the developed world the donation of organs has risen only slowly in the 1980s and plateaued since. This failure to meet the ever-increasing need caused by safer transplantation and now offered to a wider age range of patients led to many initiatives, notably the use of slightly defective "marginal" donor organs, and a return to the use of non-heart-beating donors. In liver transplantation, splitting adult livers can give two grafts instead of one.

In developing countries there was often a high level of chronic renal failure, yet these nations had poorly developed dialysis facilities, low provision of intensive care, little cultural support for brain death (in spite of helpful proclamations by religious leaders of all persuasions) and hence few or no donor kidneys, hearts, or livers from this source. This huge need for kidneys led to an unstoppable growth in payments for purchase of unrelated kidney donation, in spite of stern warnings against the procedure by the authorities in developed countries.[53]

Xenografting

Accordingly, strategies for the use of animal donors returned to the agenda. Until the 1980s, discussion of future xenografting was based on the assumption that organs from primates would be used when more powerful immunosuppression methods appeared. The emergence in other fields of methods of genetic manipulation has made the closeness of species to man irrelevant and "discordant" species of suitable size can be considered, especially now that most monkey species are under protection. The pig—a robust breeder possibly free of any disease threat to humans—was involved in the first limited success obtained by adding DNA to the pig embryo, leading to the rearing of the first transgenic animals. In a period of rapid progress in basic biology, a number of alternative strategies quickly appeared, notably the potential for obtaining and modifying stem cells and cloning thereafter.[54] Immunogenicity of such organs, however, may only be reduced and not abolished, still leaving a need for immunosuppression.

The use of cloned identical animals as organ donors meant that the antigenicity of the future donor was known and cells available. This revived the old possibility of inducing tolerance by prenatal cell insertion of future donor lymphocyte-free cell suspensions into the human fetus, particularly if future consideration for transplantation is likely, as when prenatal biliary atresia is diagnosed or guided intervention in urological obstruction is carried out.

Imaging and intervention is, and will always be, the crucial partner of surgical organ transplantation.

■ *Summary points:*

Pioneer kidney transplants:

- Lyon 1906 – human xenograft attempt by Jaboulay
- Carrel's experimental transplants gain Nobel Prize 1912
- Ukraine 1933 – Voronoy's human allograft attempt for acute renal failure
- Boston and Paris in early 1950s – unimmunosuppressed human allografting
- Mid-1950s – Boston success with transplants between twins
- Late 1950s – Boston and Paris use radiation for immunosuppression
- From 1963 – success with Starzl's combined azathioprine and steroid regimen
- Late 1970s – Calne's introduction of cyclosporin A

Early radiology and the kidney:

- Macintyre in Glasgow in 1896 detects kidney stone with "Roentgen rays"
- Bismuth and collargol used in 1910s for bladder and ureteric imaging
- First nephrograms obtained 1923 with intravenous iodine compounds
- Mid-1950s – first urograms of functioning twin kidney transplants

Later radiology and the transplanted kidney:

- Early 1970s – isotope scanning for assessment of transplant function
- Mid 1970s – ultrasound scanning of kidney for local complications
- Early 1980s – duplex Doppler ultrasound imaging for transplant blood flow assessment
- Mid 1980s – interventional radiological management of ureteric complications

References

1. Tosatti B. Transplantation and reimplantation in the arts. Surgery 1974;75:389–97.
2. Patterson TJS. The Zeis index and history of plastic surgery, 900 BC–1863 AD. Baltimore: Williams & Wilkins; 1977.
3. Gnudi MT, Webster JP. The life and times of Gaspare Tagliacozzi. Milan: Hoepli; 1939.
4. Martin CE. John Hunter and tissue transplantation. Surg Gyn Obstet 1970;131:306–10.
5. Freshwater MF, Su CT, Hoopes JE. Joseph Constantine Carpue – first military plastic surgeon. Mil Med 1977;142:603–6.
6. Reverdin H. Jaques-Louis Reverdin (1842–1929). Aarau: Sauerlander; 1971.
7. Klasen HJ. History of free skin grafting: knowledge or empiricism? Springer-Verlag: Berlin; 1981.
8. Watts SH. The suture of blood vessels. Bull Johns Hopkins Hosp 1907;18:153–78.
9. Hamilton D. Alexis Carrel and the early days of tissue transplantation. Transplant Rev 1987:2;1–15.
10. Little CC. James Bumgardner Murphy. Biog Mem Natl Acad Sci 1960;34:183–203.
11. Hamilton D, Reid WA.Yu Yu Voronoi and the first human kidney allograft. Surg Gyn Obstet 1984;159:289–94.
12. Hamilton D. The monkey gland affair. London: Chatto and Windus; 1986.
13. Loeb L. The biological basis of individuality. Springfield: Thomas; 1945.
14. Medawar PB. Peter Gorer. Biog Mem Fell Roy Soc 1961;7:9–109.
15. Macintyre J. Photography of renal calculus. Lancet 1896;ii:118.
16. Bruwer AJ. Classical descriptions in diagnostic roentgenology. Springfield: Thomas; 1964.
17. Rogers BO. John Marquis Converse 1909–1981. Ann Plast Surg 1982;8:342–58.
18. Simonsen M. Biological incompatibility in kidney transplantation in dogs. II: Serological investigations. Acta Pathol Microbiol Scand 1953;32:1–84.
19. Dempster WJ. Kidney homotransplantation. Br J Surg 1953;40:447–65.
20. Starzl TE. France and the early history of organ transplantation. Perspect Biol Med 1993;37:35–47.
21. Hume DM, Merrill JP, Miller BF, Thorn GW. Experiences with renal homotransplantation: report of nine cases. J Clin Invest 1955;34:327–82.
22. Billingham RE, Lampkin GH, Medawar PB, Williams HL. Tolerance of homografts, twin diagnosis and the freemartin condition in cattle. Heredity 1952;6:201–12.
23. Ford WL. The lymphocyte. In: Wintrobe MM, editor. Blood, pure and eloquent. New York: McGraw; 1980.
24. Murray JE, Merrill JP, Harrison JH. Kidney transplantation between seven pairs of identical twins. Ann Surg 1958;148:343–59.
25. Barnes DWH, Loutit JE. Protective effects of implants of splenic tissue. Proc R Soc Med 1953;46:251.
26. Calne RY. The rejection of renal homografts: inhibition in dogs by 6- mercaptopurine. Lancet 1960;i:417–18.
27. Calne RY. The development of immunosuppressive therapy. Transplant Proc 1981;13(suppl 1):44–49.
28. Starzl TE. Experience in renal transplantation. Philadelphia: Saunders; 1964.
29. Starzl TE. Experience in hepatic transplantation. Philadelphia: Saunders; 1969.
30. Hughes K, Adams FG, Hamilton D. Radiology of haemodialysis access devices. Clin Radiol 1980;31:489–96.
31. Brent L. A history of transplantation immunology. London: Academic Press, 1977.
32. Barnard CN. The operation. A human cardiac transplant: an interim report of a successful operation performed at Groote Schuur Hospital Cape Town. S Afr Med J 1967;41:1271–4.
33. Scarce medical resources. Columbia Law Rev 1969;69:620–92.
34. A definition of irreversible coma. Report of the Ad Hoc Committee of the Harvard Medical School to examine the definition of brain death. JAMA 1968;205:337–40.
35. Cadaveric organs for transplantation. A code of practice drawn up by a working party on behalf of the Health Departments of Great Britain and Northern Ireland. HMSO 1979 (revised 1983).
36. Jamieson SW, Stinson EB, Shumway NE. Cardiac transplantation in 150 patients at Stanford University. Br Med J 1979;i:93–5.
37. Kissmeyer-Nielsen F, Olsen S, Peterson VP, Fjeldborg O. Hyperacute rejection of kidney allografts. Lancet 1966;ii:662–5.
38. Petrak J, Tilney NL, Smith EH, Williams JS, Vineyard GC. Ultrasound in renal transplantation. Ann Surg 1977;185:441–7.
39. Morley P, Barnett E, Bell PRF, Briggs KJ, Calman KC, Hamilton DN, Paton AM. Ultrasound in the diagnosis of fluid collections following renal transplantation. Clin Radiol 1975;26:199–207.
40. Morris PJ, Yadav RVS, Kincaid-Smith P, Anderton J, Hare WS, Johnson N, et al. Renal artery stenosis in renal transplantation. Med J Aust 1971;1:1255–8.
41. Harrington KD, Murray WR, Kountz SL, Belzer FO. Avascular necrosis of bone after renal transplantation. J Bone Joint Surg Am 1971;53A:203–15.
42. Davidson JK, Tsakiris D, Briggs JD, Junor BJR. Osteonecrosis and fractures following renal transplantation. Clin Radiol 1985;36:27–35.
43. Calne RY, White DJG, Thiru S, Evans DB, McMaster P, Dunn DC, et al. Cyclosporin A in patients receiving renal allografts from cadaveric donors. Lancet 1978;ii:1323–7.
44. McWhinnie DL, Bradley JA, Briggs JD, Galloway DJ, Kyle KF, Hamilton DN, et al. Early detection of obstructed ureter by ultrasound following renal transplantation. Proc Eur Dial Transplant Assoc 1983;20:320–4.
45. Lieberman RP, Glass NR, Crummy AB, Sollinger HW, Belzer FO. Nonoperative percutaneous management of urinary fistulas and strictures in transplantation. Surg Gynecol Obstet 1982;155:667–72.
46. Smith TP, Hunter DW, Letourneau JG. Urinary obstruction in renal transplants: diagnosis by antegrade pyelography and results of percutaneous treatment. AJR Am J Roentgenal 1988;151:507.
47. Stahelin H. Ciclosporin: historical background. Prog Allergy 1986;38:19–27.
48. Wood RFM, Nasmyth DG. Doppler ultrasound in the diagnosis of vascular occlusion in renal transplantation. Transplantation 1982;33:547–51.
49. Fobbe F, Dietzel M, Schwietzer G, et al. Monitoring of the transplanted kidney with angiodynography. Radiology 1987;165:100.
50. Baxter GM, Ireland H, Moss JG, Harden PN, Junor BJ, Rodger RS, Briggs JD. Colour Doppler ultrasound in renal artery stenosis: which Doppler index? Clin Radiol 1995;50:618–22.
51. Quinn RO, Hamilton D, Briggs JD, Junor BJ, Semple PF. Transluminal dilatation of transplant renal artery stenosis. Br Med J 1980;ii:196–8.
52. Greenstein S, Verstandig A, McLean G, Dafoe DC, Burke DR, Meranze SG, et al. Percutaneous transluminal angioplasty. Transplantation 1987;43:29–32.
53. The Council of the Transplantation Society. Commercialisation in transplantation: the problems and some guidelines for practice. Lancet 1985;ii:715–16.
54. Malouin R. Surgeons' quest for life: the history and the future of xenotransplantation. Perspect Biol Med 1994;37:416–28.

Chronic Renal Failure and Pretransplantation Assessment

R.S.C. Rodger and G.M. Baxter

Presentation and Investigation of Renal Failure

Renal failure is defined as a reduction in the excretion of nitrogenous waste products from the kidney. The measurement of urea and creatinine in a blood sample is a routine investigation carried out in most patients presenting to their doctor with an unknown illness. This is often how underlying renal failure is discovered, and it should be followed by referral to a nephrologist for further assessment. Usually such patients will be seen within a few weeks of referral, but monitoring is advisable during this period to ensure that renal function is not deteriorating further. The cause of the underlying renal disease can often be determined from the patient's medical history. Physical examination of the urinary tract is usually less rewarding. Thus, the patient who has a creatinine concentration of 200 µmol/l with symptoms of prostatism and an enlarged bladder, or with a family history of polycystic kidney disease and palpable kidneys, who can be referred directly for ultrasound confirmation of the diagnosis is a rare, albeit satisfying case to meet in clinic (Figs. 2.**1**–2.**4**). Whilst it is important to exclude obstructive uropathy and polycystic kidneys, most renal diseases lead to loss of renal volume as the kidneys progressively shrink in size due to fibrosis. Cyst formation or acquired cystic disease (Fig. 2.**5**) is relatively common in patients with long-standing advanced

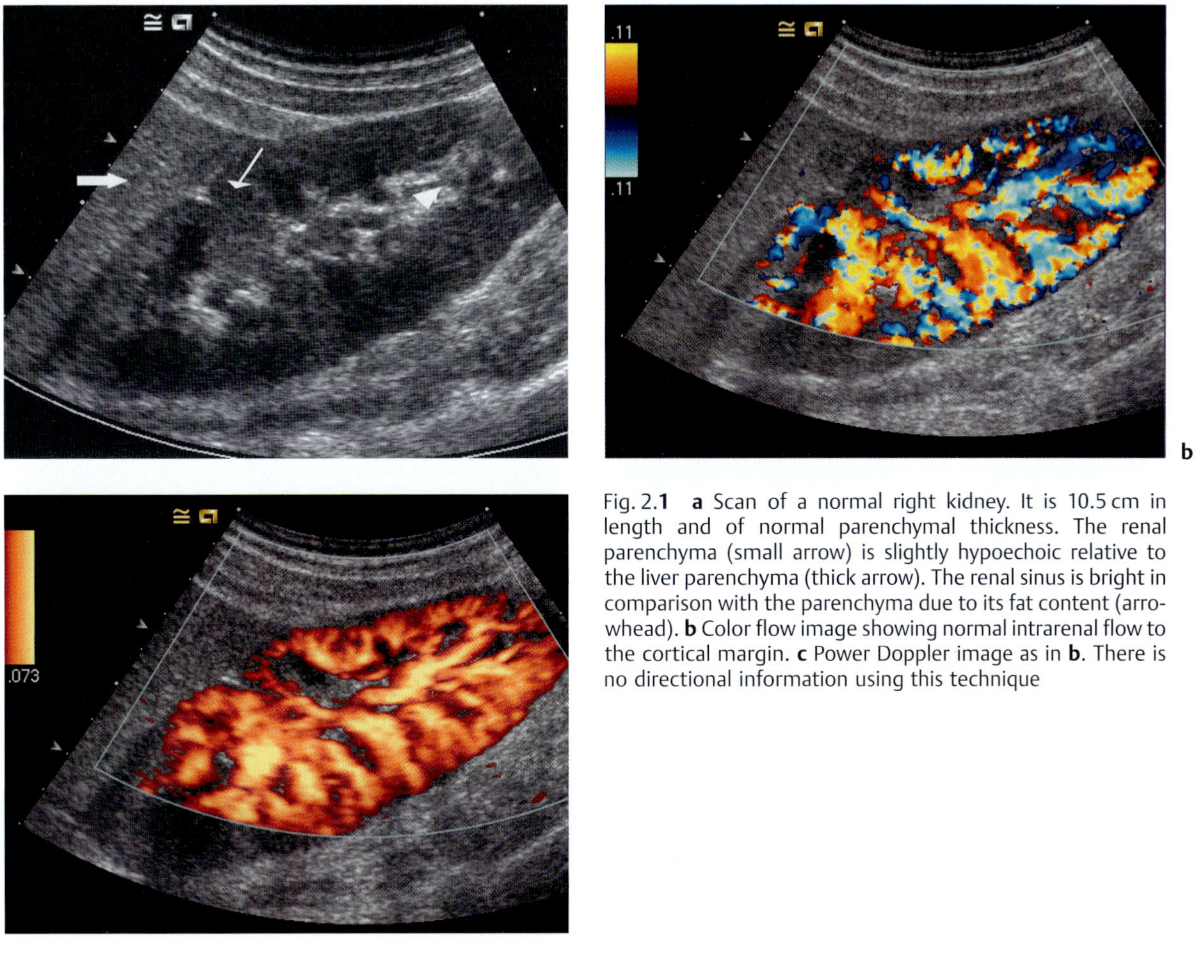

a b c

Fig. 2.**1** **a** Scan of a normal right kidney. It is 10.5 cm in length and of normal parenchymal thickness. The renal parenchyma (small arrow) is slightly hypoechoic relative to the liver parenchyma (thick arrow). The renal sinus is bright in comparison with the parenchyma due to its fat content (arrowhead). **b** Color flow image showing normal intrarenal flow to the cortical margin. **c** Power Doppler image as in **b**. There is no directional information using this technique

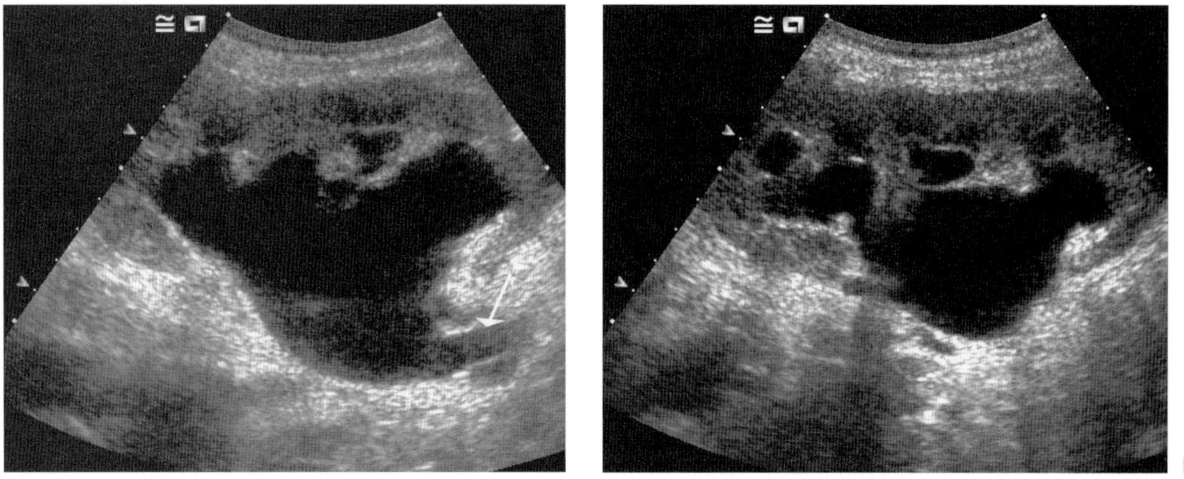

a b

Fig. 2.2 Ultrasonograms of the **a** right and **b** left kidney showing bilateral hydronephrosis. There is effacement of the renal sinus due to calyceal dilatation. The proximal ureter on the right (arrow) is dilated but could not be followed more distally. Renal cortical thickness is maintained, implying the obstruction is more acute than chronic. The most common reason for this appearance is bladder outlet obstruction secondary to prostatic hypertrophy

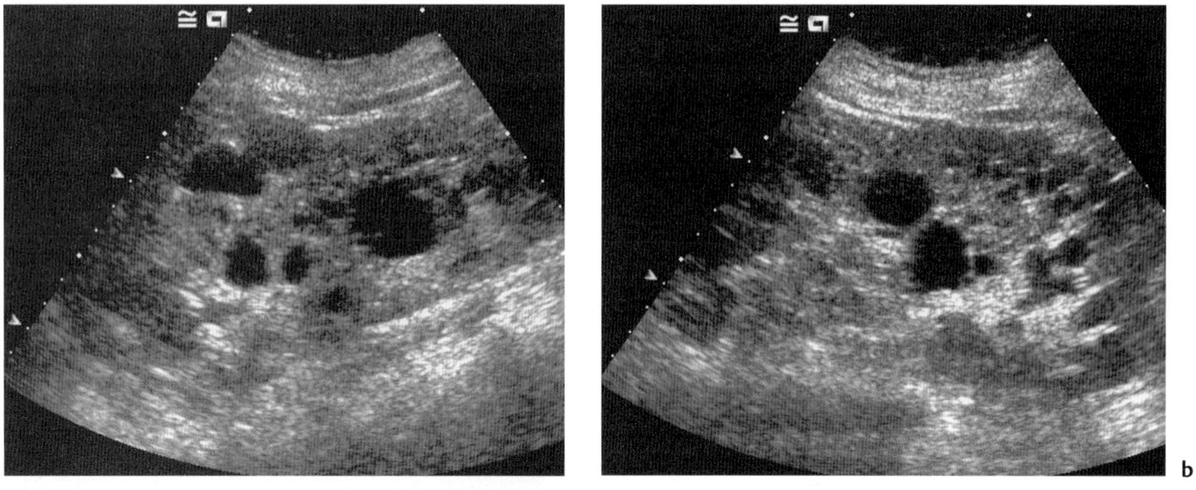

a b

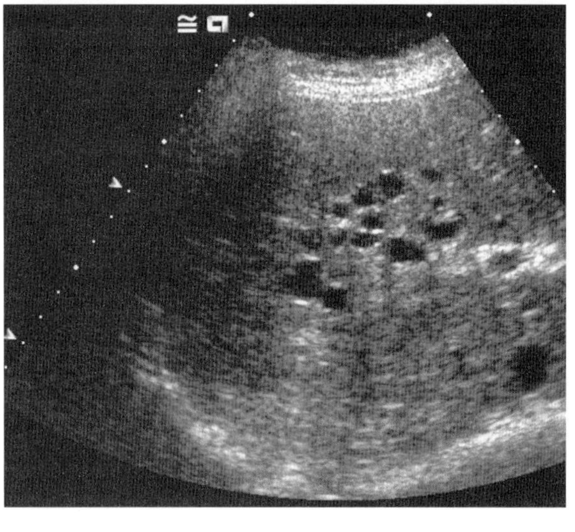

c

Fig. 2.3 **a** Right and **b** left kidneys from a patient with adult polycystic kidney disease (APKD). Both kidneys are markedly enlarged at 15 cm in length; however, both renal outlines are still just discernible. Both kidneys contain cysts of variable size and the above features are pathognomonic of this condition. **c** A gray-scale image of the liver in the same patient showing multiple small cysts of variable size. The liver may also be affected in this condition, as may the spleen and, rarely, the pancreas

Fig. 2.5 A mixture of kidneys showing the slightly different appearances of small chronically diseased kidneys. All kidneys are below 8 cm in length and have only a very thin rim of tissue remaining. **a** Small echogenic chronically diseased right kidney (compare with liver). Some parenchymal tissue remains. The left kidney was similar. **b** An echogenic kidney compared with the liver, with tiny, peripherally situated cysts. Cortical tissue is absent. **c** A kidney with a similar echogenicity to the liver. No cysts were seen. **d** Multiple larger, peripherally based cysts are seen in this small chronically diseased kidney ▷

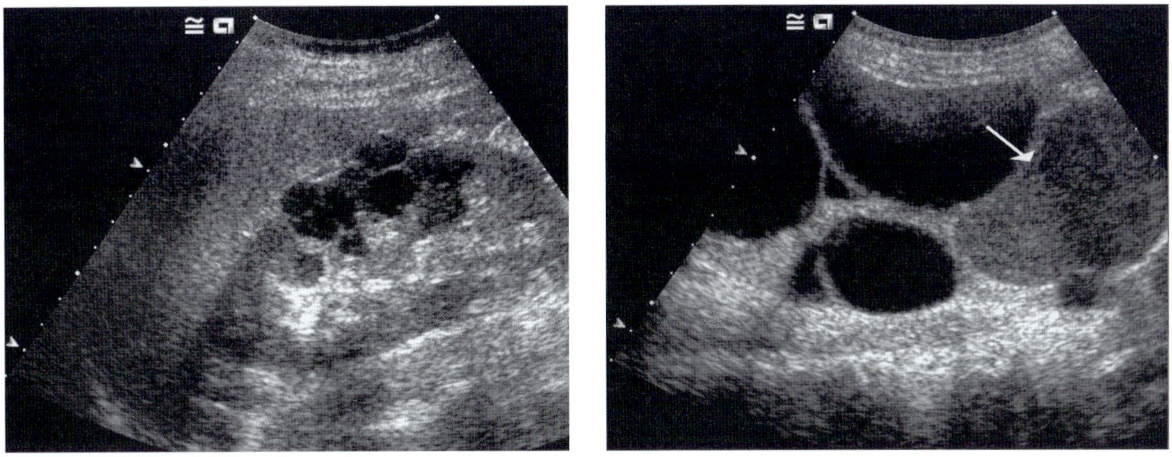

a b

Fig. 2.**4** Two different patients with APKD at either ends of the clinical spectrum. **a** Scan of the right kidney in a young patient being screened because of a family history of adult cystic disease. The kidney is normal in size and appearance except that it contains multiple small cysts. The left kidney was similar. These appearances represent the earliest ultrasonic manifestations of APKD. **b** Scan of the left kidney in a patient with longstanding APKD. There is no renal outline, just a huge conglomerate of cysts. One cyst contains more solid echoes (arrow), probably related to previous hemorrhage

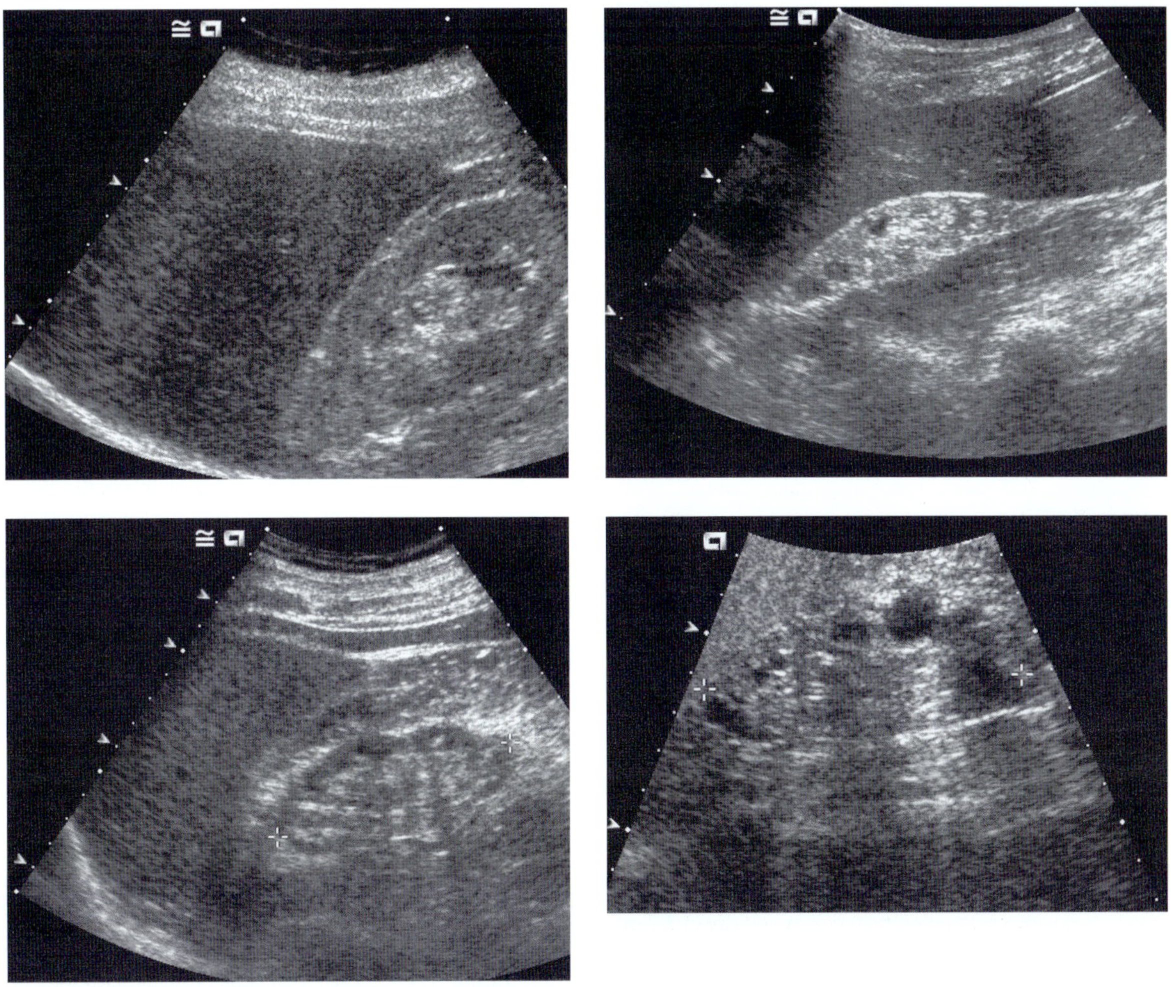

a b c d

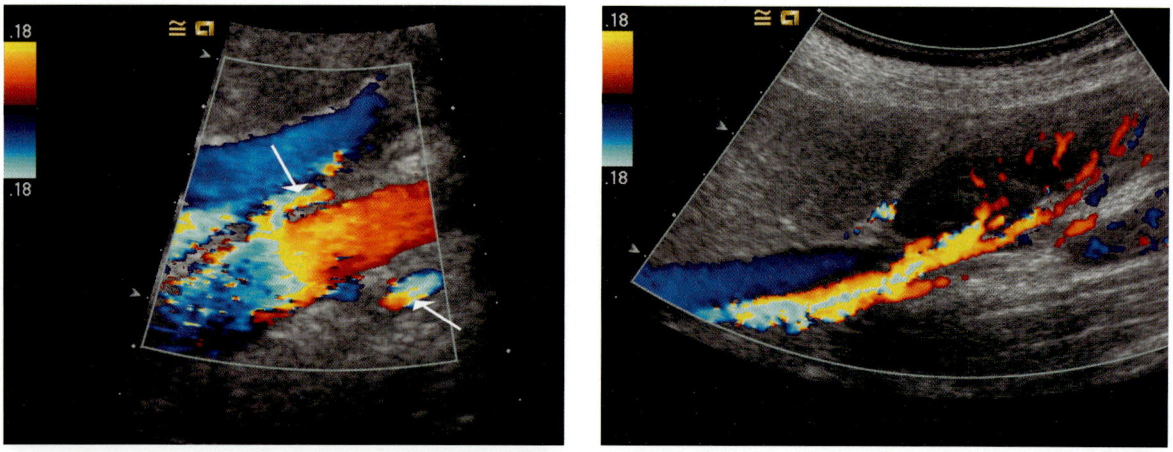

a b

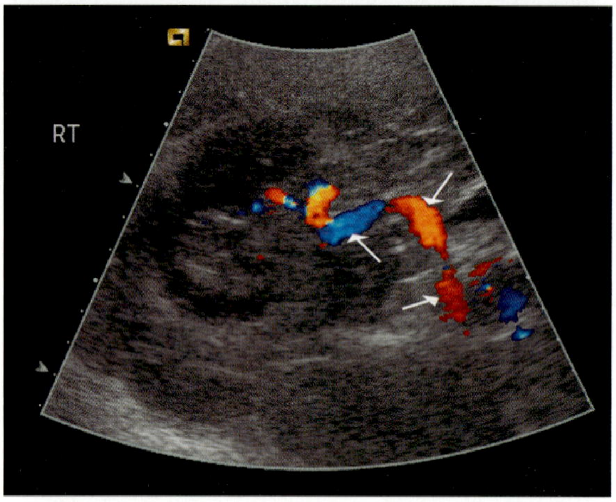

c

Fig. 2.**6** Color flow images of normal renal vessels. **a** Longitudinal axis of the upper abdominal aorta showing the origin of the renal vessels (arrows). This image is very difficult to obtain in all but the most cooperative of patients. **b** Image of the more distal aspects of the renal artery towards hilum level. The renal artery (in red) lies adjacent to the vein (in blue). **c** Transverse image of a tortuous right renal artery (arrows)

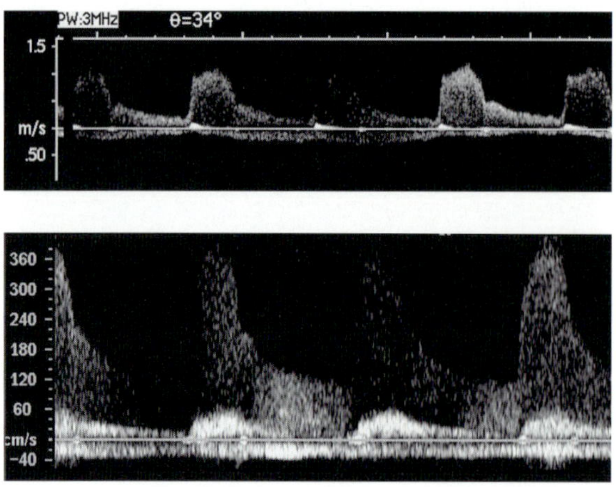

a b

Fig. 2.**7** **a** Normal Doppler waveform from the origin of the right renal artery with a peak systolic velocity of just over 1.0 m/s (normal < 1.8 m/s). **b** Spectral waveform from the left renal artery with a markedly elevated peak velocity of 3.7 m/s with associated spectral broadening. The appearances are those of renal artery stenosis

renal failure[1], and malignant transformation of such cysts has occasionally been reported.[2]

Ischemic nephropathy or renovascular disease, either due to a stenosis of the renal artery or to small vessel disease, is increasingly recognized as an important cause of renal failure, particularly in the elderly.[3] Such patients often have a history and/or signs of multisystem vascular disease. Where there is proximal renal artery disease, constriction of the postglomerular arteriole is needed to preserve glomerular filtration, and so the use of angiotensin converting enzyme (ACE) antagonists, which reduce postglomerular arteriolar tone, can precipitate a further deterioration in renal function.[4] Other pointers towards renovascular disease as the precipitating cause of renal failure include normal urinalysis results (or minimal proteinuria) and asymmetrically sized kidneys on ultrasonography.

What the best method might be for screening and diagnosis of renovascular disease has been the subject of controversy for many years.[5] Whilst Doppler ultrasonography (Figs. 2.**6**, 2.**7**) has the advantage of safety, it is time-consuming and operator-dependent,

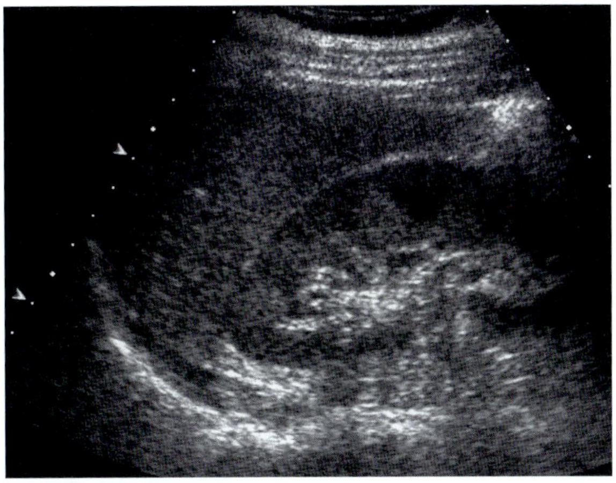

a

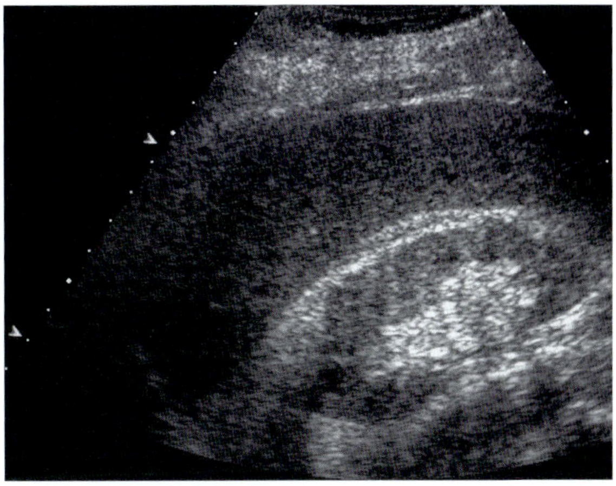

b

Fig. 2.**8** The appearances of the diabetic kidney are often unremarkable and appear normal on ultrasonography in the earlier stages of the disease. As the disease progresses and renal function deteriorates, the kidneys tend to reduce in size and become more echogenic, becoming ultrasonically indistinguishable from kidneys with pathologies of other origins. **a** Image of the right kidney in a diabetic patient with nephrotic syndrome. The kidney measures over 10 cm in length and is normal. **b** Kidney in a diabetic patient with nephropathy and a creatinine concentration of 300 µm/l. The kidney is still a reasonable size at 9 cm, and has some generalized reduction in parenchymal thickness which is only slightly more echogenic than the liver

and it is most likely that magnetic resonance imaging (MRI) techniques will become established as the diagnostic technique of choice in the future. Controversy also surrounds the place of radiological intervention in the treatment of renovascular renal failure, and prospective randomized trials are currently trying to determine whether the advantages of protecting major renal vessels from occlusion with angioplasty and stenting outweigh the side effects of the procedure.[6]

Renal failure in the patient with diabetes most commonly occurs due to microvascular disease, which initially causes glomerular hyperfiltration with microalbuminuria, progressing to frank proteinuria and ultimately glomerulosclerosis. Good diabetic control, treatment of hypertension, and protection against hyperfiltration injury by ACE inhibitors are the cornerstones of treatment.[7] Thus, ultrasound examination of patients with classical diabetic nephropathy often shows normal-sized or enlarged kidneys (Fig. 2.**8**). Other causes of renal failure in patients with diabetes should be considered, such as coexistent glomerulonephritis, to which they are more susceptible.[8] Ultrasound may be useful in detecting papillary necrosis with obstructive uropathy or renovascular disease if there are asymmetrically sized kidneys.

Chronic pyelonephritis, which is most commonly associated with vesicoureteric reflux, neurogenic bladder, or renal calculi, remains an important cause of renal failure in adults. The place of ultrasound screening alongside isotope renography and micturating cystography to detect reflux in utero or in early childhood is well recognized, and with appropriate surgical treatment and antibiotic prophylaxis progressive renal failure should be preventable.[9] Unrecognized cases presenting in adult life are now less common but may be suggested by a history of enuresis or urinary infection in childhood. Ultrasound examination should be an adequate screening test to detect previously undiagnosed adult cases, which can be confirmed by intravenous urography looking for chronic changes of scarring rather than reflux itself. Renal failure caused by excessive consumption of simple analgesics is also less common. Patients with renal failure associated with the long-term use of nonsteroidal anti-inflammatory drugs are now a much commoner clinical scenario.[10]

Ultrasound examination should provide adequate screening, especially in the most severe cases, although CT scanning to look for "lumpy, bumpy kidneys" is replacing intravenous urography for confirmatory imaging.[11] It is most important to establish a diagnosis of analgesic nephropathy, as withdrawal of analgesics and nonsteroidal anti-inflammatory drugs will halt the progression of renal failure.

Glomerulonephritis is still the most common cause of end-stage renal disease treated by dialysis or renal transplantation. Clinical presentation is very variable; some patients may present with symptoms associated with nephritis or the nephrotic syndrome, whilst others are in renal failure or have an abnormal urinalysis at a routine medical examination. Not all cases of suspected glomerulonephritis need to be confirmed by renal biopsy, as this is a potentially hazardous investigation, and it should be borne in mind that most cases of glomerulonephritis will not be responsive to immunosuppressive therapy. However, it is most important to identify treatable cases, particularly those with rapidly progressive glomerulonephritis or vasculitic conditions. Immunological screening tests such as those using immunoglobulins, complement levels, antineutrophil cytoplasmic antibodies, antinuclear antibodies, and antiglomerular basement membrane antibodies will help decision making as to who should progress to renal biopsy.

Ultrasound screening is also necessary to confirm normal size and position of the kidneys and to exclude other renal diseases. Kidney size varies according to the size of the patient, measuring 10–12 cm in length in the normal adult.[12] Renal biopsy is generally not performed in patients with suspected glomerular disease whose kidneys have shrunk in size (<9 cm) as the risk of complications from biopsy is increased and the histological analysis is likely only to show chronic fibrotic damage, unhelpful for diagnostic purposes. Ultimately the cause of renal failure will remain undiagnosed in many patients because they have presented at such a late stage in their disease.

Summary points:

Common causes of chronic renal failure are:
- Diabetes
- Glomerulonephritis
- Renovascular disease/hypertension
- Chronic pyelonephritis
- Polycystic kidneys

Important causes of chronic renal failure to be excluded are:
- Obstructive uropathy
- Rapidly progressive glomerulonephritis/vasculitis
- Drug-induced renal disease

Treatment of Chronic Renal Failure

Whilst it is possible to halt or even reverse renal failure in some cases, many patients will follow a course of progressive loss of renal function despite optimal medical therapy and will need to be assessed for dialysis and transplantation. Optimal medical therapy should encompass a variety of aspects:
- Blood pressure control
- Diet
- Water and electrolyte balance
- Acid–base balance
- Calcium, phosphate, and bone metabolism
- Anemia management

Good control of hypertension is generally regarded as the single most important factor in slowing the progression of renal failure. Most authors believe that the use of ACE inhibitors confers additional advantages over other antihypertensive agents, particularly in patients with diabetic nephropathy, but also in patients with other forms of renal disease, especially those with heavy proteinuria. However, some caution is needed with these agents as they may cause a deterioration in renal function particularly in patients with renovascular disease (RVD) as indicated above. ACE inhibitors may also exacerbate hyperkalemia and anemia, and this may lead to their discontinuation, particularly in patients with advanced renal failure.

Whilst many aspects of dietary manipulation are important in patients with advanced renal failure, controversy still exists about the value of protein restriction. Although protein restriction has been shown to slow the progression of renal failure in some studies, the effect may be relatively small, and patient acceptability of this form of therapy varies in different countries and cultures. In addition, malnutrition is relatively common in patients with chronic renal failure and confers a poorer prognosis which can be exacerbated by further protein restriction. Other aspects of dietary therapy important in management include manipulation to control salt, electrolytes and water balance; phosphate restriction, and correction of over- and undernutrition.

Other medication which may be indicated in the management of patients with renal impairment includes loop diuretics to treat fluid retention, sodium bicarbonate to correct acidosis, sodium polystyrene sulfonate (Resonium) to prevent hyperkalemia, and vitamin D analogues, calcium salts, and other phosphate binders to maintain calcium phosphate balance and control secondary hyperparathyroidism. The anemia associated with renal failure is treated by ensuring adequate iron stores and using long-term subcutaneous erythropoietin injections once to thrice weekly. Patients with renal failure are at greatly increased risk of cardiovascular disease and so attention to risk factors other than hypertension is required.

Assessment for Renal Replacement Therapy

In those patients whose renal function is deteriorating despite optimal medical therapy, it is often possible to predict when end-stage renal failure will occur by extrapolating the results of serial reciprocal serum creatinine levels (Fig. 2.**9**). This will give an indication of the likely period of time available to plan for renal replacement therapy and the patient can be informed as to when dialysis therapy is likely to start. In discussion with the patient, the following issues should be considered.

First, which forms of dialysis are technically feasible and is either likely significantly to improve the wellbeing and longevity of the patient? Whilst most patients with end-stage renal disease will be suitable candidates for both peritoneal and hemodialysis, there may be medical reasons to recommend one rather than another—e.g., hemodialysis for a patient with a colostomy, or peritoneal dialysis for a patient with poor vessel access. Some patients with severe co-mor-

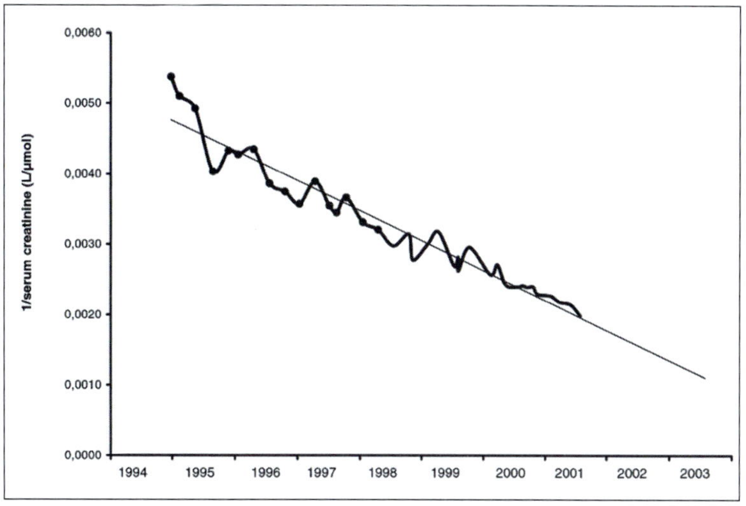

Fig. 2.**9** Progression of renal failure over five years, illustrated by a graph of reciprocal serum creatinine concentrations over time

bidity may have such a poor prognosis that it is deemed that they would not benefit from dialysis—e.g., the patient with terminal malignancy and renal failure.

Secondly, is the patient a suitable candidate for a renal transplant, and if so are there any potential living kidney donors? Suitability for transplantation is largely determined by co-morbidity (see below), and ultimately only 30–40% of the UK dialysis population are placed on the waiting list for cadaveric renal transplantation. Preemptive transplantation, i.e., transplantation before starting long-term dialysis, accounts for only a small proportion of renal transplants within Europe; however, reports from North America, where there is a larger experience, show a good outcome.[13] This form of transplantation is increasingly considered in the UK, particularly in children, and in adults where a suitable living donor can be identified.

These discussions regarding renal replacement therapy are not the sole province of the nephrologist, and a multidisciplinary team including surgeons, nurses, transplant coordinators, and others dealing with both the patient and, usually, the patient's family is preferable. The patient should have time to reflect on the information he or she has been given, and then a plan of action can be made; e.g., if the patient is unsuitable for transplantation and, having visited the dialysis unit, wishes to have hospital hemodialysis, vascular access should be arranged and a course of hepatitis B vaccinations offered. It should be pointed out, however, that unfortunately a third to a half of patients starting long-term renal replacement therapy present at a late stage of advanced renal failure requiring dialysis to be started within a week of referral. For these patients there is little opportunity for predialysis planning, and decisions have to be reached over a shorter time period.

■ *Summary points:*

Assessment for renal replacement therapy should:

- Exclude severe co-morbidity
- Consider the medical advantages of each form of dialysis
- Counsel and plan for dialysis
- Consider suitability for renal transplantation

Assessment for Cadaveric Renal Transplantation

Public awareness surrounding transplantation is such that most patients will have considered this option as a possible treatment for their renal failure at the time of diagnosis and before the subject is raised by their doctor. For suitable patients, transplantation is a better long-term treatment than dialysis as it is more cost-effective, improves quality of life, and there is some evidence, though not from controlled trials, that it also improves life expectancy.[14] The main disadvantages of renal transplantation are related to the hazards of surgery and the side effects of long-term immunosuppression, and it is these factors which should be borne in mind when assessing a patient's suitability for this form of treatment.

Cadaveric kidneys for transplantation are a scarce resource, and the number of patients on the renal transplant waiting list considerably outweighs the numbers of organs available for transplantation. Within the United Kingdom in 2000 there were less than 1400 cadaveric kidneys transplanted, whilst the number of patients on the waiting list was almost 5000. For this reason it is important that the allocation of cadaveric kidneys, which for the UK is organized from a control center in Bristol, is equitable. Kidneys are currently allocated according to nationally agreed guidelines which take account of blood group and tissue type matching, waiting time, donor and recipient age, and other factors.

For a patient to be suitable for surgery there must be access to relatively healthy iliac vessels to which the transplanted renal artery and vein can be anastomosed. The recipient should also have a normal bladder. Patients may be unsuitable for transplantation if they are very obese, because of difficulties this can create in accessing their iliac vessels, or if they have severe peripheral vascular disease. Vascular thrombosis, though rare, is the commonest cause of early graft failure and is much more likely in these circumstances. In patients who do not have normal bladder function, further urological assessment is needed before the patient is accepted for transplantation. Options such as the creation of an ileal conduit before the patient goes on the waiting list, or the use of a ureterostomy or self-catheterization in the post-transplantation period, may have to be considered.

In order to be fit for anesthesia the patient should have adequate cardiorespiratory function and no contraindication to intubation, such as an unstable cervical spine. Cardiovascular disease occurs in the renal failure population at greatly increased frequency to the general population and may be asymptomatic until unmasked by the stress of surgery. For this reason many patients undergo noninvasive cardiac investigations such as echocardiography or exercise testing prior to acceptance on the waiting list. More invasive assessment, including coronary angiography and corrective treatment by cardiac surgery where indicated, should be considered prior to acceptance on the waiting list.[15]

Unlike most other patients undergoing surgery, renal transplant recipients will also receive long-term immunosuppressive treatment, which will predispose them to infective complications and also make them more susceptible to develop cancer. For these reasons patients with chronic infection such as AIDS or malignancy will not benefit from renal transplantation. Patients with a history of malignancy that has been treated effectively are generally advised to wait for a period of two to five years depending on the tumor type[15]. Active viral hepatitis B and C carriers who do not have significant liver disease will benefit more from transplantation than from staying on long-term dialysis, although their outcome may be worse than that of noncarriers. Patients with acute infections should be temporarily suspended from the active waiting list until they have recovered. In those patients who have a source of chronic sepsis, this should be removed (e.g., by nephrectomy) prior to their being considered for transplantation.

Although recurrence of the primary disease in the transplanted kidney is not uncommon in various forms of glomerulonephritis and also in diabetes, this only rarely affects the short-term outlook. An exception to this is the rare condition of oxalosis, where recurrence is such a frequent and early complication that combined hepatorenal transplantation is often chosen to overcome the problem.

Finally, when assessing patients' suitability for renal transplantation, the risk of noncompliance should be considered. Noncompliance is suspected to account for a large proportion of late graft failures, but it is difficult to provide accurate and reliable data on this issue. Risk factors for noncompliance include younger-aged recipients, those developing cosmetic side effects from medication, such as hirsutism with cyclosporine, and patients with drug dependency, including alcohol abuse. In the latter category of patients it is usually recommended that a period of abstinence of at least six months be achieved before acceptance onto the waiting list. The dangers of not taking immunosuppressive medication regularly must be clearly explained at the time of assessment for transplantation and reinforced regularly for all patients in the post-transplantation period.

■ *Summary points:*

Assessment for renal transplantation should take into account:

- Contraindications to surgery
- Contraindications to immunosuppression
- Likelihood of early recurrence of primary renal disease
- Likelihood of noncompliance

Assessment for Live Donor Transplantation

With regard to the recipient, the assessment for suitability for live donor transplantation is very similar to that for a cadaveric transplant. As the benefits of transplantation over dialysis have emerged and the shortage of cadaveric kidneys has become more acute, so the attitudes to live donor transplantation have become more liberal. Many would argue that, in a high-risk recipient, live donor kidney transplantation is more acceptable than a cadaveric kidney transplantation. The reason for this is that live donor transplantation is a planned rather than an emergency procedure, as it is in cadaveric transplantation, and so the recipient's general condition can be optimized in preparation for surgery. Furthermore, this allows the severely restricted number of cadaveric kidneys to be used for low-risk patients, who will have a longer-term benefit. Overall, live donor transplantation still represents a minority of the renal transplants performed in the UK, although it is increasing. For example, 267 live donor kidney transplants were performed in 1999 and 297 in 2000, compared with around 1400 cadaveric kidney transplants per year. The reasons for the increase in live donor transplantation include the shortage of cadaveric kidneys and the excellent results a 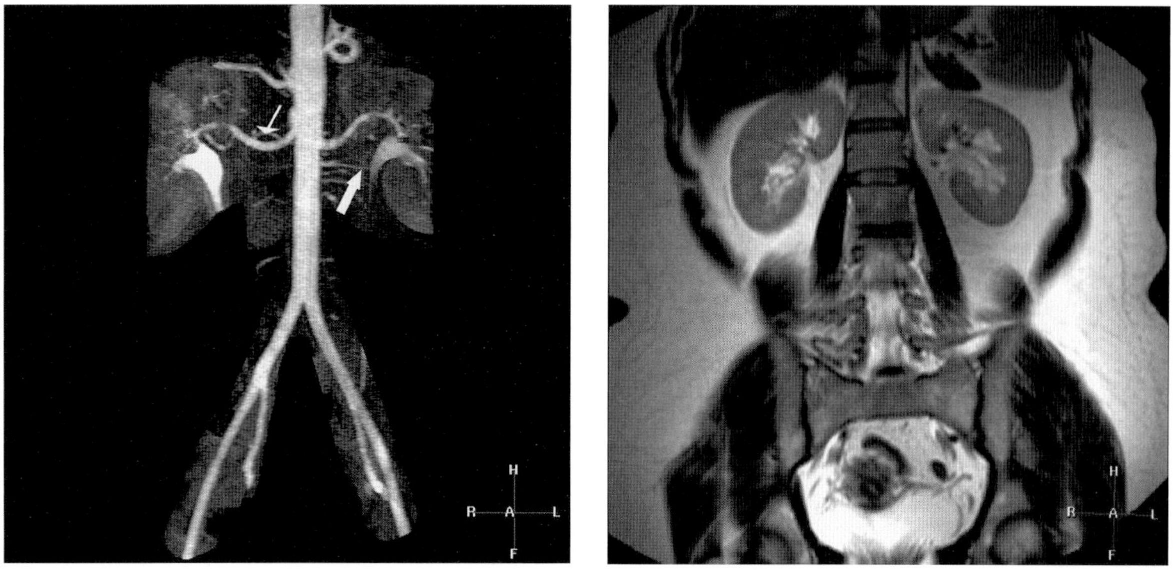 b

Fig. 2.**10** **a** Gadolinium-contrast-enhanced MR angiogram of the aorta and renal vessels in a potential live related renal donor. Early division of the right renal artery is noted (thin arrow), and an accessory lower pole renal artery to the left kidney (thick arrow) can also be seen. **b** T2-weighted MR image showing normal renal morphology. (Courtesy of Dr. G. Roditi, Dept. of Radiology, Royal Infirmary, Glasgow, UK)

achieved using both related and unrelated live organs, which are possibly better than the cadaveric graft survival figures.[16]

Assessment of the Live Kidney Donor

Guidelines for the assessment of living kidney donors have been produced by the British Transplantation Society in association with the UK Renal Association.[17] It is the role of the evaluation process to ensure that the offer to donate is "altruistic without coercion or reward" and that the donor is fully informed about the potential short-term risks of donation, with a perioperative mortality of 3–6/10 000, principally due to pulmonary emboli and cardiovascular events and a variety of postoperative complications such as wound and chest infections, pneumothorax, and wound pain, which will delay the full recovery of the donor. In the long term there is little evidence of risk from living kidney donation: mortality and the likelihood of developing end-stage renal disease are not increased, although there may be a slightly higher incidence of hypertension and proteinuria than in the general population.[18] Potential living kidney donors should be aged over 18 years and genetically or emotionally related to the recipient. They should be ABO blood-group-compatible, and the recipient should not have preformed antibodies against the donor. A negative donor/recipient cross-match test between recipient serum and donor T and B lymphocytes using appropriate techniques is required and should exclude the possibility of hyperacute rejection occurring in the early postoperative period.

A full medical assessment should be undertaken to detect renal disease and to identify other contraindications to organ donation. Imaging should be performed to confirm renal anatomy using ultrasound, differential isotope renography, and conventional or MR angiography. Conventional angiography has a small but significant complication rate, and MR angiography in appropriately experienced hands is becoming the preferred final imaging investigation to visualize the renal vasculature (Fig. 2.**10**). Although a donor kidney with a single renal artery is preferred, reconstruction of an organ with multiple vessels is usually possible and will allow the transplant operation to proceed.

For the United Kingdom, legislation controlling living donor transplantation is set out in the Human Organ Transplantation Act (1989) and associated regulations. Where a close genetic relationship cannot be established by an approved tissue typing laboratory, or in the case of an unrelated donor, approval is required from the Unrelated Live Transplant Regulatory Authority. It is a requirement for unrelated live donor transplantation that the donor is interviewed and assessed by an independent person, who is usually a doctor, but not one practicing in nephrology or transplantation. Many centers will use such a person for independent live related donor assessment also, although this is not mandatory.

Following donor nephrectomy, the patient can expect to be in hospital for several days and to be able to return to normal activities within a few weeks. The period of hospitalization, degree of postoperative pain, and time to full recovery can all be significantly reduced if a laparoscopic surgical technique for nephrectomy is used,[19] and it is likely that this will become the preferred method in the future. There is hope that the increased patient acceptability of this technique might contribute to an increase in the number of live donor transplants in the future.

Following uncomplicated nephrectomy, the donor should undergo an outpatient review after four to six weeks and thereafter remain under lifelong annual follow-up. The long-term review is to screen for proteinuria, renal impairment, and hypertension; however, this need not necessarily take place in the transplant unit.

Summary points:

Exclusion criteria for live kidney donor transplantation are as follows:

Absolute contraindications:

- Inability to give informed consent
- Evidence of coercion
- Hypertensive end-organ damage
- Body mass index ✱ 35 kg/m^2
- Most malignancies
- Pregnancy
- Intravenous drug abuse
- Human immunodeficiency virus or human T-cell lymphotropic virus infection
- Major respiratory or cardiovascular disease
- Other major co-morbid illness
- Thrombophilia
- Diabetes mellitus or impaired glucose tolerance
- Renal disease
- Systemic disease affecting kidneys

Relative contraindications:

- Patient aged below 18 years (but able to give informed consent)
- Patient aged over 70 years
- Patient intellectually impaired but able to give informed consent
- Obesity: body mass index of 30–35 kg/m^2
- Cigarette smoking
- Risk factors for type 2 diabetes mellitus
- Child-bearing age in female patients
- Psychiatric disorder
- Hepatitis B infection
- History of deep vein thrombosis or pulmonary embolism
- Hypertension
- Renal tract abnormality

References

1. Thomson BJ, Jenkins DAS, Atlar PL. Acquired cystic disease of the kidney patient with end-stage renal disease: a study of prevalence and aetiology. Nephrol Dial Transplant 1986;1:38–43.
2. Marple JT, MacDougall M, Chonko AM. Renal cancer complicating acquired cystic kidney disease. J Am Soc Nephrol 1994;4:1951–6.
3. Scoble JE, Maher ER, Hamilton G, Dick R, Sweney P, Moorhead JF. Atherosclerotic renovascular disease causing renal impairment—a case for treatment. Clin Nephrol 1989;31:119–22.
4. Kalra PS, Mamtora H, Holmes AM, Waldek S. Renovascular disease and renal complications of angiotension-converting enzyme inhibitor therapy. Q J Med 1990;76:1013–8.
5. Breyer JA, Jacobson HR. Ischemic nephropathy. Curr Opin Nephrol Hypertens 1993;2:216–24.
6. Harden PN, MacLeod MJ, Rodger RSC, et al. Effect of renal-artery stenting on progression of renovascular renal failure. Lancet 1997;349:1133–6.
7. Lewis EJ, Hunsicker LG, Bain RP, Rohde RD. The effect of angiotensin-converting-enzyme inhibition on diabetic nephropathy. N Engl J Med 1993;329:1456–62.
8. Richards NT, Greaves I, Lee SJ, Howie AJ, Adu D, Michael J. Increased prevalence of renal biopsy findings other than diabetic glomerulopathy in type II diabetes mellitus. Nephrol Dial Transplant 1992;7:397–9.
9. Smellie JM, Tamminem-Mobius T, Olbing H, et al. Five year study of medical or surgical treatment in children with severe reflux. Pediatr Nephrol 1992;6:223–30.
10. Pugliese F, Cinotti GA. Non steroidal anti-inflammatory drugs (NSAIDs) and the kidney. Nephrol Dial Transplant 1997;12:386–8.
11. Elseviers MM, Waller I, Nenoy D, et al. Evaluation of diagnostic criteria for analgesic nephropathy in patients with end stage renal failure: results of the ANNE study. Nephrol Dial Transplant 1995;10:808–14.
12. Dalla-Palma L, Bazzocchi M, Cressa C, Tommasini G. Radiological anatomy of the kidney revisited. Br J Radiol 1990;63:680–90.
13. Mange KC, Joffe MM, Feldman HI. Effects of the use or non use of long term dialysis on the subsequent survival of renal transplants from living donors. N Engl J Med 2001;344:726–31.
14. Wolfe RA, Ashby VB, Miford EL et al. Comparison of mortality in all patients on dialysis, patients on dialysis awaiting transplantation and recipients of a first cadaveric transplant. N Engl J Med 1999;341:1725–30.
15. EBPG Expert Group on Renal Transplantation. European Best Practice Guidelines for Renal Transplantation. Nephrol Dial Transplant 2000;15:Suppl 7.
16. Terasaki PI, Cecka JM, Gjertson DW, Takemoto S. High survival rates of kidney transplants for spousal and living unrelated donors. N Engl J Med 1995;333:333–6.
17. United Kingdom guidelines for living donor kidney transplantations. London: British Transplantation Society/Renal Association; 2000..
18. Saran R, Marshall SM, Madsen R, Keavey P, Tapson JS. Long term follow up of kidney donors: a longitudinal study. Nephrol Dial Transplant 1997;12:1615–21.
19. Kavoussi LR. Laparoscopic donor nephrectomy. Kidney Int 2000;57:2175–86.

Renal Transplant Surgery

B. C. Jaques

Introduction

Renal transplantation is the preferred treatment for selected patients requiring renal replacement therapy. Patients with successful renal transplants enjoy improved quality of life,[1] may live longer than patients undergoing dialysis awaiting transplantation,[2] and can reduce health provision expenditure when other renal replacement therapy is discontinued.[3]

In the war against early and late graft dysfunction, ultrasonography is invaluable in the diagnosis of ureteric outflow obstruction and perinephric collection, whilst color Doppler ultrasonography is helpful in the diagnosis of diminished or abnormal arterial perfusion, venous outflow obstruction, and a wide range of other abnormalities which may lead to graft failure. As an ultrasound examination is noninvasive, serial Doppler ultrasound studies of transplanted renal grafts have become routine and are incorporated into many units' standard patient follow-up protocols.

■ ***Summary point:***

- Renal transplantation is the preferred treatment for patients requiring renal replacement therapy.

Donor Kidney

The blood supply to the developing kidney comes from the great vessels, which lie in close proximity to the kidneys during embryological growth. Initially, early in development, the kidneys lie in the pelvis, but as the embryo grows they are seen to migrate such that they occupy progressively higher positions within the abdomen. To begin with, the renal blood supply is derived from branches of the middle sacral and common iliac arteries. As the kidneys ascend, the blood supply originates from sequential arteries extending from the lateral aspect of the elongating aorta, until, in most individuals, definitive single renal arteries supplying all of the kidney and the first 10–15 cm of the ureter form just adjacent to the superior mesenteric orifice. It is not surprising however, that 25% of kidneys are found to have multiple renal arteries, a variation which reflects the manner in which the blood supply continually changes during the ascent from the pelvis to the abdomen. A single lower polar accessory vessel supplying up to 40% of the lower kidney and the first 10–15 cm of the ureter, or a single upper polar accessory vessel supplying less than 10% of the upper pole of the kidney are the most common of the polar variants. Dual and triple polar variations, however, are also encountered.

Usually, when cadaveric renal grafts are used for transplantation, polar vessels are left on the aortic patch so that only one arterial anastomosis is fashioned during the transplant operation. In some circumstances, however, this may not always be possible, because as part of the bench work to clear the kidney of unwanted fat prior to transplantation, accessory vessels may need to be reconstructed onto the main renal artery or the aortic patch trimmed and re-sutured. Unfortunately, reconstruction procedures increase the likelihood of a postoperative arterial complication, and when lower polar variants are encountered, a complication of thrombosis of the accessory artery may lead to both renal infarction and ureteric necrosis.

Transplant Procedure

Transplant Wound

The side chosen to transplant on may ultimately be decided because of the presence of a previous transplant graft or asymmetry in peripheral vascular or polycystic kidney disease, but a few other factors should also be considered at the time of transplantation. With the renal vein entering the kidney superficial to the artery in the coronal plane, a right or left kidney when transplanted into the contralateral iliac fossa with the lower pole placed caudally requires the artery and vein to be crossed when the anastomoses are fashioned using the external iliac vessels (Fig. 3.**1**). This is usually not problematic, but can be easily avoided if the transplant is carried out on the side that the kidney was removed from (Fig. 3.**2**). However, if the internal iliac artery is used for the arterial anastomosis, as is commonly preferred when live donor kidneys are used, the artery and vein do not cross when situated in the contralateral iliac fossa (Fig. 3.**3**). It is interesting to note that when renal transplantation was evolving, the internal iliac artery was used in preference to the external iliac artery, and it became

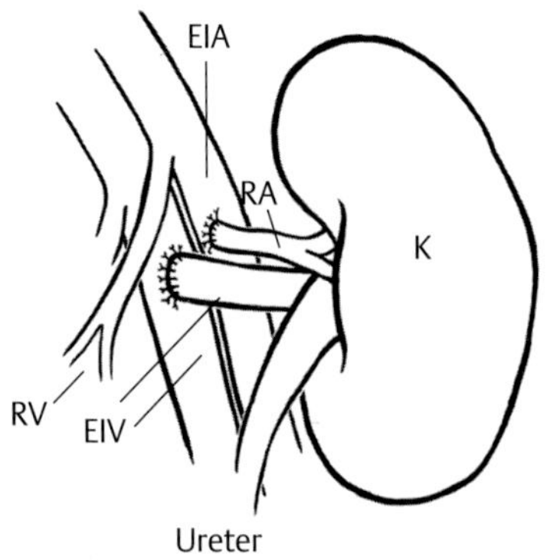

Fig. 3.**1** Contralateral renal transplant. This figure depicts the crossing of the donor renal vessels when a right kidney is transplanted into the left iliac fossa and the external iliac vessels are used for the anastomoses. In the coronal plane, the renal artery is superficial to the renal vein but the external iliac artery is lateral (i.e., deep) to the external iliac vein. Note, however, that the ureteric pelvis is superficial and more accessible to percutaneous intubation in this orientation

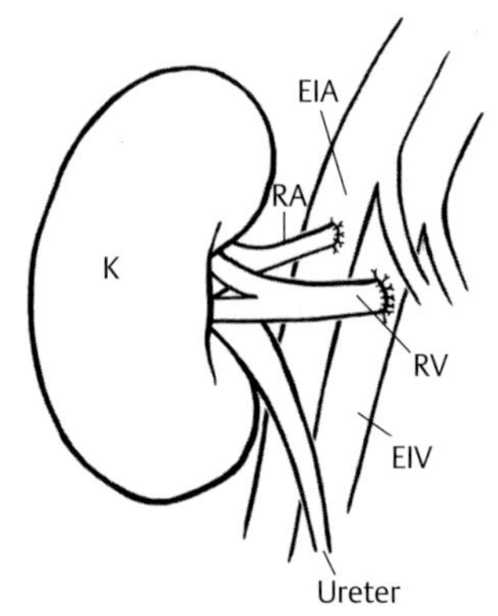

Fig. 3.**2** Isolateral renal transplant. This figure depicts a right donor kidney transplanted into the patient's right iliac fossa. Note in this orientation that the donor renal vessels do not cross each other when the external iliac vessels are used for the anastomoses. In the coronal plane, the renal vein lies superficial to the renal artery and the external iliac vein is medial (i.e., superficial) to the external iliac artery. Note that the ureteric pelvis lies deep in this orientation

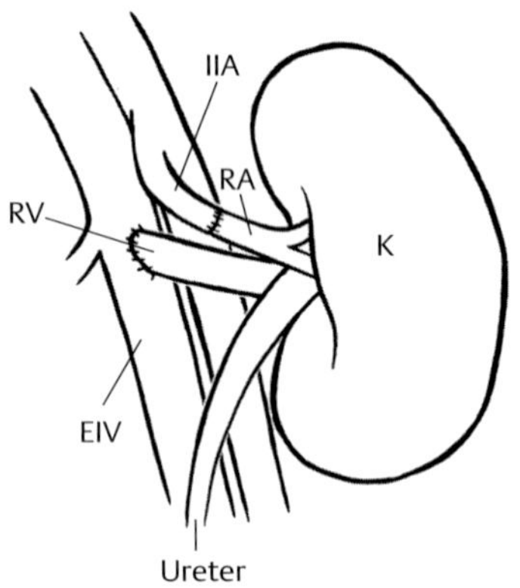

Fig. 3.**3** Contralateral renal transplant using the internal iliac artery. This figure illustrates the transplantation of a right kidney into the left iliac fossa. Note that when the internal iliac artery is used for the anastomosis with the donor renal artery, the renal artery and vein do not cross

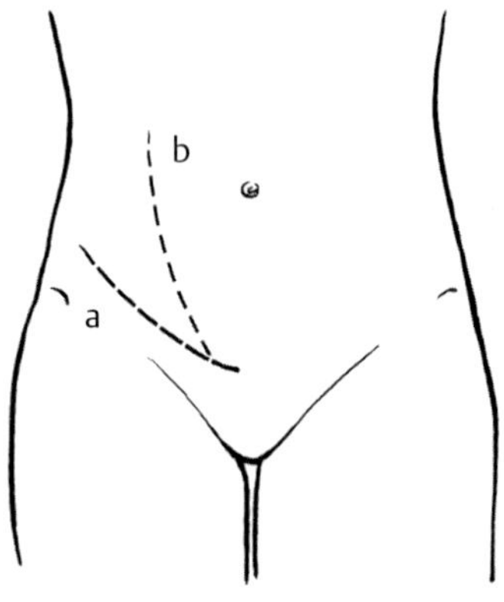

Fig. 3.**4** Typical incisions for renal transplant. **a** The curvilinear incision preferred by the author. **b** The more vertical incision preferred by some other surgeons

conventional and incorporated into surgical dogma that kidneys should always be placed on the contralateral side!

After preparation of the donor kidney and choosing the side for the transplant, a curvilinear incision is made in the iliac fossa. The present author prefers an almost horizontal skin crease incision starting in the midline 2 cm above the pubic symphysis and extended laterally to a position 2 cm medial to the anterior iliac spine (Fig. 3.**4a**). The length of the incision is generally governed by the size of the recipient and the donor kidney. When using this incision, to allow adequate exposure of the iliac vessels, the rectus muscle is also divided transversely in the medial wound. Alternatively, some surgeons prefer to leave the rectus muscle intact and use an incision that starts in the midline but takes a much more acute vertical course, extending 2 cm lateral to the rectus sheath border (Fig. 3.**4b**). This incision frequently results in neurological denervation of the "preserved" lower rectus muscle with wasting and incisional hernia formation because of interruption of the sequential terminal branches of the intercostal nerves supplying the rectus abdominis.

In opening the wound, care should be taken to avoid opening the peritoneum, which can be swept cranially, exposing the round ligament/spermatic cord and external iliac vessels below. The round ligament can be divided between ligatures and the spermatic cord mobilized, allowing insertion of any variety of retractor systems for maximum vascular exposure. Hemostasis

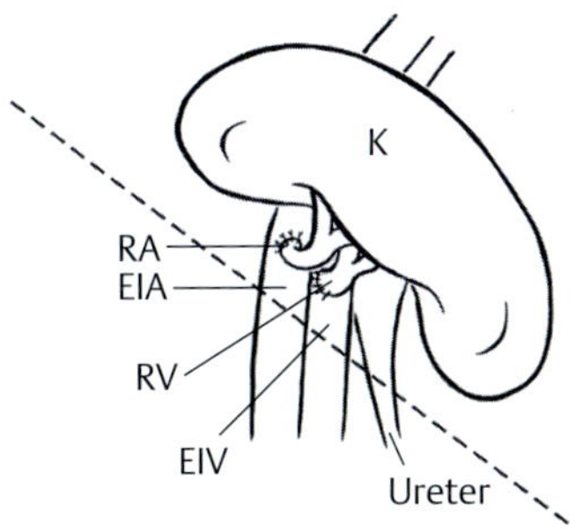

a

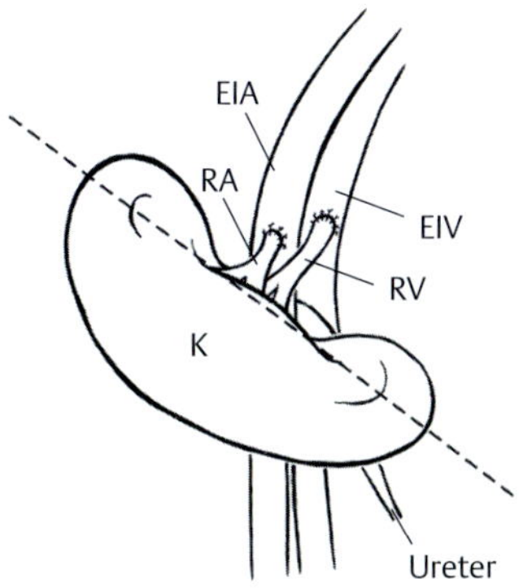

b

Fig. 3.5 "Folding" of the transplant kidney during wound closure: **a** cranial, **b** caudal. The drawings show how transplanted kidneys lie with their long axis parallel to the wound and can be "folded" in the coronal plane through an arc of 180°. The broken line depicts the wound in the right iliac fossa. In **a** a transplanted kidney is folded cranially such that the outer convex surface faces medially, and in **b** the fold is caudal, whereby the outer convex border of the kidney faces laterally

should be controlled meticulously to avoid retroperitoneal hematoma formation, which may lead to a number of complications including hypovolemia, infection, renal venous–arterial occlusion, or even colonic pseudo-obstruction, for example.

Vascular Anastomoses

Prior to fashioning the anastomoses, the connective tissue is cleared from both the external iliac vessels, allowing mobilization from the origin of the common iliac to the inguinal ligament. The external iliac artery should be devoid of branches, but, conversely, the vein often has a deep posterior tributary proximal to the confluence with the internal iliac vein which, when ligated and divided, allows lifting of the external iliac vein into the wound and an easier anastomosis for the surgeon. Both the vascular anastomoses are usually fashioned in an end-to-side manner using a continuous suturing technique with a fine nonabsorbable Prolene suture. Alternatively, the anterior and posterior divisions of the internal iliac artery may be ligated and the internal iliac artery used for an end-to-end anastomosis with the renal artery. In either event, following the vascular anastomoses, the vascular clamps are released and the joys of performing renal transplantation are realized with revascularization of the graft and the immediate production of urine.

Ureteric Anastomosis

Attention is then focused on the ureteric anastomosis. In the male patient, the shortened and spatulated transplant ureter is placed below the spermatic cord, a problem not encountered in the female as the round ligament has already been divided. There are two main techniques for fashioning the ureterovesical anastomosis. As neither of the techniques described below is any better or worse at preventing ureteric reflux,[4] and as the first technique is relatively simple to perform and the second technique dogged by unwanted postoperative hematuria, the present author's preferred method will be described first. This technique is based on the Lich antireflux extravesical ureteroneocystostomy[5] and involves dividing the bladder muscle layer until the mucosa balloons out into the cystostomy wound. The mucosa is then opened at the distal end of the cystostomy and the spatulated ureter anastomosed using interrupted 4.0 or 5.0 polydioxinone absorbable sutures. The opened muscle layer is then closed over the ureteric anastomosis, making an extravesical tunnel before the transplant ureter empties into the bladder. The second well-described technique is that of Politano and Leadbetter[6] and involves making a formal anterior cystostomy to gain access into the bladder. Via a separate incision through the bladder muscle, the transplant ureter is pulled through a submucosal tunnel before opening into the mucosa of the bladder. The spatulated ureter is then fixed in the corners using fine absorbable sutures. The anterior cystostomy is closed separately.
Stenting the ureteric anastomosis with a removable double J stent has become common practice in many units. Routine placement of such stents in all patients is still somewhat controversial. A major criticism of routine stenting remains the burden of having to remove the stents some six to eight weeks following surgery. Against this, stents can be easily removed using local anesthetic by fiberoptic cystoscopy or ultrasound-guided snare, and as an ever-growing proportion of patients receive renal replacement therapy via peritoneal dialysis, patients with in-dwelling continuous ambulatory peritoneal dialysis catheters (which will have to be removed) can usually have both the Tenckhoff catheter and the double J stent removed at the same sitting. Additionally, after performing a prospective study involving over 300 patients, the author's current unit found the ureteric complication rate to be lower when double J stents were employed than when they were not,[7] and changed their policy accordingly.

Wound Closure

When closing the transplant wound, the kidney is "folded" cranially or caudally in its coronal plane, allowing unimpeded blood flow to and from the transplant (Fig. 3.**5**). The long axis of the kidney usually follows the wound, making percutaneous biopsy both possible and a relatively safe procedure. Most surgeons prefer to close the wound over a surgical drain to minimize the tamponade effect of collecting blood or lymph on renal perfusion.

Summary points:

- Transplantation is usually performed in the iliac fossa by fashioning anastomoses using the end of the renal artery and vein onto the side of the external iliac artery and vein respectively. Alternatively, the internal iliac artery may be used for an end-to-end anastomosis with the renal artery.
- The ureteric anastomosis is performed by suturing the end of the ureter onto the dome of the bladder, often over a removable silicon stent.
- The orientation of the long axis of the transplanted kidney is usually parallel to the wound incision. However, the outer convex surface of the kidney may face laterally or medially depending on the size of the kidney or recipient and/or the site of the anastomoses.

Postoperative Considerations

Postoperative management of the transplant patient must insure that all reversible causes of graft dysfunction are avoided or minimized. As well as adequate immunosuppression, all patients should receive intravenous fluid therapy sustaining a systolic blood pressure of greater than 100 mmHg in the perioperative period and have their vital signs and urine output recorded hourly. Acute anuria or oliguria may not be the result of acute tubular necrosis, but of, for example, a blocked urinary catheter, urinary leak, or other obstructive uropathy. Common things are common, and fortunately transplanted kidneys function more commonly than not! When there is delay in function, hypovolemia, bleeding, catheter blockage, ureteric leak or obstruction, and vascular compromise must all be excluded as a matter of urgency if the graft is to be saved. Noninvasive Doppler ultrasound examination can aid in the diagnosis of these complications and is an invaluable tool in the management of the transplanted patient.

Summary point:

- Ultrasound can aid in the diagnosis of a number of renal transplant complications.

References

1. Cameron JI, Whiteside C, Kate J, Devins GM. Differences in quality of life across renal replacement therapies: a meta-analytic comparison. Am J Kidney Dis 2000;35:629–37.
2. Wolfe RA, Ashby VB, Milford EL, Ojo AO, Ettenger RE, Agodoa LY, et al. Comparison of mortality in all patients on dialysis, patients on dialysis awaiting transplantation, and recipients of a first cadaveric transplant. N Engl J Med 1999;341:1725–30.
3. Laupacis A, Keown P, Pus N, Krueger H, Ferguson B, Wong C. A study of the quality of life and cost-utility of renal transplantation. Kidney Int 1996;50:235–42.
4. Thrasher JB, Temple DR, Spees EK. Extravesical versus Leadbetter–Politano ureteroneocystostomy: a comparison of urological complications in 320 renal transplants. J Urol 1990;144:1105–9.
5. Lich R, Haverton LW, David LA. Recurrent urosepsis in children. J Urol 1961;86:554–9.
6. Politano VA, Leadbetter WF. An operative technique for the correction of vesicoureteral reflux. J Urol 1968;79:932–9.
7. Pleass HCC, Clark KR, Rigg KM, Reddy KS, Forsythe JL, Proud G, et al. Urological complications after renal transplantation: a prospective randomized trial comparing different techniques of ureteric anastomosis and the use of prophylactic ureteric stents. Transplant Proc 1995;27:1091–2.

Ultrasound Imaging in Renal Transplantation

G. M. Baxter

The number of patients with end-stage renal disease continues to rise and is unlikely to plateau before the middle of this century. This has tremendous implications in terms of public health resources, in terms of diagnosis, treatment, and long-term surveillance in an ever increasingly elderly population.[1] Prognosis for these patients has generally improved, especially for those with co-morbidity disease processes such as diabetes mellitus.[2]

A number of treatment options are available, including peritoneal and hemodialysis, but there is no doubt that the optimum treatment option is renal transplantation. There are limitations, namely the continuing shortage of suitable donor kidneys[3]; however, improvements in outcome due to better donor–recipient matching[4] and the use of more potent immunosuppressive regimens has meant that the one-year and five-year graft survival rates in Europe now stand at 77–82% and 57–64% respectively.[5] In order to improve on these figures further, early recognition and appropriate treatment of a variety of transplant insults and complications is required.

Transplantation is undoubtedly the treatment of choice for many patients with chronic renal failure. A well-functioning transplant will provide a glomerular filtration rate (GFR) of 50–60 ml/h, which is sufficient to return most patients to a much more independent life pattern. Leaving aside the significantly improved quality of life, in the harsh world of health economics, the cost benefit of a functioning successful transplant outweighs that of failure and hence many resources are targeted throughout the pre-, peri-, and post-transplant period to ensure high success rates are achieved. Currently the average normal life expectancy of a transplant kidney is 7–10 years, increasing to 15–20 years when a live donor organ is used.

Whilst a number of different modalities are used in imaging the renal transplant, there is no doubt that ultrasound fulfils a very useful role in both the early postoperative period, as a noninvasive indicator of transplant dysfunction, and in the long-term follow-up of these patients. This chapter will highlight the value and application of this technique.

Indications and Contraindications

There are few absolute contraindications to renal transplantation, which should be considered for all patients with end-stage renal disease severe enough to require dialysis. Patients unsuitable for transplantation are generally those who are for whatever reason, generally unfit for anesthesia or surgery, e.g., because of severe arteriopathy or severe cardiac or respiratory disease. In addition, the known hazards of immunosuppression in the context of preexisting infection or malignancy must be considered, as should the risk of disease recurrence, e.g., in patients with oxalosis or active vasculitis.

Donor Supply

Sources of organ transplantation include cadaveric, brain-dead, ventilated organ donors and live related donors. In developed countries, the majority are cadaveric in origin, whilst live related donor transplantations are favored in developing countries. Although there are some small technical differences in surgical technique and recipient outcome, the overall management of the recipient should be regarded similarly for transplants of either origin.

Histocompatibility Testing

In order to reduce the risk of rejection, especially hyperacute rejection, the presence of donor-specific antibodies in the lymphocyte cross-match test is a contraindication to transplantation. Graft acceptance in transplant patients with a negative lymphocyte cross-match test depends upon the degree of matching between the donor and the recipient giving lymphocytic antigens (HLA). There are three classes of HLA, all of which are located on chromosome 6.[6,7] All are recognized targeted antigens for T cells. HLA status is determined for all donors and recipients at the HLA A, B, and C locations. The importance of this is reflected in the improved graft survival of an HLA-matched graft $T_{1/2}$ = 17.3 years, compared with an HLA-mismatched graft survival of 7.8 years.[8] This improved survival was also demonstrated in another study, where a 17% improvement in five-year graft survival was noted in patients who received matched HLA B and DR kidneys compared to those who did not.[9]

Preoperative Management

Transplantation should be carried out within 24 hours of organ retrieval if possible, and at worst within 48 hours. During this period, a suitable recipient will have been chosen and appropriately prepared for the operating room, i.e., screened for infection and cardiorespiratory reserve, and additional dialysis given if necessary to correct any fluid or metabolite imbalance.
A live related donor, who may be a family member or a close friend, is screened by means of a thorough history, clinical examination, and HLA status assessment. Tests vary from center to center but will include a 24-hour creatinine clearance test, virology, liver function tests, and the choice of intravenous urogram, DMSA scan, arteriography, or computed tomography and/or magnetic resonance imaging to assess the kidneys.

Surgery

The standard method of surgery is a retroperitoneal iliac approach in which the transplant renal vessels are anastomosed to the external iliac vessels in the case of a cadaveric transplant and the internal iliac vessels in the case of a live related transplant. In patients receiving a third transplant, an intraperitoneal approach to the iliac vasculature is often used. The vesicoureteric anastomosis is performed by attaching the shortened donor ureter to the dome of the bladder. As a result of this procedure, the lower end of the ureter is prone to ischemic insult and secondary stricture formation, which may be functionally significant. (For more surgical details, see Chapter 3.)
Postoperative complications vary from center to center but include bleeding (less than 1 %), major vascular occlusion of the artery or vein (1–2 %), wound infection (1.6–6.3 %), and urological complications, including anastomotic leak, obstruction, and hematuria (1.3–7 %).[10–13]

Immunosuppression

The underpinning aim of immunosuppression is to prevent rejection without infectious complications or serious drug toxicity. A number of treatment options are now available and these include regimes of drugs such as cyclosporine (cyclosporin A) or tacrolimus[14] and steroids with either azathioprine or mycophenolate.[15] Antibody therapy with anti-interleukin-2 agents is effective and less toxic than with the older humoral agents including OKT3 and antithymocyte globulin. Newer developments, including rapamycin as a replacement for azathioprine or mycophenolate, are currently the subject of clinical trials. Standard immunosuppressive regimes are variable; however, our local regimen includes a combination of prednisolone, mycophenolate, and cyclosporine.
The treatment for established acute rejection is normally high-dose oral or intravenous steroids and, in more difficult cases, immunodepletion with antibody therapy or tacrolimus. There is no effective treatment for hyperacute or chronic rejection.

■ *Summary points:*

- The one-year and five-year graft survival rates are now 77–82 % and 57–64 %
- Contraindications to transplantation are few
- The risk of disease recurrence after transplantation is high in patients with oxalosis or active vasculitis
- Negative HLA cross-matching is essential for a favorable outcome

Imaging the Transplant Kidney

B Mode Ultrasound

The transplant kidney can normally be easily visualized in either iliac fossa a number of centimeters or so beneath the skin surface. Although its orientation may be variable due to the surgical technique, it is normally possible to obtain views of the transplant kidney that are perpendicular to each other. As for any other ultrasound technique, image resolution will depend on a number of factors, including patient build, the depth of the transplant below the skin surface and the presence or absence of postoperative edema. Generally a 4-MHz probe will give a good overall gray-scale assessment of the transplant kidney and is best suited to the detection of peritransplant collections and the assessment of the iliac and transplant vasculature. A higher-frequency probe, i.e., 7 MHz, will give excellent near-field resolution and good anatomical detail of the kidney, but except in the thinnest of patients, will not allow visualization of the deeper-situated vascular structures.
Morphologically the transplant kidney is very similar to the native; any apparent differences being attributable to the better ultrasonic resolution in the former. In essence, there is a well-defined renal parenchyma peripherally with a bright echogenic sinus centrally (Fig. 4.**1a**). The renal pyramids are more commonly visualized in the transplant kidney than in the native, are hypoechoic relative to the parenchyma, and bear a constant relationship to the medulla, being regularly spaced with no communication between (Fig. 4.**1b**), this being a useful differential feature from dilated calyces. Mild hydronephrosis maybe visualized with the "normal" transplant kidney, this being most common in the early transplant period when postoperative edema at the lower end of the vesicoureteric anasto-

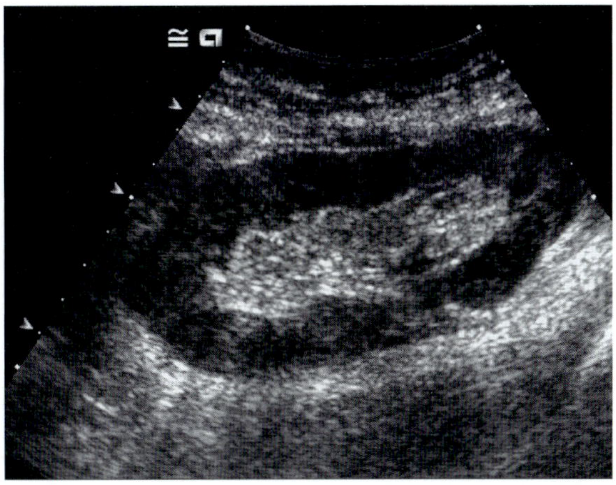

a

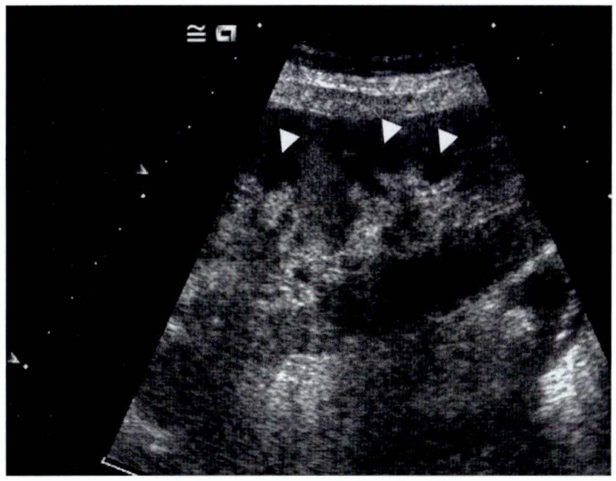

b

Fig. 4.1 **a** Ultrasound image of a normal transplant kidney. The features are similar to those of a native kidney, but detail is improved due to the more superficial position of the transplant. **b** The normal pyramids (arrowheads) are slightly more hypoechoic than the adjacent cortex, are regularly spaced, and bear a constant relationship to the medulla

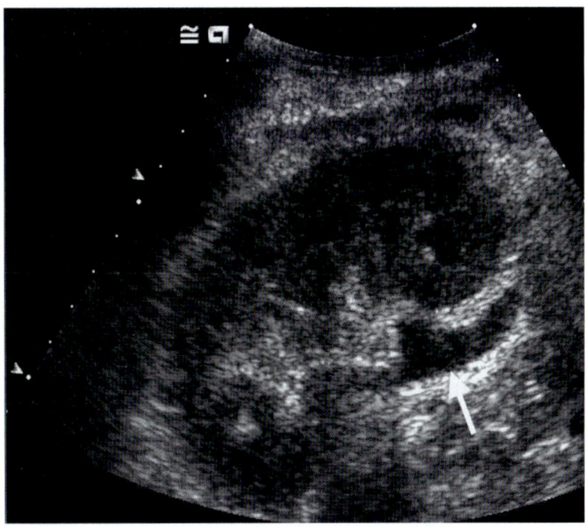

a

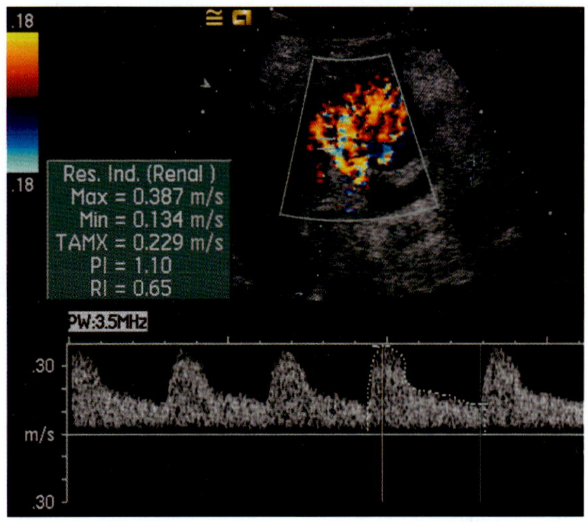

b

Fig. 4.2 **a** Ultrasound image of a 5-day-old live related renal transplant showing mild hydronephrosis with some dilatation of the proximal ureter (arrow). **b** Color Doppler image of the same patient showed excellent renal perfusion and a normal intrarenal spectral Doppler waveform with a pulsatility index (PI) of 1.10. The transplant was functioning normally and therefore the hydronephrosis was simply noted and followed on subsequent studies

mosis may be responsible. This may resolve with time. Assuming renal function to be normal, any minor degree of hydronephrosis is normally documented to act as a baseline scan against which to evaluate subsequent studies (Fig. 4.**2**).

The transplant vessels at the renal hilum should not be confused with a slightly dilated or prominent renal pelvis, and can easily be differentiated with the use of color or power Doppler ultrasound. The iliac vessels are normally identified with the color Doppler technique, although spectral Doppler is required for quantitative information. The bladder should be routinely visualized when possible and should be echofree. If turbid echoes are present, this may indicate either infection or hemorrhage, depending on the clinical setting.

Color Doppler Ultrasound

Color Doppler imaging provides an instantaneous assessment of the intrarenal vasculature and a global impression of transplant perfusion, and also identifies the transplant artery, vein, and iliac vessels (Fig. 4.**3**). Such information is purely qualitative and spectral Doppler is required for quantification. This technique is similar to that used elsewhere, i.e., a suitable in-

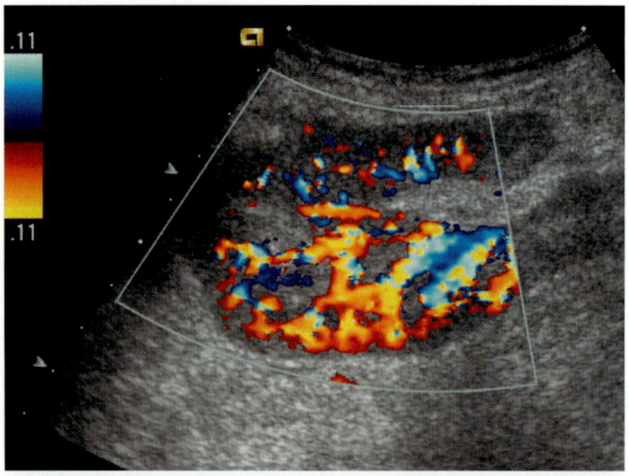

a

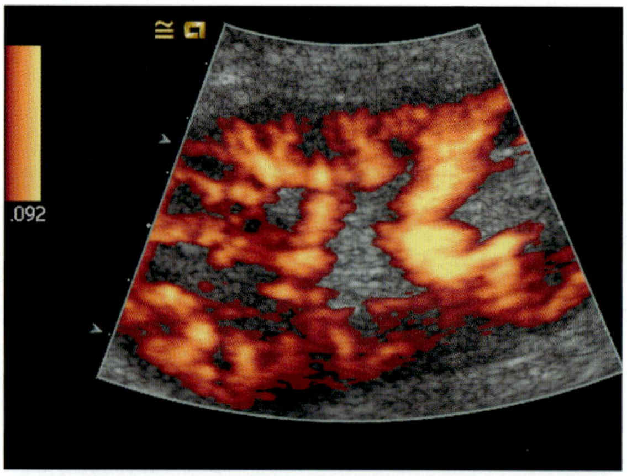

b

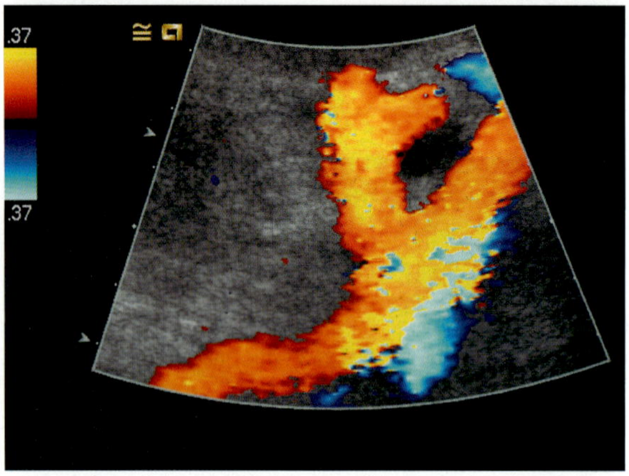

c

Fig. 4.**3** **a** Color Doppler image showing normal perfusion of the transplant kidney. **b** Power Doppler scan of **a**. This technique is more sensitive to flow detection, but all information with regard to flow direction is sacrificed. **c** Color flow image demonstration of the origin of the transplant renal artery (thick arrow) arising from the external iliac artery (thin arrow)

trarenal vessel is identified with color flow (normally an interlobar artery), the spectral gate is placed over the vessel, and a Doppler tracing is obtained. The normal Doppler tracing is a low-resistance waveform similar to that seen in the native kidney and hepatic artery. It has previously been described as having a "ski-slope" appearance with diastolic flow normally contributing up to a third or a half of the peak systolic value. Any reduction in end-diastolic flow may reflect a pathological process. For color Doppler ultrasound to be used effectively, sequential studies are required. It is generally accepted that the value of a single isolated examination is limited, and our practice is to perform transplant studies every second day in the early transplant period until renal function is satisfactory.

Many different indices have been used in an attempt to quantify "flow." These include pulsatility index (PI), resistive index (RI), systolic–diastolic ratio (SDR), and diastolic–systolic ratio (DSR). The most commonly used indices are the PI and RI; there is no specific advantage of one over the other (Fig. 4.**4a**).

With regard to the transplant artery, this can be a difficult vessel to study as it is extremely tortuous. As with other Doppler studies, an angle of less than 60° is required for accurate velocity determination, and within the transplant artery a range of normal peak systolic velocity values up to 2.5 m/s have been published.[16–18] At our center the cut-off value is 2.5 m/s; values below this level are regarded as normal (Fig. 4.**4b**) whilst those above are taken to represent a significant stenosis. The numerous twists and turns of the vessel in combination with a requirement for precise angle correction and thus velocity readings make this a meticulous and demanding examination.

There are no specific velocity values for flow in the transplant renal vein; however, often the prime consideration is simply the presence or absence of flow.

It is always of paramount importance to identify both the iliac artery (Fig. 4.**4c**) and the iliac vein in order to distinguish these from the renal vessels, and to exclude a more proximal lesion, e.g. a stenosis in the iliac artery, which may contribute to or be the cause of adverse renal function.

Summary points:

- A 4-MHz ultrasound probe gives the best overall assessment of the transplant kidney
- Mild hydronephrosis is "normal" in the early postoperative transplant period
- Serial measurements with color Doppler ultrasonography can monitor transplant dysfunction

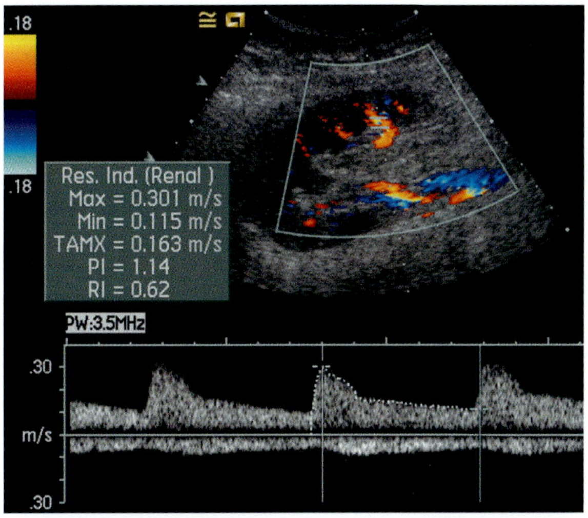

a

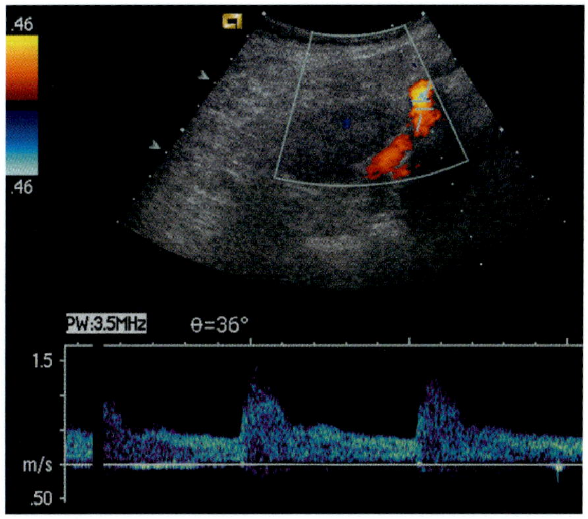

b

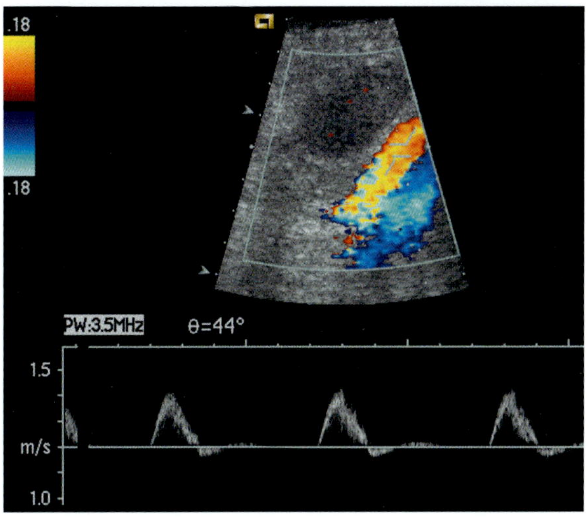

c

Fig. 4.**4** **a** Normal intrarenal spectral Doppler waveform. There is normal flow throughout diastole, this being reflected in the PI of 1.14 (RI 0.62). The PI is derived by the formula

$$PI = \frac{\text{peak systolic velocity–end diastolic velocity}}{\text{time averaged mean velocity}},$$

whilst the resistive index

$$RI = \frac{\text{peak systolic velocity–end diastolic velocity}}{\text{peak systolic velocity}}.$$

b Normal Doppler waveform from the origin of the transplant renal artery. The peak systolic velocity is 1.0 m/s. **c** Normal spectral Doppler waveform from the iliac artery just proximal to the origin of the transplant artery. The waveform is triphasic and the peak systolic velocity is 1.0 m/s

- Both the transplant and the iliac vessels should always be identified to avoid confusion
- The pulsatility index (PI) and resistive index (RI) are the most commonly used Doppler indices

Early Complications

A number of complications are recognized in the early transplant period; these include parenchymal insults, i.e., acute tubular necrosis (ATN), acute rejection, or both; vascular occlusions; obstruction; hemorrhage; urinary leak; collections; infection; and drug toxicity related to the antirejection treatment itself. Many of these complications can be differentiated on the basis of a combination of clinical history, bacteriology. and ultrasound. Very often, however, the main differential diagnosis is between acute rejection and ATN, and this may be difficult clinically as symptoms are often absent. Since the two entities require different treatment, early accurate diagnosis is essential. It is not possible to distinguish between these pathological entities with color Doppler ultrasonography—histology is required. Nevertheless, ultrasound is useful in its dual role of not only monitoring transplant dysfunction but also assessing response to therapy.

Acute Tubular Necrosis

ATN is common in the early transplant period; as many as 10–30% of patients require dialysis in the early stages. Delayed graft function, rare when a live related donor is used, is principally related to both the donor and the donor kidney, particularly the warm ischemic time. In patients with established ATN requiring dialysis, recovery usually occurs within one to two weeks following transplantation, although on rare occasions it may be delayed for up to three months.

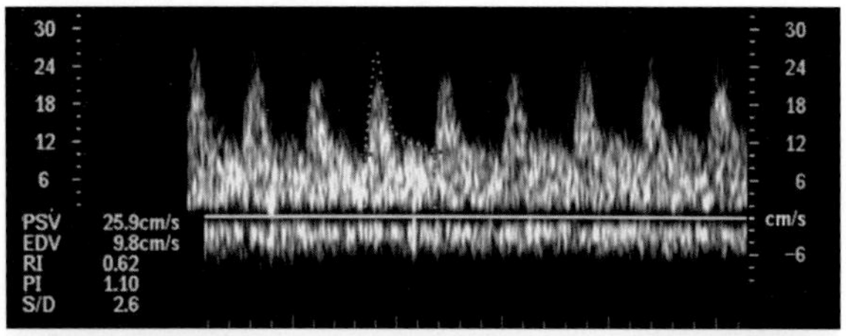

a

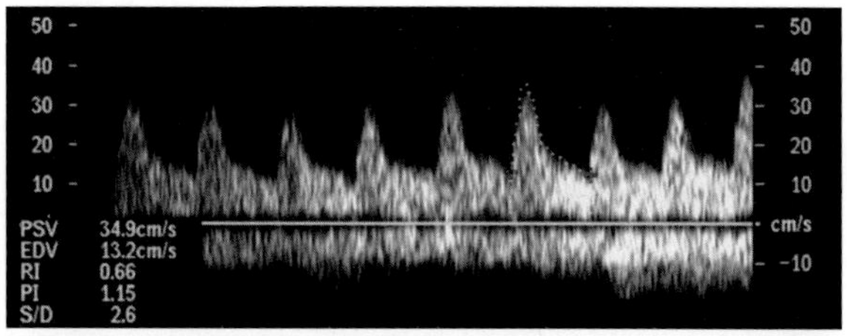

b

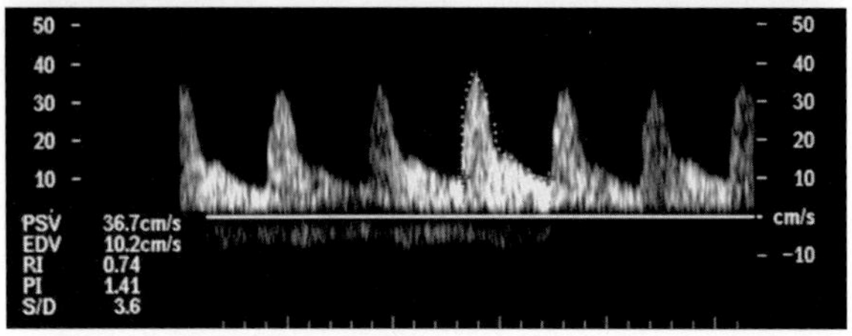

c

Fig. 4.**5 a–c** Series of spectral Doppler images performed over the course of five days in a patient with delayed function. Normal diastolic flow is demonstrated on all three scans with normal PIs of 1.10, 1.15, and 1.41 respectively. The presumptive diagnosis was acute tubular necrosis (ATN), biopsy was withheld, and the kidney began to function one day after the last scan. There had been no change to the immunosuppressive regime in that time

Acute Rejection

Biopsy is required for the diagnosis of acute rejection and in experienced hands is generally safe; complications of postbiopsy bleeding requiring blood transfusion or pain requiring opiate analgesia occur at a frequency of less than 5%.[19] Acute rejection may affect up to 40% of patients, peaking at one to three weeks following transplantation. Assuming it is promptly recognized, it is normally treated with high-dose steroids or antibody therapy. It is normally asymptomatic, but rarely may be accompanied by flu-like symptoms, pyrexia, and graft tenderness. It should be excluded in patients with deteriorating renal function, and the diagnosis is often difficult, especially in patients with nonfunctioning grafts. Unfortunately, its occurrence is an adverse long-term prognostic indicator.[20]

Role of Ultrasound in Delayed Function

A number of studies were performed in the 1980s to assess the value of Doppler ultrasonography in differentiating acute rejection from ATN in a search for an accurate noninvasive test to supplant biopsy. Initial results were confusing and contradictory. A number of well-recognized factors are now known to be responsible for this, including inhomogeneous study populations, poorly defined end points, and differing diagnostic criteria between the different study groups. In retrospect, the expectation of differentiating ATN from acute rejection with Doppler was, to say the least, hopeful; however, Doppler ultrasonography continues to have a role as a monitoring tool in patients with delayed function (Fig. 4.**5**).

B Mode Ultrasound

Although the B mode ultrasound appearances of acute rejection are well documented, the reports include many different arbitrary observations[21]: reduction in corticomedullary differentiation, reduction in renal sinus echoes, increased and reduced renal parenchymal echoes, increased cortical reflectivity, and so on have all been described. These appearances are largely of historical interest and should no longer be observed, certainly within the early transplant period. They occur late, well after the onset of acute rejection, and are so arbitrary and inconsistent that they are of limited value. It is of interest to note, however, that observations including increased renal length[22] and cross-sectional area[23] have been reported during rejection. ATN can cause renal length to increase minimally in comparison with acute rejection; however, suffice it to say that none of these last measurements have been adopted for clinical use.

Color Doppler Ultrasound

Color Doppler is utilized in the early transplant period and provides both an overall qualitative impression of renal perfusion and then—more specifically on interrogation of individual vessels with spectral Doppler—quantitative serial measurements. Scanning is normally performed three times per week until function is established. As mentioned previously, the technique cannot differentiate ATN from acute rejection,[24,25] despite earlier claims to the contrary[26,27]; however, serial measurements of PI or RI in conjunction with clinical and biochemical findings are useful in the early transplant period and guide the clinician as to whether to refrain or to proceed to biopsy. A PI of less than 1.5 or RI less than 0.7 is normal, whilst a PI greater than 1.8 or RI greater than 0.7 should be regarded as pathological. Although both acute rejection and ATN can cause both ratios to increase, as the ratios rise the likelihood of the process being due to acute rejection becomes greater (Table 4.**1**). Complete absence of diastolic flow or flow reversal is due to acute rejection in the majority of cases. Once the diagnosis has been confirmed histologically the response to treatment can be followed

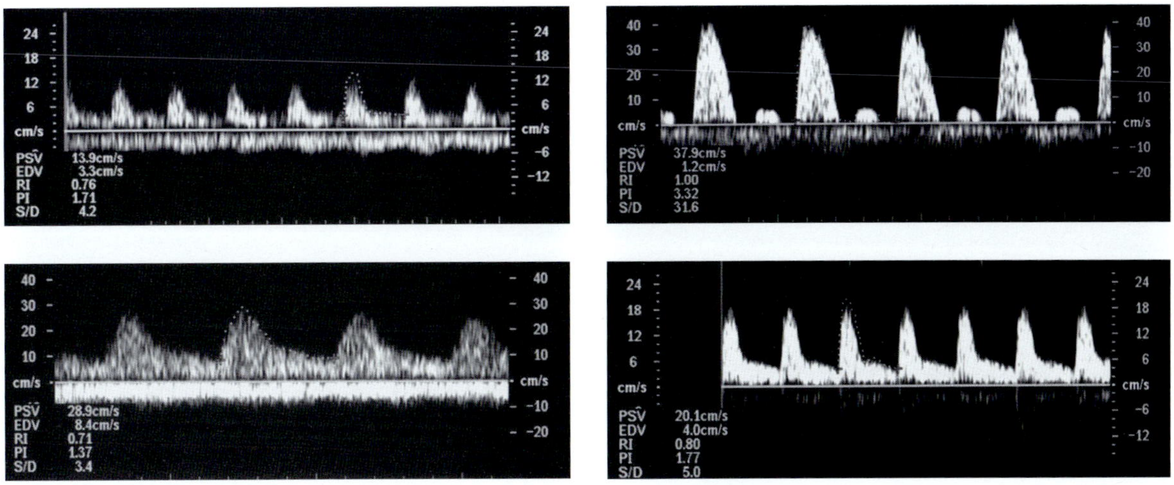

Fig. 4.**6** **a–d** Series of spectral Doppler traces in a patient with delayed function. The initial scan (**a**) demonstrated normal diastolic flow with a PI of 1.71; however, the scan two days later (**b**) showed only a small blip of diastolic flow and an elevated PI of 3.32. Biopsy was performed and this confirmed the suspicion of acute rejection. Antirejection therapy was begun and the scan two days later (**c**) showed a significant improvement with restoration of normal diastolic flow and a PI of 1.37. A subsequent scan five days later (**d**) showed good maintenance of diastolic flow and a PI of 1.77

with serial ultrasound studies (Fig. 4.**6**). Power Doppler can be used in addition to or even instead of color Doppler imaging; however, there are no studies to date to show any improved benefits of doing so, and indeed the loss of directional information may actually be disadvantageous.

Some recently published work looking at the use of the acceleration time in the early transplant period has shown interesting results. It was shown that a short acceleration time on day 1 was associated with a longer duration of delayed function, whilst an acceleration time of less than 90 milliseconds at day 5 was associated with a high risk of rejection. The authors felt that these results were more sensitive than conventional RI measurements[28]; however, the results remain to be substantiated.

Table 4.**1** Resistive index in relation to distribution of diagnosis

RI	RI and Distribution of Diagnosis Rejection (%)	Normal (%)	ATN (%)	Other (%)
<0.65	0	61	25	14
0.65–0.79	25	39	22	14
0.80–0.89	70	5	25	0
≥0.90	100	0	0	0

ATN, acute tubular necrosis

Thrombosis

Arterial Thrombosis

Arterial thrombosis is rare, occurs in the early transplant period, and is often asymptomatic. It may be discovered incidentally at isotope renography or on routine Doppler examination of a nonfunctioning graft. Predisposing factors include multiple renal vessels, young pediatric donor kidneys, and atherosclerosis in either the donor or the recipient. The process is normally irreversible, resulting in graft infarction and nephrectomy. Should a transplant kidney contain multiple or accessory renal vessels, it is possible for one vessel to thrombose, resulting in segmental infarction. In this situation renal function can remain stable and satisfactory in the long term.

The ultrasound appearances are striking. There is complete absence of flow in the main transplant renal artery and intrarenal vasculature on both color flow and spectral analyses. When seen, it is important first to confirm that the appropriate ultrasound settings have been used. Absence of renal flow may be seen in patients with hyperacute rejection or renal vein thrombosis; however, in both these conditions the main transplant artery is normally patent and shows reversed diastolic flow on spectral examination.[29] Occasionally trauma may be the cause of acute arterial thrombosis; however, this normally occurs outside the early transplant period (Fig. 4.**7**).

Venous Thrombosis

Venous thrombosis is more common than arterial thrombosis and causes acute pain and swelling of the graft, normally in association with an abrupt cessation of renal function and output. A typical patient would be one with a nonfunctioning graft, normally between the third and the eighth postoperative day.[30] Measures to avoid this complication include withholding cyclos-

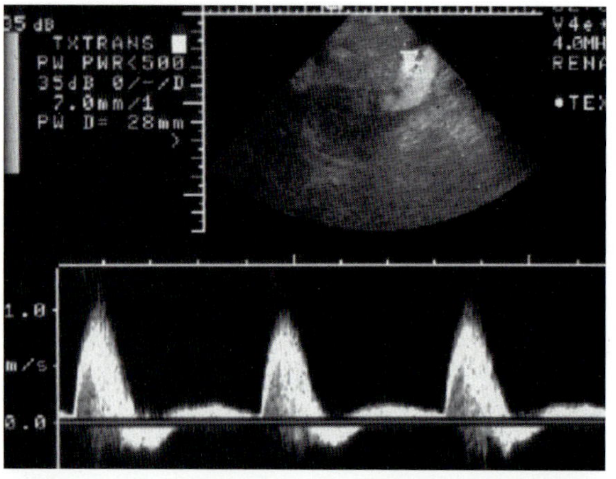

a

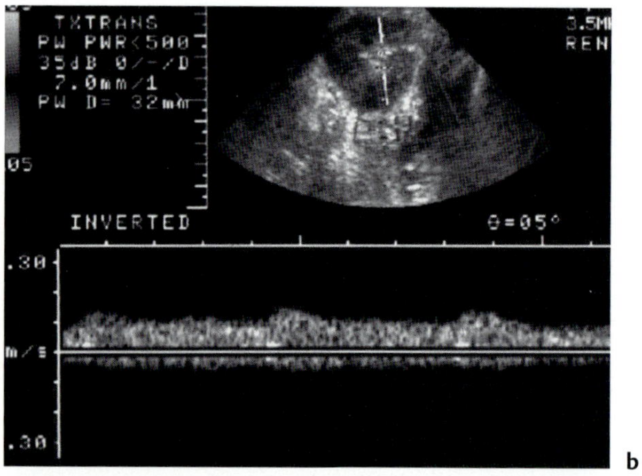

b

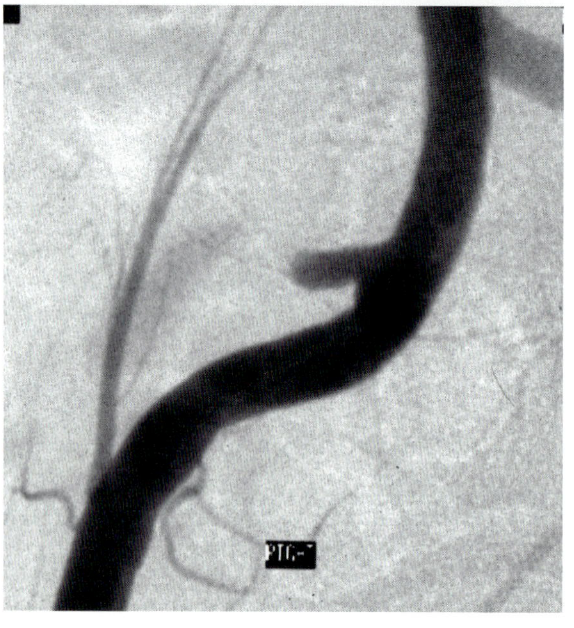

c

Fig. 4.7 A young transplant patient fell off a mountain bike, became anuric, and presented 48 hours later. **a** Color Doppler imaging demonstrated a normal iliac artery waveform, but the main transplant artery could not be identified. **b** A trace of color flow was seen at the renal hilum, and spectral examination showed a low-amplitude parvus-tardus-type waveform. No additional flow could be demonstrated within the kidney, and the overall picture was suggestive of a major proximal arterial catastrophe, i.e., an intimal dissection of the transplant artery. **c** An arteriogram was performed immediately and confirmed the suspected diagnosis. A transplant nephrectomy was performed

porine and tacrolimus in the early postoperative period and the use of subcutaneous heparin or aspirin alone. None of these options, however, have been proven in clinical trials. A low index of suspicion for venous thrombosis is required as a rapid diagnosis and intervention may salvage the kidney, although it is a fact that nephrectomy is still performed in the majority of cases.

Diagnostic criteria include a dilated transplant vein containing thrombus or thrombus within the main intrarenal venous system, absent venous flow in the transplant vein on color flow ultrasonography, and reversed diastolic flow within the intrarenal arterial system and the transplant renal artery on Doppler imaging[31,32] (Fig. 4.**8**). It is important to remember that reversed diastolic flow may also be seen in severe acute rejection.

A low-amplitude parvus tardus arterial waveform has also been described in incomplete renal vein thrombosis, some residual venous flow being noted within the intrarenal venous radicles. Only a few cases have been described and it is not clear whether prognosis is altered or is as universally poor within this subgroup[33] (Fig. 4.**9**).

Obstruction

Early obstruction within 72 hours of operation is normally due to ureteric or vesical blood clots and may be relieved by simple bladder irrigation. Obstruction thereafter may reflect a distal ureteric stenosis or external compression of the ureter by, e.g. a lymphocele. Collections, if present, may be drained percutaneously either as a temporary or as a permanent procedure. In patients with a suspected ureteric stenosis, nephrostomy drainage followed by a contrast examination is normally performed. Depending on the clinical situation, reoperation or percutaneous stenting with monitoring of renal function are normally the treatment options.

Although hydronephrosis is easily identified with ultrasound, these appearances must always be interpreted in conjunction with renal function. In addition, it is important to consider hydronephrosis as a cause of an elevated PI or RI in the early transplant period.

Hemorrhage

Bleeding can occur from either the wound site or the transplant kidney itself. Ultrasound can readily detect hematoma. Any bleeding is usually self-limiting. Reexploration is only occasionally required to identify and treat the bleeding point and subsequent hematoma. Catastrophic hemorrhage is rare and is due to either rupture or anastomotic breakdown, the most likely clinical scenario being when there is an associated deep wound infection or postbiopsy hemorrhage.

Urinary Leak

Urinary leak occurs in up to 6% of renal transplant recipients[34] and is due to disruption or breakdown of the vesicoureteric anastomosis or, indeed, necrosis of the distal ureter. Symptoms normally include increased abdominal pain, reduction of urine volumes, and, sometimes, urine leakage from the wound site. Ultrasound may show a new collection, a cystogram may show leakage from the bladder; an isotope scan may be helpful. Treatment is normally surgical repair, although a temporizing nephrostomy can be useful in certain clinical situations.

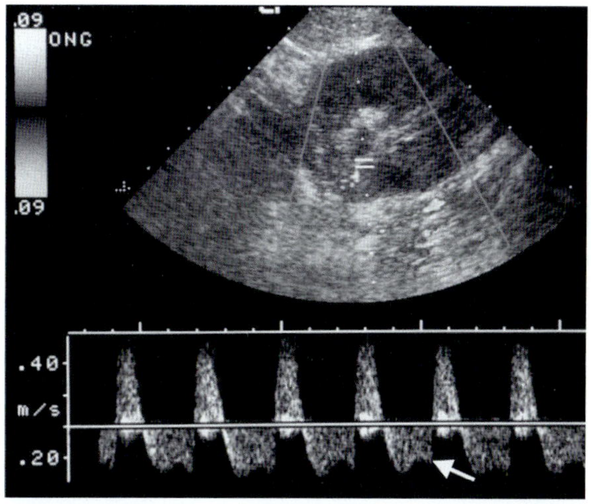

Fig. 4.**8** Intra-arterial spectral Doppler waveform from a patient with renal vein thrombosis, showing a typical reverse diastolic flow pattern with the aptly named “reverse M sign” (arrow) said to be characteristic of the condition. Venous flow was absent both within the kidney and in the transplant vein itself

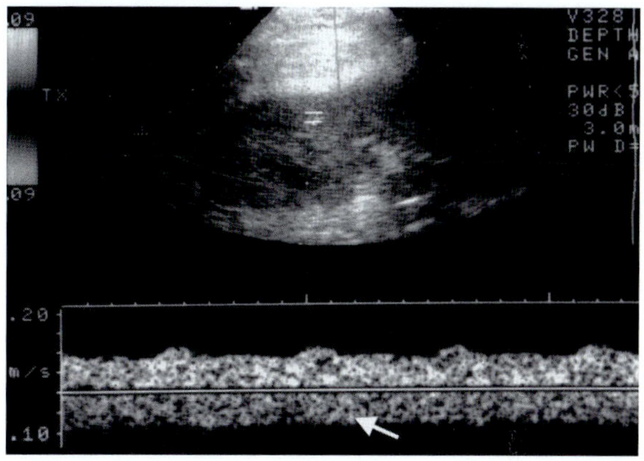

Fig. 4.**9** Intra-arterial waveform from a patient with renal vein thrombosis. In this case a little venous flow could be identified on both color and spectral analysis within the kidney. The arterial waveform is of low amplitude with a significantly reduced systolic component. Note the venous flow beneath the baseline (arrow). Surgery confirmed an incomplete renal vein thrombosis

Post-transplant Collections

Abscess, hematoma, lymphocele, and urinoma may all occur in the post-transplant period. Ultrasound can identify all, and although septations and more solid echoes may be seen in some, normally it is the clinical findings interpreted in conjunction with the ultrasound appearance that allow the nature of the collection to be recognized. If there is doubt and a definitive diagnosis is required, aspiration and drainage can be performed (Fig. 4.**10**).

Cyclosporine and Tacrolimus Toxicity

The antirejection agents cyclosporine and tacrolimus are both calcineurin inhibitors and, although they represent a major advance in organ transplantation, their nephrotoxicity remains a problem. Both produce a reversible renovascular constriction acutely and an interstitial fibrosis chronically.[35] This may delay recovery from ATN and cause irreversible damage to the transplant itself. To make a diagnosis of nephrotoxicity in the setting of a nonfunctioning graft is notoriously difficult and many would prefer to avoid the use of these drugs. Serum drug levels and renal biopsy are traditional but imperfect methods of diagnosis. Ultrasound is generally unhelpful as the nephrotoxic effects of these drugs generally do not produce any significant change in diastolic flow. Occasionally a reduction in diastolic flow has been noted.

Infection

Patients are susceptible to infections of the chest, wound, and urinary tract in the early postoperative period. Wound infections are likely to be due to *Staphylo-*

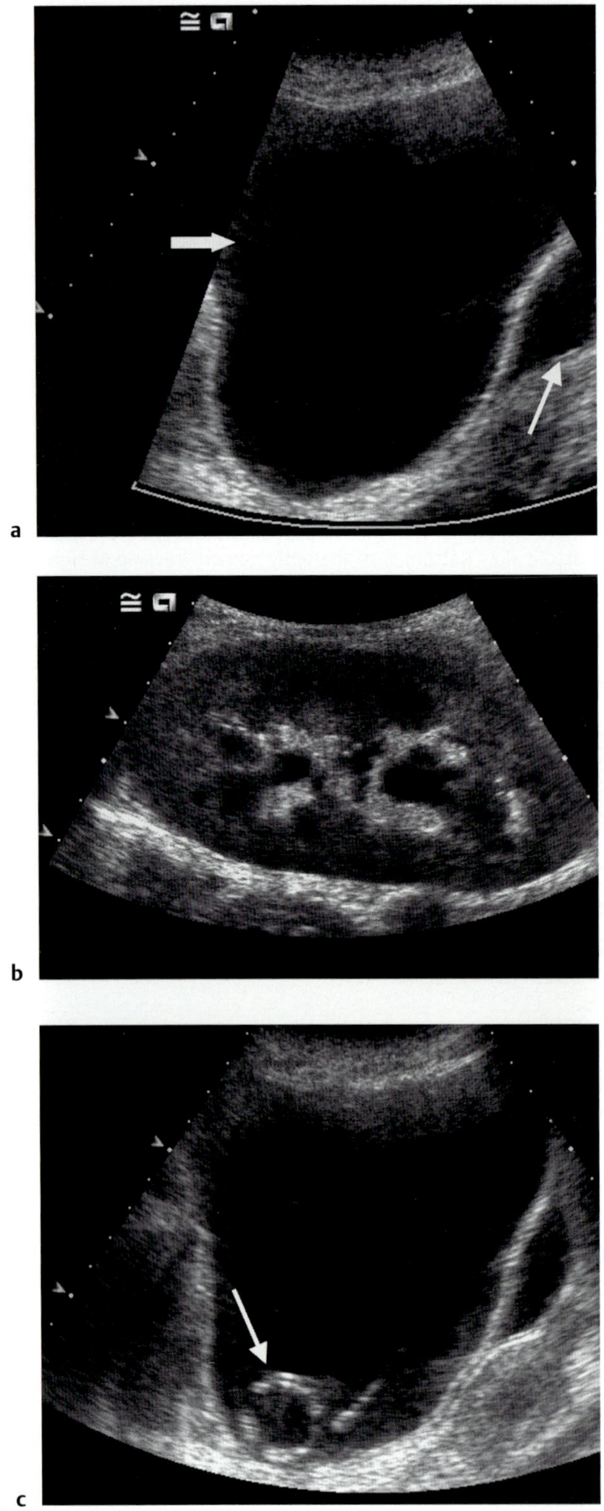

Fig. 4.**10** **a** Transverse image through the pelvis showing a large 10.5×9.0 cm cystic collection (thick arrow) displacing the bladder to the left (thin arrow). **b** A scan of the transplant kidney showed early hydronephrosis secondary to ureteric compression. **c** The fluid was drained using the Seldinger technique under ultrasound control. An 8-Fr pigtail catheter was placed into the collection (arrow) and drained a large amount of lymph

coccus aureus, whilst use of urinary catheters and reflux predisposes to urinary tract infection. This may result in a deterioration in renal function which on occasion can be indistinguishable from rejection, and occasionally pyelonephritis may be diagnosed following transplant biopsy for suspected rejection. Although, as we have said, ultrasound has little or no role in the diagnosis of infection, infection itself may adversely affect the PI or RI ratio.

■ *Summary points:*

- From 10% to 30% of patients require dialysis for acute tubular necrosis following transplantation
- Up to 40% of patients develop acute rejection following transplantation
- Gray-scale ultrasound gives anatomical information only; color Doppler imaging is necessary for graft monitoring
- Vascular occlusions, ureteric obstruction, collections, and infection can all elevate the PI and RI
- Both arterial and venous occlusions carry a poor prognosis and often result in transplant nephrectomy

Late Complications

As mentioned previously, ischemia may affect the lower aspect of the transplant ureter with secondary stricture formation, hydronephrosis, and deterioration in renal function. This is related to the surgical technique which sheds the blood supply to the lower two thirds of the ureter during transplantation, the main supply after transplantation being from the transplant renal artery. An overlong ureter is at risk of an ischemic-related stenosis at its lower end, and this has a tendency to progress insidiously, with deterioration in renal function a late event. Routine ultrasound screening should therefore detect this process early before permanent severe renal damage results (Fig. 4.**11**).

Transplant Artery Stenosis

Stenosis of the transplant renal artery can occur in 10% of cases[36] and may be found in asymptomatic patients. Clinically, however, suspicion should be raised in those patients with difficult-to-control hypertension, progressive renal impairment, or a combination of both. Deterioration in renal function following ACE inhibitor therapy is also a recognized indication for referral. Predisposing factors include renal donor atherosclerosis and small pediatric renal donors to adult patients. With regard to the best diagnostic test, opinions vary from center to center: advocates exist for isotope renography, angiography, MRI and ultrasonography.[37–39] To some extent the choice of the best will depend upon

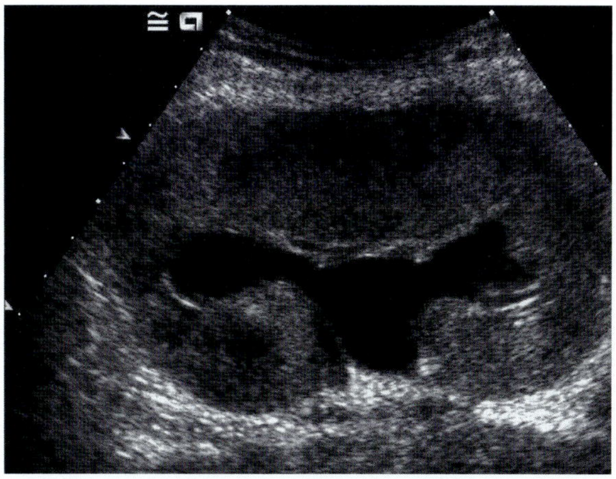

Fig. 4.11 Patient with a failed pancreatic transplant and a failing renal transplant. The cortical echogenicity is increased and there is loss of corticomedullary differentiation indicative of chronic rejection. The degree of hydronephrosis was felt to have worsened from previous scans. A nephrostomy was inserted but overall function did not improve

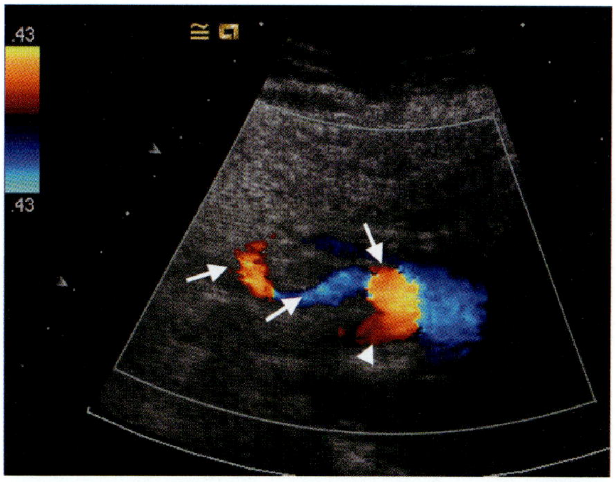

Fig. 4.12 Color Doppler image showing the tortuous nature of the transplant artery (arrows). Its origin from the external iliac artery (arrowhead) is easily appreciated

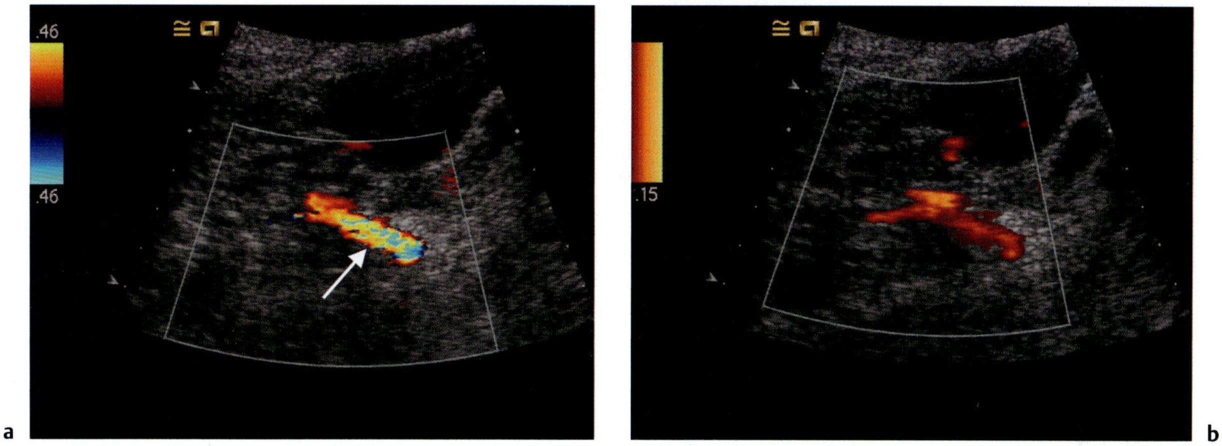

Fig. 4.13 **a** Color Doppler ultrasonography of a transplant artery showing an area of aliasing (arrow) highly suggestive of a stenosis. **b** The same area on power Doppler imaging. The stenosis is no longer visible

local expertise and the availability of technology. In our unit we use color Doppler ultrasonography, and if this confirms a stenosis, angiography is performed with a view to percutaneous angioplasty and/or stenting.

The color Doppler examination can be difficult because vessel tortuosity may result in poor Doppler angle correction and therefore incorrect velocity estimation. In addition, distinguishing between a focal stenosis and the numerous twists and turns of the transplant artery is known to be difficult and a potential pitfall, as the latter also alter local hemodynamics and thus peak velocity readings (Fig. 4.**12**). Although techniques such as power Doppler can be helpful in displaying the twists and turns more elegantly than color Doppler, a stenosis may be masked by the former technique (Fig. 4.**13**). When examining the transplant artery it is important to remember to examine the proximal iliac artery, as a stenosis in this region may also contribute to a reduction in renal function. The majority of stenotic lesions, however, occur at or close to the surgical anastomoses and result in a focal area of aliasing on color flow imaging and a peak systolic velocity greater than 2.5 m/s on spectral Doppler analysis.[38] The secondary effects of downstream turbulence, flow reversal, and spectral broadening may be seen distal to the primary stenotic site and add weight to the primary diagnostic findings (Fig. 4.**14**). The transplant renal artery can normally be visualized throughout its length, and therefore reliance upon the demonstration of secondary downstream effects (i.e., the parvus tardus effect) within the intrarenal

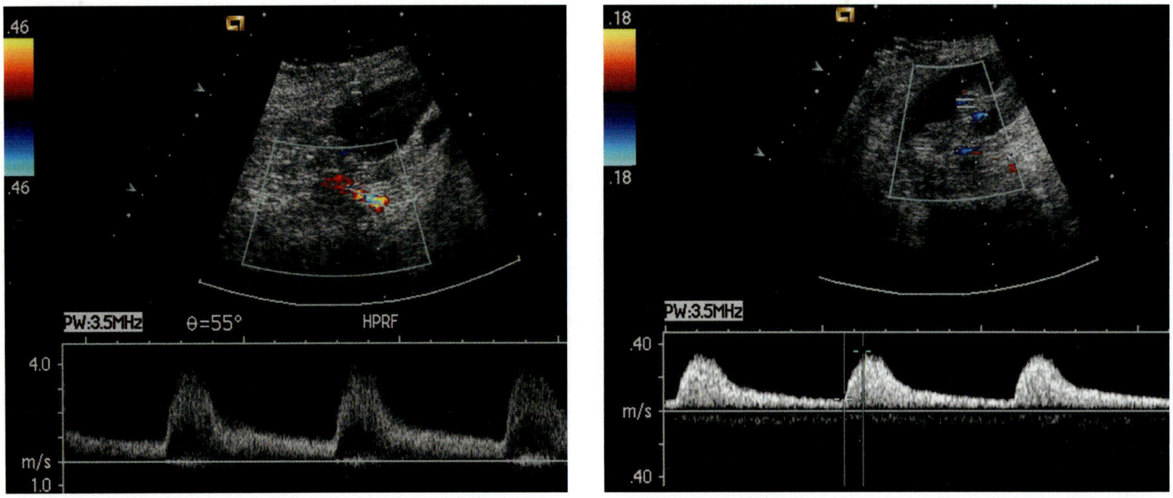

a b

Fig. 4.**14** **a** Spectral Doppler analysis of the transplant vessel in Fig. 4.**13**, showing a markedly elevated peak systolic velocity of 3.5 m/s consistent with a transplant artery stenosis. **b** Intrarenal Doppler analysis from the same patient demonstrating a very slow rise time, i.e., the parvus tardus effect, often associated with a more proximal stenosing lesion. The acceleration time was measured at 120 milliseconds (normal < 70 milliseconds)

Transplant artery

Intrarenal artery

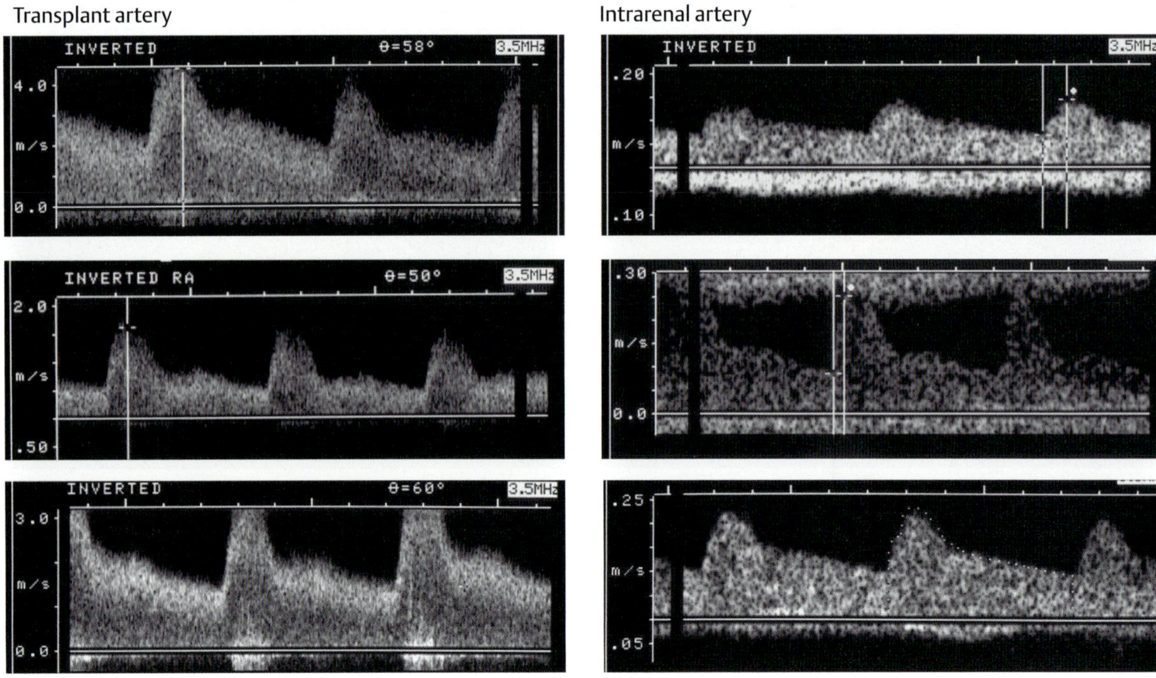

a b c

Fig. 4.**15** Serial spectral Doppler studies from a patient with a transplant artery stenosis treated by angioplasty. **a** The baseline study of the transplant artery shows an elevated peak systolic velocity of 4 m/s and a downstream intrarenal parvus tardus waveform. **b** An angioplasty was performed and examination one month later showed a normal transplant artery velocity of 1.5 m/s and a normal intrarenal waveform. **c** Seven months later, however, the transplant artery velocity had increased to 3.0 m/s and the parvus tardus waveform had returned, indicative of a recurrent stenosis

vasculature to aid diagnosis is less important than in the native kidney.[38] Branch stenoses are known to occur within the transplant kidney, but these are as difficult to visualize both with angiography and ultrasound.

Color Doppler ultrasonography may also have a role in the detection of disease recurrence in patients treated by angioplasty or stenting (Fig. 4.**15**).

Arteriovenous Fistula

Arteriovenous fistulae generally occur secondary to renal biopsy with an incidence of 1–2 %. Normally they are of little clinical significance, and most resolve spontaneously, as reflected in a study in which 10 % of patients developed an arteriovenous fistula after bi-

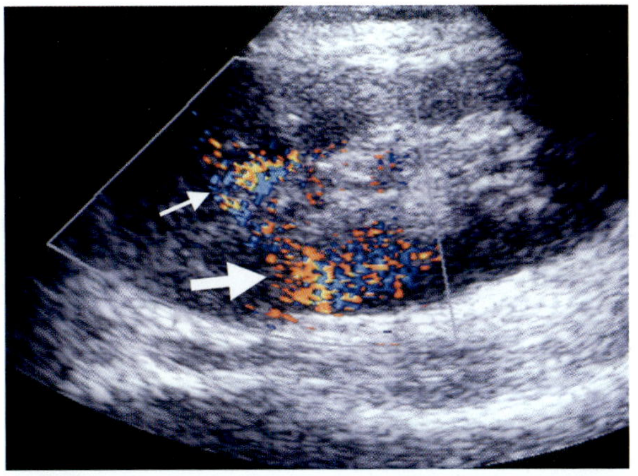

a

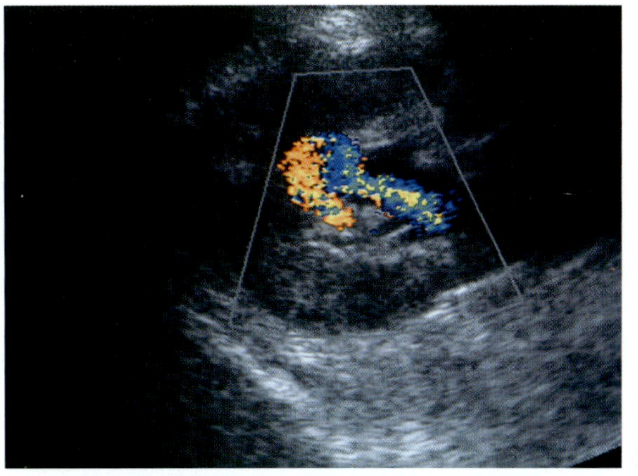

b

Fig. 4.**16** **a** Color flow image of an arteriovenous fistula (thin arrow) with surrounding tissue vibration (thick arrow). Note the absence of normal intrarenal flow. **b** A large tortuous draining vein from the fistula is easily visualized

opsy, all but one of which completely resolved.[40] Those that do persist give rise to a very spectacular pathognomonic color flow appearance. Some authors have postulated arteriovenous fistulae as a cause of hypertension and impaired renal function, although this is not common; often these lesions are simply observed. Any radiological intervention would only be considered if the fistula was bleeding or significantly increasing in size, producing a "steal syndrome" from the kidney, as in both situations the benefits of embolization would be considered to outweigh those of inactivity.

The ultrasound appearances of an arteriovenous fistula include a focal pool of color flow containing both arterial and venous components on spectral analysis. It can often be differentiated from "high flow" in other parts of the kidney by increasing the pulse repetition frequency (PRF) to a level that results in nonvisualization of normal intrarenal vasculature. At this level, only the pathologically increased flow of a fistula will be visualized. This maneuver itself is almost diagnostic. Spectral analysis showing increased systolic and diastolic flow may be noted in the affected area, with a resultant normal or reduced PI or RI ratio in comparison to the normal surrounding vessels.[41] Venous flow can be normal or turbulent in up to one third of patients. A large draining vein may also be visualized (Fig. 4.**16**).

Cyclosporine and Tacrolimus Toxicity

Both drugs have a well recognized toxic effect on renal function which may lead to progressive deterioration of graft function. This maybe difficult to distinguish from chronic rejection. A therapeutic trial of dose reduction or conversion to an alternative immunosuppressive agent may need to be considered. Following this maneuver, a small but significant number of patients will respond.

Rejection

Acute Rejection

Acute rejection is an unusual late complication; if it occurs, noncompliance with drug therapy should be considered a strong possibility. The diagnosis and treatment are as discussed previously.

Chronic Rejection

Chronic rejection is a gradual deterioration in graft function beginning at least three months after transplantation in association with the biopsy appearances of fibrous intimal thickening, interstitial fibrosis, and tubular atrophy. The most consistent predisposing factors are previous episodes of acute rejection. As there is no effective treatment for chronic rejection, all efforts are concentrated on trying to prevent episodes of acute rejection as a method of reducing chronic rejection. Some ultrasound features have been described and include increased transplant echogenicity and a reduction in the number of intrarenal vessels; however, these signs are of minimal prognostic significance and the role of ultrasound in chronic rejection is limited (Fig. 4.**17**).

Urinary Infection

Asymptomatic bacteriuria is common and has a good prognosis. Symptomatic infections are also common and may cause pyuria, pyelonephritis, and a temporary reduction in renal function. Repeated infections may be due to an underlying structural abnormality such as calculi, obstruction, or reflux. Repeated infections may occasionally lead to malakoplakia.

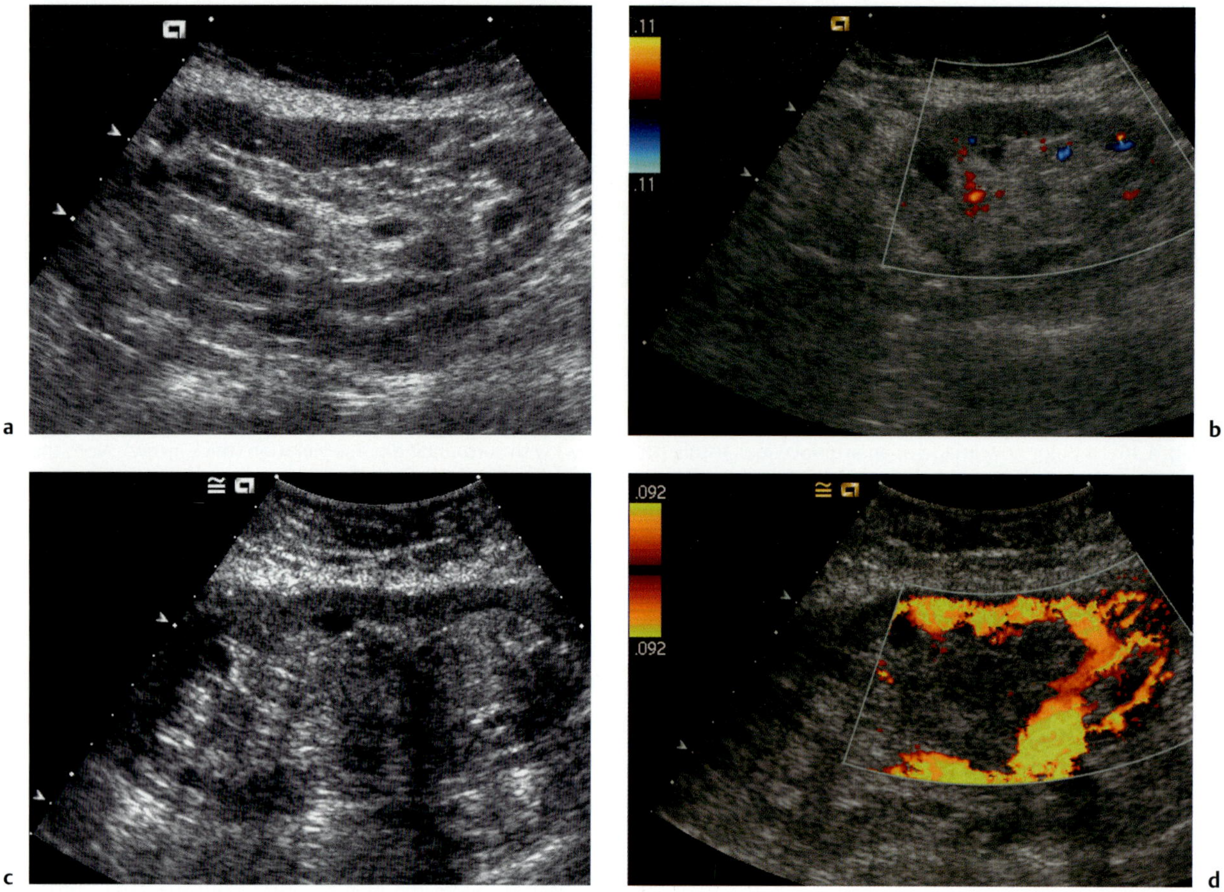

Fig. 4.**17** **a** Transplant kidney failing with chronic rejection, showing marked loss of cortical thickness. **b** Color flow analysis of **a** showed a marked reduction in flow with only a paucity of vessels within the kidney. **c** A similar-appearing kidney to that in **a** with loss of cortical thickness, this time in a 13-year-old transplant kidney with good function. **d** Color flow in this case showed excellent global perfusion, in contrast to **b**

Summary points:

- The lower end of the transplant ureter is at risk of an ischemic-related stricture
- Transplant artery stenosis occurs in up to 10% of patients
- The peak systolic velocity in the transplant renal artery is the best measurement for the detection of renal arterial stenosis. In our institution the cutoff value is 2.5 m/s
- Arteriovenous fistulae have an incidence of 1–2%. The vast majority are benign but ultrasonically interesting. Vascular steal is uncommon
- There is no effective treatment for chronic rejection
- Long-term risk factors are related to cardiovascular disease, infection, and the risk of malignancy

Long-Term Complications

Recurrent Glomerulonephritis and Recurrent Disease

Most forms of glomerulonephritis may cause recurrent disease in the transplant kidney. Early recurrence and graft failure are rare. Recurrent disease is more commonly detected in long-term recipients with diabetes mellitus, amyloidosis, and cystinosis. Of more importance in patients with oxalosis or active vasculitis is the fact that disease recurrence and renal damage are commoner in the early stages of transplantation.[42] Ultrasound has no specific role in this area apart from excluding the treatable causes of reduced renal function as discussed previously.

Other Complications

Transplant patients suffer increased morbidity and mortality from cardiovascular disease and are at increased risk of developing malignancy and infection secondary to the immunosuppressive regime. Car-

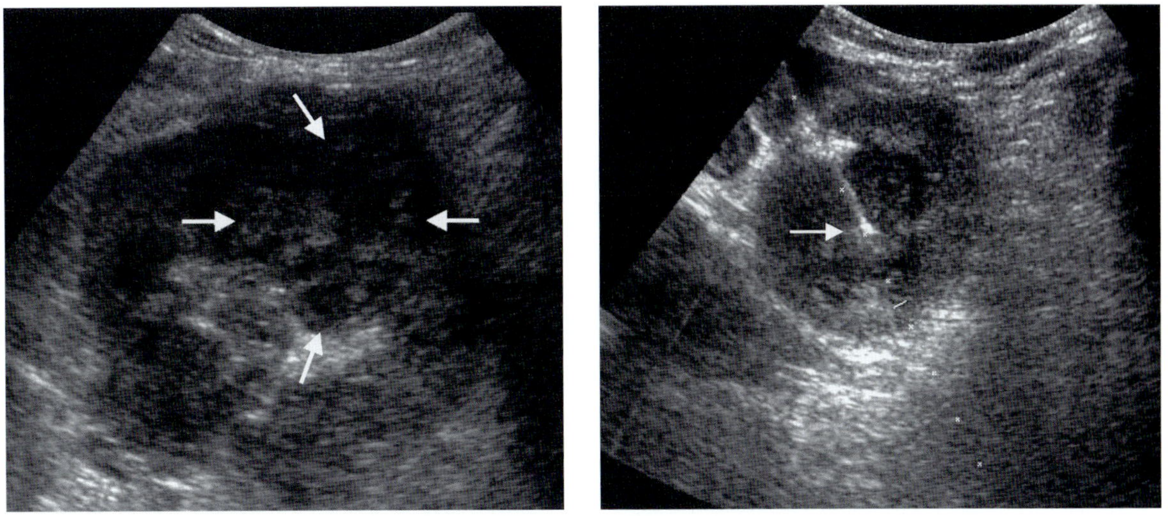

Fig. 4.**18** **a** A 4.5-cm solid mass was noted in the transplant kidney (arrows). **b** This was biopsied using an 18G Tru-Cut needle under ultrasound guidance. The needle can be easily visualized (arrow) within the mass. Histological analysis confirmed the presence of a melanoma

diovascular risk factors include hypertension, left ventricular hypertrophy, and altered liver profile, but as yet specific targeting of those areas has not resulted in any improvement in survival.

In contrast, the incidence of infection has been reduced significantly by the improvement in immunosuppression and by an increased awareness of the different types of infection leading to specific targeted therapy.

The most common malignancies are skin-related, cervical cancer, and non-Hodgkin lymphoma, and careful supervision of the transplant population is required. It is hoped that earlier diagnosis will result in the best prognosis for each of these disorders[43] (Fig. 4.**18**).

Summary

Renal transplantation is the best treatment option for chronic renal failure, with improvements in social activity, work, and family life. It is an extremely cost-effective procedure when successful. Ultrasonography plays a major role in the imaging of these patients, and color Doppler is helpful to the transplant physician in the detection of graft dysfunction and peritransplant collections, some of which may be drained under ultrasound guidance. It is also helpful in the diagnosis of chronic vascular complications, including transplant artery stenosis and arteriovenous fistula, although it has no specific application in the diagnosis of chronic rejection.

References

1. Valderrabano F, Jones EHP, Mallick NP. Report on the management of renal failure in Europe XXIV, 1993. Nephrol Dial Transplant 1995;10(Suppl 51):1–25.
2. Charra B, Calemerd E, Ruffet M, et al. Survival as an index of the adequacy of dialysis. Kidney Int 1992;41:1286–91.
3. Gore SM, Cable DJ, Holland AJ. Organ donation from intensive care units in England and Wales—two year confidential audit of deaths in intensive care. Br Med J;304:349–55.
4. Takemoto S, Terasaki PI, Cecka JM, Chong YW, Gjertson DW. Survival of nationally shared HLA-matched kidney transplants from cadaveric donors. N Engl J Med 1992;327: 834–9.
5. Berthoux FC, Jones EHP, Mehls O, Valderrabano F. Transplantation report: report on management of renal failure in Europe, XXV, 1994. Nephrol Dial Transplant 1996;11(Suppl 1):37–40.
6. Robinson MT, Kindt TJ. Major histocompatibility complex antigens and genes. In: Paul W, editor. Fundamental immunology. New York: Raven Press; 1989. p. 489–539.
7. Krensky AM. Transplant immunobiology. In: Paediatric nephrology. 3rd ed. Baltimore: Williams & Wilkins; 1993. p. 1373–89.
8. Jamison RL, Wilkinson R. The pretransplant selection and evaluation of donor and recipient. In: Nephrology 1997; Chapman & Hall, p. 1072–82.
9. Opelz G. Correlation of HLA matching with kidney graft survival in patients with or without cyclosporine treatment. Transplantation 1985;40:240–3.
10. Robles J, Errasti P, Abad J, et al. Surgical complications in renal transplantation: determinant factors. Transplant Proc 1995;27:2258–59.
11. Lai M, Huang C, Chu S, et al. Surgical complications in renal transplantation. Transplant Proc 1994;26:2165–66.
12. Gruber s, Chavers B, Payne W, et al. Allograft renal vascular thrombosis—lack of increase with cyclosporin immunnosuppression. Transplantation 1989;47:475–8.
13. Hakim N, Benedetti E, Pirenne J, et al. Complication of uterovesical anastomosis in kidney transplant patients: the Minnesota experience. Clin Transplant 1994;8: 504–7.

14. Vincenti F, Laskow DA, Neylan JF, Mendez R, Matas AJ. One year follow up of an open label trial of FK506 for primary kidney transplantation. Transplant 1996;61:1576–81.
15. European Mycophenolate Mofetil Cooperative Study Group. Placebo controlled study of mycophenolate mofetil combined with cyclosporin and corticosteroids for prevention of acute rejection. Lancet 1995;345:1321–5.
16. Duda SH, Erley CM, Wakat JP, et al. Post transplant renal artery stenosis—outpatient intraarterial DSA versus color aided duplex Doppler sonography. Eur J Radiol 1993;16:95–101.
17. Snider JF, Hunter DW, Moradian GP, Castaneda-Zuniga WR, Letourneau JG. Transplant renal artery stenosis: evaluation with duplex sonography. Radiology 1989;172:1027–30.
18. Taylor KJW, Morse SS, Rigsby CM, Bia M, Schiff M. Vascular complications in renal allografts: detection with duplex Doppler US. Radiology 1987;162:31–8.
19. Wilczek HE. Percutaneous needle biopsy of the renal allograft. Transplant 1990;50:790–7.
20. Pirsch JD, Ploeg RJ, Gange S, et al. Determinants of graft survival after renal transplantation. Transplant 1996;61:1581–5.
21. Cochlin DLL, Wake A, Salaman JR, Griffin PJA. Ultrasound changes in the transplant kidney. Clin Radiol 1988;39:373–6.
22. Pozniak MA, Kelcz F, D'Alessandro A, Oberley T, Stratta R. Sonography of renal transplants in dogs: the effect of acute tubular necrosis, cyclosporin nephrotoxicity and acute rejection on resistive index and renal length. Am J Radiol 1992;158:791–7.
23. Parvin SD, Rees Y, Veitch PS, et al. Objective measurement by ultrasound to distinguish cyclosporin A toxicity from rejection. Br J Surg 1986;73:1009–11.
24. Genkins SM, Sanfilippo FP, Carroll BA. Duplex Doppler sonography of renal transplants: lack of sensitivity and specificity in establishing pathologic diagnosis. Am J Radiol 1989;152:535–9.
25. Kelzc F, Pozniak MA, Pirsch JD, Oberly TD. Pyramidal appearance and resistive index: insensitive and nonspecific indicators of acute renal transplant rejection. Am J Radiol 1990;155:531–5.
26. Rifkin MD, Needleman L, Pasto ME, et al. Evaluation of renal transplant rejection by duplex doppler examination: value of the resistive index. Am J Radiol 1987;148:759–62.
27. Rigsby CM, Taylor KJW, Weltin G, et al. Renal allografts in acute rejection: evaluation using duplex sonography. Radiology 1986;158:375–8.
28. Merkus JWS, Hoitsma AJ, van Asten WNJC, Koene RA, Scotnicki SH. Doppler spectrum analysis to diagnose rejection during post transplant acute renal failure. Transplantation 1994;58:570–6.
29. Kaveggia LP, Perella RR, Grant EG, et al. Duplex Doppler sonography in renal allografts: the significance of reversed flow in diastole. AJR Am J Roentgenol 1990;155:295–8.
30. Penny MJ, Nankivell BJ, Disney APS, Blyth K, Chapman JR. Renal graft thrombosis: a survey of 134 consecutive cases. Transplant 1994;58:565–9.
31. Baxter GM, Morley P, Dall B. Acute renal vein thrombosis in renal allografts: new Doppler ultrasonic findings. Clin Radiol 1991;43:125–7.
32. Reuther G, Wanjura D, Bauer H. Acute renal vein thrombosis in renal allografts: detection with duplex Doppler ultrasound. Radiology 1989;170:557–8.
33. MacLennan AC, Baxter GM, Harden P, Rowe PA. Renal transplant vein occlusion; an early diagnostic sign? Clin Radiol 1995;50:251–3.
34. Nargund VH, Cranston D. Urological complications after renal transplantation. Transplant Rev 1996;10:24–33.
35. Myers BD, Sibley R, Newton L, et al. The long term course of cyclosporin associated chronic nephropathy. Kidney Int 1988;33:590–600.
36. Gray DWR. Graft renal artery stenosis in the transplanted kidney. Transplant Rev 1994;8:15–21.
37. Erley CM, Duda SH, Wakat JP, et al. Noninvasive procedures for diagnosis of renovascular hypertension in renal transplant recipients and prospective analysis. Transplantation 1992;54:863–7.
38. Baxter GM, Ireland H, Moss J G, et al. Colour Doppler ultrasound in renal transplant artery stenosis: which Doppler index? Clin Radiol 1995;50:618–22.
39. Gedroye WM, Negus R, al Kautoubi A, et al. Magnetic resonance angiography of renal transplants. Lancet 1992;339:789–91.
40. Merkus JWS, Zeebregts CJAM, Hoitsma AJ, van Asten WNJC, Koene RAP, Skotnicki SH. High incidence of arteriovenous fistula after biopsy of kidney allografts. Br J Surg 1993;80:310–12.
41. Renowden SA, Blethyn J, Cochlin DLL. Duplex and color flow sonography in the diagnosis of post biopsy arteriovenous fistulae in the transplant kidney. Clin Radiol 1992;45:233–7.
42. Matthew TH. Recurrent disease after transplantation. Transplant Rev 1991;5:31–45.
43. Penn I. Cancer is a complication of severe immunosuppression. Surg Gynaecol Obstet 1986;162:603–10.

Pediatric Renal Transplantation

H. Maxwell

The incidence of end-stage renal failure in children under the age of 15 years is estimated to be 5–8 per million children, and is commoner in males by nearly two to one.[1] The incidence in adolescents between the ages of 15 and 18 years is more difficult to determine because of referral practices, but is thought to be higher.[1]

Etiology of Chronic Renal Failure

The causes of renal failure in childhood are very different from those in the adult population and are outlined in Table 5.**1**. The majority of patients, particularly younger patients, suffer from congenital structural anomalies of the urinary tract. These conditions are often complicated by poor urinary concentrating ability and polyuria. Commonly, bladder function as well as kidney function is abnormal, and the management of end-stage renal failure must also involve the investigation and treatment of abnormal bladder function prior to transplantation.

Table 5.**1** Etiology of chronic renal failure in childhood (% of total). (From Lewis[1])

Renal dysplasia and related conditions	28
Obstructive uropathy	20
Glomerular disease	17
Reflux nephropathy and chronic renal failure of uncertain etiology	9
Primary tubular and interstitial disorders	7
Congenital nephrotic syndrome	7
Renal vascular disorders	5
Metabolic diseases	3
Polycystic disease	2
Malignant and related disorders	2

Management of Chronic Renal Failure

For most children with chronic renal failure, progression to end-stage renal failure is a slow process. Conservative management is aimed at maintaining fluid, electrolyte, and acid–base balance, controlling blood pressure, providing an adequate calorie intake, and preventing anemia and renal osteodystrophy. This can be difficult in uremia, as a greater calorie requirement is needed to achieve normal weight gain.[2] This last, coupled with anorexia and vomiting due to abnormal gut motility, compounds the problem. In some children this is further aggravated by excessive thirst due to marked polyuria. Often an enteral feed, either with a nasogastric tube or with a gastrostomy tube, is the only way of ensuring a sufficient calorie intake.

Children with oligoanuria will need fluid restriction, but many children with chronic renal failure pass significant quantities of urine. The enteral route allows the provision of adequate fluid and electrolyte supplements and can correct metabolic acidosis. Anemia of chronic renal failure can be corrected with recombinant human erythropoietin once sufficient iron stores have been achieved, and activated vitamin D and phosphate restriction prevent renal osteodystrophy.

Peritoneal Dialysis

Peritoneal dialysis is the treatment modality of choice in childhood. Although less efficient than hemodialysis, it is better tolerated in children. Furthermore, automated peritoneal dialysis can be carried out overnight at home, with little disruption to schooling. Even very small infants can tolerate peritoneal dialysis, but it is a huge undertaking to dialyze a baby from birth, and it is a treatment which can be fraught with complications. In general, the success of peritoneal dialysis in small infants is related to the presence of residual renal function and the lack of nonrenal co-morbid factors.[3]

The main complications of peritoneal dialysis are exit site infections and peritonitis, particularly in infants and children who are still in diapers. The presence of a coexisting gastrostomy tube does not increase the incidence of peritonitis, but insertion of a gastrostomy tube once dialysis has been established does increase the risk of peritonitis.[4] Prolonged periods of time on peritoneal dialysis can result in membrane failure or, more rarely, sclerosing peritonitis.

Hemodialysis

In patients who have undergone extensive abdominal surgery, or those who have suffered from peritoneal membrane failure, hemodialysis is required. In all but the older child, double-lumen indwelling cannulae are used. Hemodialysis is more disruptive in terms of schooling, and may be poorly tolerated in the younger child, in whom achievement of fluid balance is more difficult.

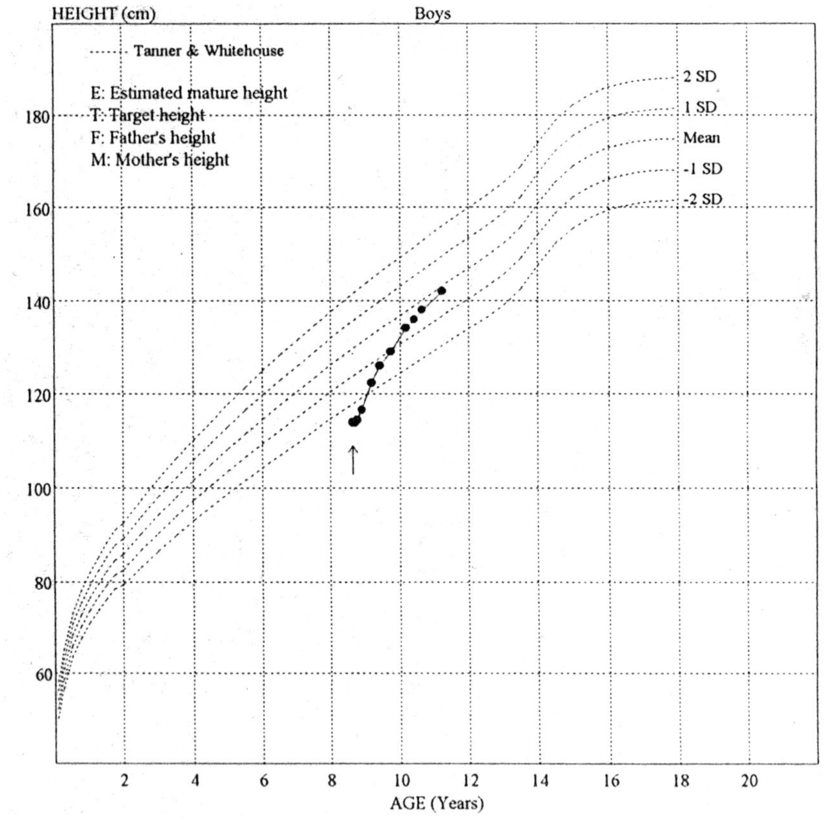

Fig. 5.**1** Growth chart showing substantial catch-up growth after renal transplantation (arrow) in a boy aged 8.7 years at the time of transplantation. Growth prior to transplantation, whilst the child was on peritoneal dialysis, had been below but parallel to the lower limit of the normal range

Transplantation

In addition to offering more effective renal replacement therapy, transplantation offers better physical and psychological well-being and social rehabilitation. In the case of children this includes better growth and nutrition (Fig. 5.**1**), and in infants better neurological development.[5] Following transplantation, children are more likely to have a better attendance record at school and to partake in normal childhood activities.[6] Increasingly, children are receiving transplants without first undergoing dialysis (so-called pre-emptive transplantation), which avoids disruption to schooling, periods of ill health on dialysis, and poor growth.[6] Graft survival data for pediatric patients are now as good as for adults; three-year graft survival for both pediatric and adult cadaveric transplant recipients is 77 %.[7]

Living Related Donation

The decision as to cadaveric versus living related donor transplantation depends on the individual patient's circumstances. The results for living related donor kidneys are superior to those of cadaveric transplantation at all ages (Fig. 5.**2**), but the difference is most marked in young recipients.[8,9] Living related donation generally involves parents, but grandparents, aunts, uncles, and older siblings can all be considered. Living unrelated donation can be performed with adopted parents.

The incidence of living related donation varies from country to country. In the United Kingdom the figure is 16 %,[10] whereas in North America 49 % of pediatric transplants are from living donors,[9] and in Scandinavia the figure is as high as 86 %.[11] The variation is due to differences in organ-sharing programs and to geographical and cultural factors.

For many families, an advantage of living related donation is that it allows a degree of control over the timing of surgery. It also allows all required personnel to be present at the operation and both child and donor to be in the best possible health. Other advantages of living related donation are that preemptive transplantation is more easily performed, the incidence of acute tubular necrosis is reduced,[12] and graft survival is improved.[12,13] The disadvantage of living related donation is that one of the child's carers becomes a patient, leaving the other carer with two dependants to look after in addition to any other siblings.

Preemptive Transplantation

The decision to start renal replacement therapy depends upon biochemical factors as well as clinical parameters. Failure of conservative management to con-

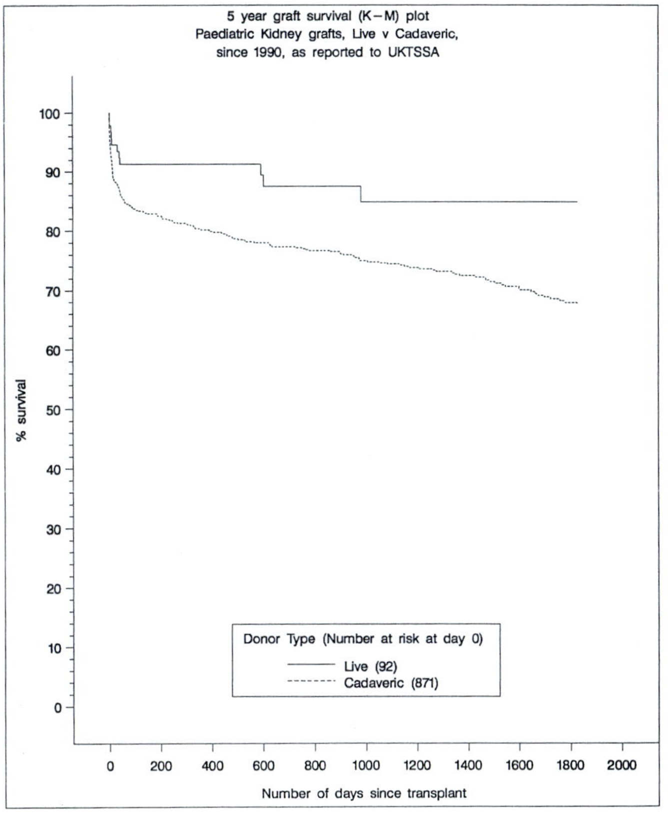

Fig. 5.**2** Kaplan–Meier plot of five-year graft survival in pediatric renal recipients since 1990 comparing cadaveric and living related donor renal transplantation. Living related graft survival was 85 % (CI 76–94 %) and cadaveric graft survival 67 % (CI 64–71 %). (These statistics were prepared by UK Transplant from the National Transplant Database maintained on behalf of the UK transplant community)

trol acidosis, hyperkalemia, or fluid overload, as well as failing growth, failure to thrive, and the inability to manage a full day at school are taken into account. In general at this stage, the glomerular filtration rate is between 5 and 10 ml/min per 1.73 m^2.[14] Living related donation allows greater control over the timing of transplantation, but cadaveric preemptive transplantation is also possible.

At present between 20 and 25 % of transplants are performed preemptively.[14,15] Children who go directly to transplantation are generally healthier, and many of them have no experience of inpatient admission. The perioperative time can therefore be a very difficult time. Concern has been expressed that preemptive transplantation does not allow patients to experience how unwell they can feel on dialysis and therefore appreciate the benefits of transplantation. There is no evidence in pediatric practice that this is the case, however[14]; indeed there is preliminary evidence that preemptive transplantation has a beneficial effect, with improved graft survival in living donor recipients.[15]

The Young Recipient

Infants with chronic renal failure often have developmental delay as well as failure to thrive. Dialysis does little to improve development and growth in infants,[16] but following transplantation impressive catch-up growth is seen,[17] and, more importantly, there is an improvement in the indices of mental and motor development.[5]

Early results of transplantation in young recipients were poor, especially for cadaveric grafts.[12] Vascular thrombosis and technical difficulties are important causes of graft loss in the under-5 age group.[18–20] At this age the immune system is more active,[21] and there is increased metabolism and more variable absorption of cyclosporine.[22] However, there have been improvements in graft survival in young recipients (Fig. 5.**3**) related to the use of more living related donors and the avoidance of young donor organs.[8,19,23] Excellent long-term graft survival and graft function have been described in this age group,[24] which is no different to those seen in older recipients.[25]

Within the under-5-year age group, results for the under-2-year-olds do not differ from those for children over 2 years,[19,25,26] although transplantation of the very young recipient is best carried out in specialized centers. Fluid management is critical in this group, particularly when the donor organ is relatively large in proportion to the recipient. In this situation elective post-operative ventilation aids management. The use of a living donor organ provides the best option[25]; a body weight of 7–8 kg has been suggested as the minimum necessary for receiving an adult-sized kidney.[26]

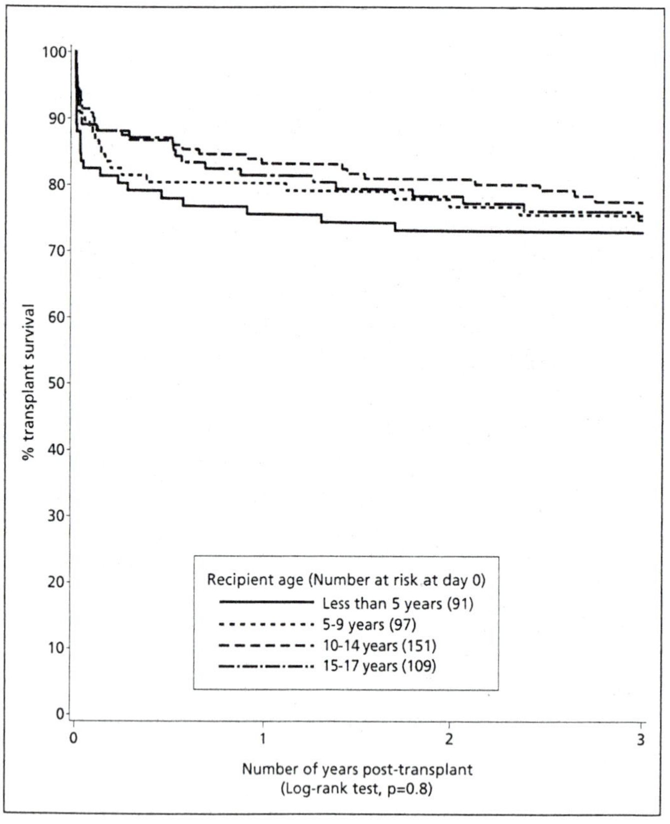

Fig. 5.**3** Kaplan–Meier plot of three-year graft survival after first pediatric cadaveric renal transplant, 1990–1997, by recipient age. Graft survival for the under-five-year-olds is now approaching that seen in older children. (These statistics were prepared by UK Transplant from the National Transplant Database maintained on behalf of the UK transplant community)

Summary points:

- More likely to have underlying structural anomalies of the renal tract
- More likely to receive a larger donor kidney
- Operative fluid management critical
- More likely to have acute tubular necrosis
- Higher incidence of early graft loss

Contraindications to Transplantation

In contrast to adults, the majority of children with end-stage renal failure will be suitable for transplantation; contraindications are the presence of malignancy within the previous two years, HIV infection, and elevated circulating anti-glomerular basement membrane antibodies. Renal transplantation is not carried out in the presence of ABO blood group incompatibility, nor in the presence of cytotoxic antibodies against donor antigens. Consideration needs to be given to the quality of life following transplantation, therefore multiple organ failure and severe brain damage will in general preclude transplantation. Transplantation should be delayed for several months if there is ongoing active disease such as hemolytic uremic syndrome or rapidly progressive glomerulonephritis. Patients with hepatitis B or C can proceed with transplantation in the absence of active liver involvement.

Work-Up for Transplantation

To optimize the chances of success, it is important to investigate the child thoroughly before transplantation. Several areas require attention.

Sensitization

Anti-HLA antibodies may be formed during blood transfusions or as a result of a previous graft. These are screened for prior to transplantation, and if any are detected, the relevant antigen should be avoided in the donor.

Viral Infections

It is also important to screen for prior exposure to viral infections (cytomegalovirus [CMV], Epstein–Barr virus [EBV], varicella, hepatitis B, and hepatitis C). Antiviral prophylaxis is given to CMV-seronegative recipients who receive CMV-positive grafts, and varicella vaccination is performed in those children who have not been exposed to varicella.

Urinary Tract

Imaging of the native kidneys and bladder should be performed (Table 5.**2**). It is important to determine whether the child can empty the bladder completely as residual urine is a risk factor for urinary tract infection, as is the presence of marked reflux into large dilated ureters. Large-capacity bladders which do not empty

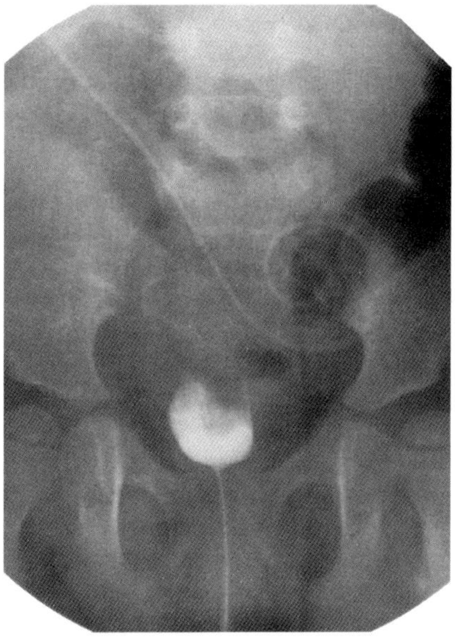

Fig. 5.**4** Cystogram showing a very small capacity bladder with a maximum volume of only 20 ml

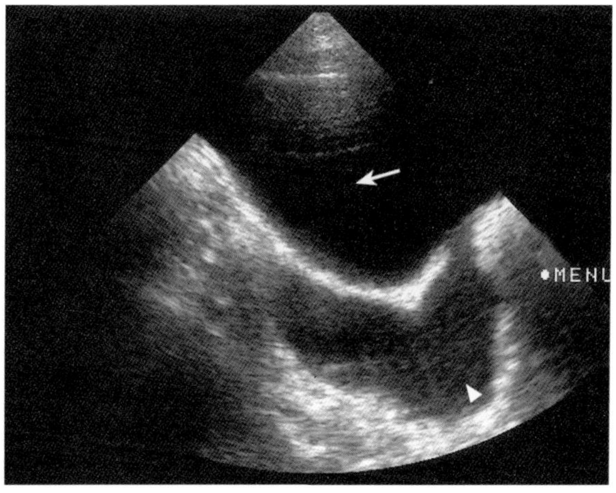

Fig. 5.**5** Ultrasound scan of the bladder (arrow) showing a dilated left ureter (arrowhead) at the level of the bladder. After voiding, a significant postvoid residue was observed. A cystogram showed the presence of gross left-sided vesicoureteric reflux

completely may be helped with intermittent catheterization either per urethra or via a Mitrofanoff stoma. Small bladders which are under high pressure can result in damage to the transplanted kidney, and bladder augmentation may be required prior to surgery. If the bladder capacity is inadequate, a transplant ureterostomy is necessary (Fig. 5.**4**).

Initial imaging with ultrasound can show bladder wall thickness, ureteric abnormalities, and bladder emptying (Fig. 5.**5**). For those with known bladder abnormalities, a micturating cystogram will give more information on bladder capacity and reflux (Fig. 5.**6**). In those found to have an abnormal bladder, formal urodynamic studies should be performed. Initial results of transplantation into recipients whose renal failure was due to a posterior urethral valve were poor,[27] with grafts becoming scarred from a combination of functional obstruction and infection. More recent data report similar graft survival data for bladder outlet obstruction as compared to other causes of chronic renal failure in childhood.[28]

Native Nephrectomy

Up to 24% of children undergo native nephrectomies prior to transplantation.[12] The main indications include recurrent urinary tract infections, severe hypertension, persistent nephrotic state, and massive enlargement of polycystic kidneys causing respiratory or gastrointestinal compromise.

Vasculature

Large kidneys transplanted into small children require a greater blood flow than smaller kidneys. These grafts are placed onto the aorta and inferior vena cava rather than the iliac vessels. It is helpful to know the size and patency of the major vessels prior to transplantation.[26]

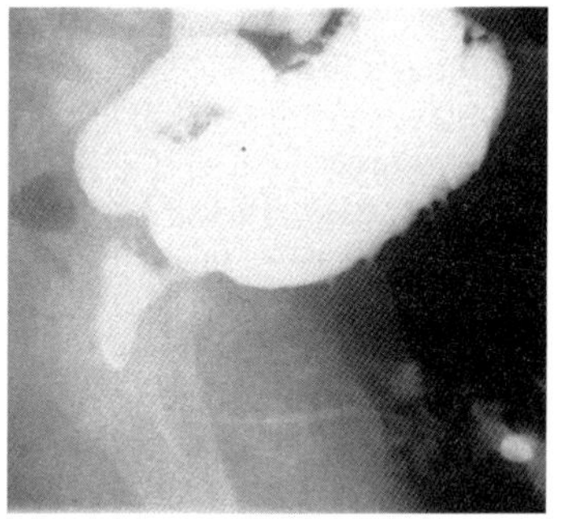

Fig. 5.**6** Micturating cystourethrogram showing the presence of a posterior urethral valve with dilatation of the posterior urethra. The bladder is cone-shaped with multiple diverticula

Table 5.**2** Imaging in pediatric renal transplantation

Pretransplant:
Native urological tract:
Ultrasound/MCU/urodynamics
Patency of abdominal vessels:
Doppler ultrasound imaging
Perioperative:
DTPA perfusion scan
Doppler ultrasound imaging
Postoperative:
Ultrasound/DTPA at times of graft dysfunction
Contrast studies through stent
MCU

Doppler ultrasonography may be sufficient, but if there is doubt as to the question of patency, angiography or magnetic resonance angiography may be appropriate. The children at particular risk of vascular thrombosis are those who are small (body weight < 15 kg), those with a constellation of congenital anomalies, and those who are predisposed to thrombosis (congenital nephrotic syndrome, focal segmental sclerosis, clotting abnormalities).

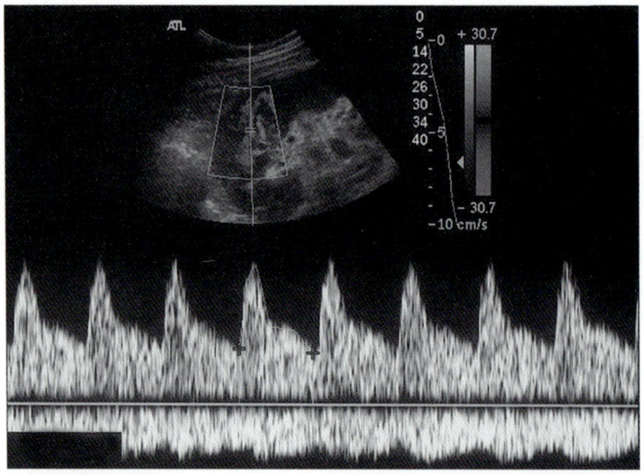

Fig. 5.**7** Postoperative renal Doppler ultrasound scan confirming good perfusion of the graft with a spectral Doppler waveform

Transplant Surgery

Many centers will have a minimum size requirement of 10 kg or a minimum age requirement of 21–24 months for children undergoing transplantation; however, guidelines vary and some centers will undertake transplantation in younger patients.[25,26] In general, in recipients of less than 15–20 kg body weight—especially when the donor organ is of adult size—an intraperitoneal approach is preferred, with anastomosis of the graft vessels to the aorta and inferior vena cava respectively.[26] This approach carries a greater risk of postoperative ileus.[26] The extraperitoneal approach is used in recipients over 15 kg, but has been used in some younger recipients with good results.[23]

Early Postoperative Management

Aggressive fluid management is required after transplantation, particularly where the donor graft is proportionally bigger than the recipient, and is used to higher perfusion pressures. A greater blood flow reduces the risk of thrombosis. Many children, particularly those receiving preemptive transplants, have a considerable native urine output which continues postoperatively.

Imaging

Postoperatively it is helpful to assess blood flow to the transplant, particularly in the absence of primary function. Doppler ultrasonography or isotope scanning with DTPA or MAG3 are used routinely (Fig. 5.**7**) (Table 5.**3**).

Immunosuppression

The majority of children receive standard triple immunosuppression therapy with azathioprine, cyclosporine, and steroid.[9] Increasingly, cyclosporine is being replaced by tacrolimus, and azathioprine by mycophenolate mofetil.[9] Both of these agents have been shown in trials in adult renal transplant recipients to reduce the incidence of acute rejection. The perceived benefit of these drugs in pediatric patients is that the incidence of rejection is higher in children than adults. The use of these agents may also allow a reduction in the dose of steroid, with a potential for improved growth.[29] Cessation of steroid use, however, has been associated with acute rejection,[30] while normal growth has been observed in patients on steroids, particularly in the young.[19] The use of alternate-day steroids is also helpful.[31]

Complications of Transplantation

Bleeding

Postoperative bleeding may occur either from the site of the vascular anastomosis or from the donor vessels. This manifests as signs of intravascular volume depletion with poor peripheral perfusion, tachycardia, and other signs of shock. There may be abdominal distension and evidence of graft dysfunction. Treatment is aimed at maintaining intravascular volume, with surgical intervention where necessary.

Graft Thrombosis

Up to 13 % of graft failures are due to renal artery or vein thrombosis.[12] The risk factors include young cadaveric donor age, young recipient age, prolonged cold ischemia time, and acute tubular necrosis.[20] Screening for prothrombotic tendencies,[32] the use of thromboprophylaxis,[33] and the avoidance of young donor organs, particularly for young recipients, have all been employed in an effort to reduce this incidence. Thrombosis of the renal artery may be related to technical difficulties during donor nephrectomy, organ perfusion, or vascular anastomosis.[34] This results in complete nonfunction of the graft, and investigation by Doppler ultrasonography or isotope perfusion scan will demonstrate the absence of renal blood flow. Renal artery thrombosis usually results in graft loss.

Renal vein thrombosis may be the result of the technical difficulties outlined above. There is often a more gradual loss of function, graft swelling, and gross hematuria. Doppler ultrasonography will show absence of blood flow in the renal vein. Thrombectomy may be useful, but again graft loss often ensues.[20,34]

Renal Artery Stenosis

Renal artery stenosis of the graft is manifest clinically by marked and persistent hypertension and deteriorating graft function. The diagnosis is often evident on Doppler ultrasonography or isotope perfusion scan and can be confirmed by angiography. Percutaneous transluminal angioplasty or surgical correction are therapeutic options. Only 1 % of graft failures are due to renal artery stenosis.[12]

Acute Tubular Necrosis

Approximately 20% of pediatric cadaveric renal transplants suffer primary nonfunction, defined as the need for dialysis in the first post-transplant week.[12] The comparative figure for living related donor transplants is 6%. In cadaveric grafts, acute tubular necrosis is more likely with prolonged cold ischemia time (24 hours), in patients with prior transplants, and in patients with no HLA-DR match. With living donor grafts, a recipient age under two years and prior transplantation are risk factors.[12] The long-term outcome for grafts with acute tubular necrosis is worse than that for grafts with primary function; at three years 74% of cadaveric grafts with primary function are still functioning, compared with 51% of grafts for which dialysis had been necessary during the first week.[12]
Patients with prolonged primary nonfunction may require renal biopsy to exclude the presence of rejection.

Graft Dysfunction

There are several reasons why the serum creatinine level may not fall or may even increase postoperatively (Table 5.**3**). There may be a degree of acute tubular necrosis as discussed above. The patient may be intravascularly depleted; this is not uncommon in small recipients of large kidneys or in patients with large native urinary losses.
Several of the drugs commonly used after transplantation are nephrotoxic (e.g., ganciclovir, aciclovir, aminoglycosides) and may cause an increase in creatinine. Both tacrolimus and cyclosporine have a narrow therapeutic window and are themselves nephrotoxic at higher doses. Other drugs can potentiate the nephrotoxicity of tacrolimus and cyclosporine (e.g., nonsteroidal anti-inflammatory drugs), whilst drugs such as erythromycin or fluconazole inhibit the metabolism of these agents, causing an increase in plasma levels.
The creatinine may also be elevated due to infection, obstruction, urinary leak, or acute rejection.

Rejection

Diagnosis of Acute Rejection

Creatinine levels are used to monitor for rejection. As discussed above, a raised creatinine level may be caused by a number of different factors including infection, urinary tract obstruction, dehydration, drug nephrotoxicity, or rejection. Rejection may also be accompanied by fever, fluid retention, hypertension, and graft tenderness. In general, a sustained increase in creatinine concentration of greater than 10% or a rapidly rising concentration is suggestive of rejection. The rise in creatinine may be late in small recipients with relatively larger grafts.[35] In these patients a low threshold of suspicion is required; clinical signs of rejection such as fever and graft tenderness may precede signs of impaired graft function by some time.[35]
The definitive diagnosis of rejection is made by renal biopsy. Color Doppler ultrasonography may show reduced blood flow generally with a reduction in end-diastolic flow on spectral Doppler examination. It will also exclude or confirm the presence of a dilated obstructed collecting system (Fig. 5.**8**). A DTPA scan is helpful in assessing graft perfusion.
Where possible, rejection should be confirmed by biopsy. Treatment of rejection is with intravenous methylprednisolone or high-dose oral steroid. Rejection resistant to steroid boluses is increasingly being treated with a switch to a more potent immunosuppression regime rather than the use of anti-T-cell preparations.[36] Even if the creatinine responds favorably to steroid treatment, baseline immunosuppression is usually increased to prevent further rejection.

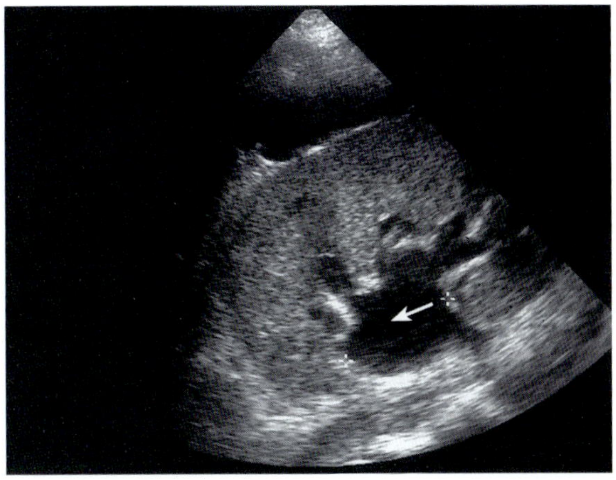

Fig. 5.**8** Renal transplant ultrasound scan showing dilatation of the renal pelvis (arrow), in this case due to extrinsic compression of the transplant ureter

Table 5.**3** Reasons for graft dysfunction

Early (< 30 days)	**≥Late (30 days)**
Poor renal perfusion	Intravascular volume depletion
Low cardiac output	Renal artery stenosis
Low central venous pressure (CVP)	Acute rejection
Renal artery thrombosis	Chronic rejection
Renal vein thrombosis	Drug toxicity
Acute tubular necrosis	Infection
Rejection	Urinary tract infection
Nephrotoxicity	Cytomegalovirus
Obstruction	Epstein–Barr virus
Ureter	Recurrence of primary disease
Foley catheter	De novo renal disease
Stent	Ureteric stenosis
Urine leak	Vesicoureteric reflux
Lymphocele	

Renal Transplant Biopsy

In all but the oldest children, renal transplant biopsy is performed under intravenous sedation. An extraperitoneal graft is generally easily palpated and biopsy should not present too much difficulty. Abdominally sited organs may be more difficult to biopsy, but adult-sized kidneys are often easily palpated in the right flank. Ultrasound guidance is normally used to assess the position of the graft, and allows accurate positioning of the biopsy needle. Generally a biopsy gun or disposable needle is used. An 18-cm 18G needle is usually sufficient in all but the biggest children.

The amount of tissue required depends upon the reason for biopsy. In a biopsy performed for suspected rejection, one good core of tissue for light microscopy is required. The Banff criteria for rejection are commonly used, i.e., sufficient tissue needs to be obtained to allow accurate staging of the severity of rejection. If the cause of graft dysfunction is in dispute, further tissue will be required, e.g., for detection of CMV or Epstein–Barr virus, or for immunofluorescence and electron microscopy studies if disease recurrence is thought likely (see below).

Recurrence of Disease

Recurrence of the original disease is responsible for approximately 5–6% of graft failures in pediatric series.[37]

Focal Segmental Glomerulosclerosis

Focal segmental glomerulosclerosis presents in childhood with a nephrotic syndrome that is resistant to or only partially sensitive to steroid treatment. Approximately 30% of cases will progress to renal failure, and in 20–30% of this subgroup the disease will recur in the graft when they undergo transplantation.[38] Factors predictive of recurrence after transplantation are rapid deterioration of native renal function in less than two years from the time of diagnosis, and the presence of mesangial hypercellularity on the native renal biopsy.[39]

Recurrence of focal segmental glomerulosclerosis can occur within hours of transplantation and is heralded by the presence of profound proteinuria. The graft loss from recurrence is high at 60%,[40] and the risk of recurrence in a second graft is as high as 80%.[39] It is because of these poor statistics that increasingly powerful regimes of post-transplantation treatment with plasma exchange, cyclophosphamide,[41] and high-dose intravenous cyclosporine[42] have been tried, with some success.

Atypical Hemolytic Uremic Syndrome

Hemolytic uremic syndrome is a heterogeneous group of conditions, comprising typical (diarrhea-associated) and atypical forms. The latter category can be further divided into familial, relapsing, and secondary forms. It is children with atypical hemolytic uremic syndrome rather than the more common diarrhea-associated form who are at risk of disease recurrence after transplantation. Recurrence rates between 0 and 25% have been reported from different centers.[43] Graft loss from recurrent disease is high.[43]

Membranoproliferative Glomerulonephritis

Membranoproliferative glomerulonephritis is an uncommon cause of nephrotic syndrome in childhood.[44] Untreated, nearly 50% of patients will progress to end-stage renal failure; however, alternate-day steroid therapy reduces proteinuria, improves renal function, and prolongs renal survival.[45] Two types of membranoproliferative glomerulonephritis are distinguished by their appearance on electron microscopy of renal biopsy material, types I and II (dense deposit disease). Recurrence of type I membranoproliferative glomerulonephritis after transplantation results in graft loss in about 20% of patients.[46] Recurrence occurs in up to 85% of children with type II disease, but for most of these patients the disease is not clinically apparent, and graft loss is rare.[46]

Oxalosis

In type I primary hyperoxaluria there is overproduction of oxalate, which accumulates in the tissues and causes renal failure.[47] Renal transplantation alone does not cure the condition as oxalate continues to be deposited in the transplanted kidney. Combined liver and kidney transplantation[48] or indeed preemptive liver transplantation before renal failure occurs[49] are now the treatments of choice.

Infection

Infection is an important complication of renal transplantation, responsible for significant morbidity and mortality; 34% of post-transplant deaths are infection-related.[12]

Bacterial Infection

Bacterial infection is most likely in the early post-transplant period. The common sites are wound, chest, and urinary tract infections, and sepsis associated with indwelling catheters. Urinary tract infection occurs frequently,[50] and may be related to indwelling catheters or stents and abnormalities of the native kidneys and ureters, resulting in stasis or reflux of urine or poor bladder emptying. Venous access is often difficult, particularly in the young recipient, and central venous lines are common.

Intravenous antibiotics are used in the early post-transplant period, and prophylactic antibiotics are often given until the urinary catheter is removed. Patients with abnormal bladders and poor bladder emptying or significant vesicoureteric reflux usually remain on antibiotic prophylaxis.

Viral Infection

Compared with adults, a high proportion of pediatric transplant patients will not have been exposed to common viral infections including CMV and Epstein–Barr virus. Viral infections usually occur later than bacterial infections, classically one to two months after transplantation.

Cytomegalovirus

Those most at risk of CMV are children who are seronegative for CMV and who receive an organ from a seropositive donor.[51] Reactivation of latent infection can also occur, so that seropositive recipients can also be at risk. The risk is further increased when additional immunosuppression is used to treat rejection. CMV infection (when patients seroconvert) may be asymptomatic, but CMV disease with fever, anemia, thrombocytopenia, and abnormal liver function is more serious. Tissue-invasive disease with pneumonia, esophagitis, or other gastrointestinal involvement may be fatal. Treatment is with intravenous ganciclovir and, where possible, a reduction in immunosuppression.[51] CMV is itself immunosuppressive and can predispose to other infections such as *Pneumocystis carinii* pneumonia. Co-trimoxazole prophylaxis against *Pneumocystis* is often given during treatment of CMV infection.

Epstein–Barr Virus

Most children are seronegative for Epstein–Barr virus at the time of transplantation and virtually all will seroconvert afterwards, especially if they receive an organ from a seropositive donor.[52] Their Epstein–Barr viral infection may be asymptomatic or may appear as a flu-like illness. Most patients will recover, but in the presence of heavy immunosuppression, especially with the use of anti-T-cell preparations, continued B-cell proliferation may occur—the so-called post-transplant lymphoproliferative disorder.[52,53] First-line treatment is a reduction in immunosuppression; more aggressive disease will require additional therapy.[53]

Post-transplant Lymphoproliferative Disorder

Post-transplant lymphoproliferative disorder can occur at different sites, including in the graft itself, the nasopharynx, central nervous system, chest, or gastrointestinal tract (Fig. 5.**9**). Investigation may include abdominal ultrasound and CT of the chest, abdomen, and brain if necessary. A bone marrow aspiration should also be performed.

Other Infections

Other infections may occur after transplantation. Varicella can be severe in immunosuppressed patients and so varicella status should be determined prior to transplantation, and varicella vaccine administered if necessary.[54] Those who are seronegative who are exposed to varicella after transplantation should receive zoster immune globulin, and if they develop clinically apparent chickenpox should also receive aciclovir. Herpes simplex infection is not uncommon and can be treated with oral or topical aciclovir. Fungal and other atypical infections can occur in the first few months following transplantation; a high index of suspicion is necessary when investigating fever or ill-health in these patients.

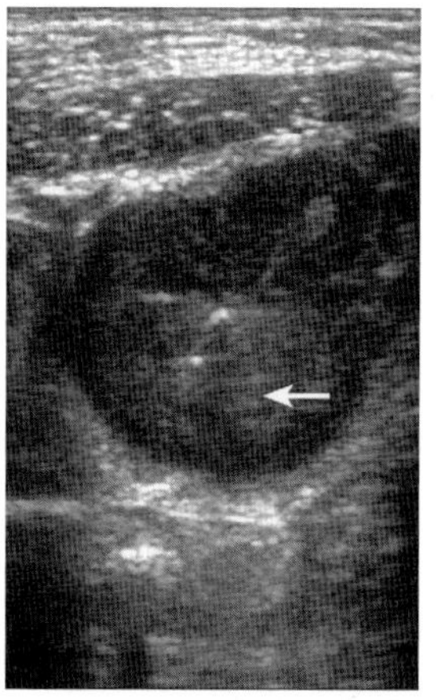

Fig. 5.**9** Abdominal ultrasound scan in a five-year-old child presenting with abdominal pain eight months after renal transplantation. There is a 3×2 cm heterogeneous mass in the left iliac fossa (arrow). Laparotomy revealed inflamed ileum and enlarged mesenteric lymph nodes. Histopathological and viral studies confirmed a diagnosis of post-transplant lymphoproliferative disorder related to Epstein–Barr virus infection

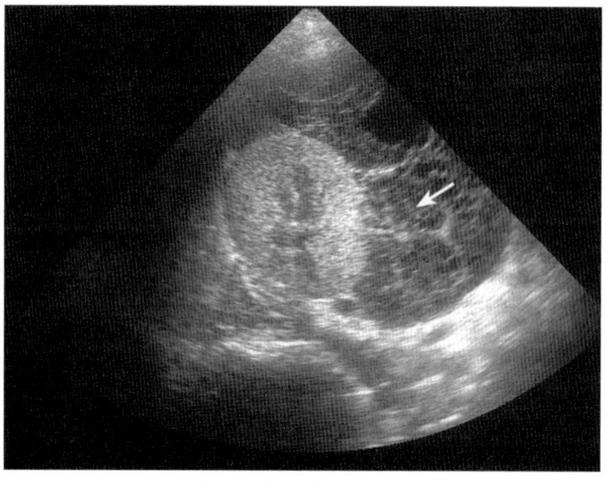

Fig. 5.**10** Large peritransplant lymphocele (arrow)

Malignancy

Malignancy is an uncommon problem following pediatric renal transplantation, with an incidence of 1.4–2%.[9,12] In this North American series, in which data have been collected since 1987, approximately 70% of these malignancies were post-transplant lymphoproliferative disorders.[9] An earlier analysis from the Cincinnati Transplant Tumor Registry, with longer follow-up, reveals that 31% of the reported tumors were lymphomas, 29% skin and lip cancers, and the rest a mixture of primary liver tumors (6%), sarcomas (5%), and others.[55] The category of lymphoma includes post-transplant lymphoproliferative disorder; the higher incidence of this problem in more recent years may reflect the use of newer, more potent immunosuppressants.[9]

Urological Complications/Obstruction

A urine leak can result from necrosis of the distal ureter, or from the pressure of a distended bladder, e.g., after the urinary catheter is removed. Urine output will be reduced and the creatinine may rise. An isotope scan will demonstrate the leak. Obstruction may also result from extrinsic pressure on the ureter, e.g., from a lymphocele (Fig. 5.**10**) or hematoma.

Post-transplant bladder dysfunction may result in urinary tract infections or obstruction due to incomplete bladder emptying. A later complication is ureteral stenosis; this may occur at the level of the anastomosis or at the PUJ. Ultrasound will be helpful in showing upper tract dilatation. Renal stones are an uncommon cause of obstruction.

Hypertension

In the early post-transplant period, up to 70–80% of children will be hypertensive requiring treatment,[56,57] 48% having been hypertensive prior to transplantation.[57] The main causes of hypertension after transplantation are fluid overload, steroids, cyclosporine and tacrolimus, and rejection. By one year the figure for the use of antihypertensives is lower at 63%, and at 2 years it is 59%.[57] The causes at this late stage are chronic rejection, renal artery stenosis, hypoperfused failing grafts, disease recurrence, and urinary tract obstruction.[56]

Outcome of Pediatric Renal Transplantation

In pediatric renal transplantation, graft and patient survival have improved with the passage of time.[7,9] In the United Kingdom, the five-year graft survival after first cadaveric transplantation improved from approximately 60% between 1984 and 1990 to 78% between 1990 and 1993.[10] In Paris, the five-year graft survival following cadaveric transplantation has improved from 64% between 1987 and 1990 to 90% between 1990 and 1996.[58] The same group reported an improvement in living related transplantation during the same time period from 68% to 87%.[58]

Data collection in North America is more complete than in Europe. Living donor graft survival rates at one, three, and five years are 92%, 85%, and 80% respectively.[9] For comparison, cadaveric graft survival rates at the same intervals are 83%, 73%, and 65%.[9] Calculation of graft half-life (time to which 50% of grafts survive) gives a slightly different perspective of long-term graft survival; graft half-life is 11.2 years for living donor transplants and 9.8 years for cadaveric grafts.[8]

These improvements have been attributed to the use of stronger immunosuppressants, improvements in molecular techniques used in tissue typing allowing more accurate matching, and the avoidance of young donor grafts, especially in young recipients.

Graft Loss

The principal causes of early renal allograft loss in children are chronic rejection (30% of early graft losses), acute rejection (18%), thrombosis (14%), death (11%), and recurrent disease (6%).[12] Late graft loss (after the first year) is due mainly to chronic rejection, patient death, and noncompliance.

Chronic allograft nephropathy is a complex process that most probably involves both immunological and nonimmunological processes.[59] The presence of acute rejection is one predisposing factor to chronic allograft nephropathy, although the relationship is not absolute.[12] Effort is directed at reducing the incidence of acute rejection in an attempt to prolong graft survival, but other factors, such as the response to treatment of acute rejection, are also important. Newer immunosuppressants have been shown in adult and pediatric studies to reduce the incidence of acute rejection, but it is too early to say whether this will prolong graft survival.

Graft Function

Perhaps a more informative measure than graft survival is the degree of graft function as determined by the measurement of glomerular filtration rate (GFR). This is generally measured by the clearance of exogenous chromium[51] EDTA, or DTPA, or by endogenous creatinine clearance. Absolute GFR has been shown to remain static for several years, but GFR corrected for body surface area falls as the child grows.[24, 26] Functional adaptation of the graft depending on the size of the donor and recipient has been demonstrated.[26,60] With time, and presumably the effect of chronic allograft nephropathy, mean GFR in any given cohort of patients declines, but some individuals can maintain good graft function for up to 25 years.[61]

References

1. Lewis M. Report of the Paediatric Renal Registry 1999. Chapter 15. The UK Renal Registry, Renal Association, 1999.
2. Chantler C, Lieberman E, Holliday MA. A rat model for the study of growth failure in uraemia. Pediatr Res 1974;8:109.
3. Ellis EN, Pearson D, Champion B, Wood EG. Outcomes of infants on chronic peritoneal dialysis. Adv Perit Dial 1995;11:266–69.
4. Ramage IJ, Harvey E, Geary DF, Hebert D, Balfe JA, Balfe JW. Complications of gastrostomy feeding in children receiving peritoneal dialysis. Pediatr Nephrol 1999;13:249–52.
5. Davis ID, Chang P-N, Nevins TE. Successful renal transplantation accelerates development in young uraemic children. Pediatrics 1990;86:594–600.
6. Krmar RT, Eymann A, Ramirez JA, Ferraris JR. Quality of life after kidney transplantation in children. Transplantation 1997;64:540–1.
7. Renal Transplant Audit 1990–1998, UK Transplant Bristol, 2001.
8. Schurman SJ, McEnery PT. Factors influencing short-term and long-term pediatric renal transplant survival. J Pediatr 1997;130:455–62.
9. Seikaly M, Ho PL, Emmett L, Tejani A. The 12th report of the North American Pediatric Renal Transplant Cooperative Study: renal transplantation from 1987 through 1998. Pediatr Transplant 2001;5:215–31.
10. Renal Transplant Audit 1984–1993, UKTSSA Bristol, 1995.
11. Ehrich JHH, Loirat C, Brunner FP. Report of management of renal failure in children in Europe. Nephrol Dial Transplant 1992;7:36.
12. Warady BA, Hebert D, Sullivan EK, Alexander SR, Tejani A. Renal transplantation, chronic dialysis, and chronic renal insufficiency in children and adolescents. The 1995 Annual Report of the North American Pediatric Renal Transplant Cooperative Study. Pediatr Nephrol 1997;11:49.

13. Broyer M, on behalf of the EDTA registry committee. Kidney transplantation in children. Data from the EDTA registry. Transplant Proc 1989;21:1985.
14. Fine RN, Tejani A, Sullivan EK. Preemptive renal transplantation in children: report of the North American Pediatric Renal Transplant Cooperative Study. Clin Transpl 1994;8:474.
15. Vats AN, Donaldson L, Fine RN, Chavers B. Pretransplant dialysis status and outcome of renal transplantation in North American children: A NAPRTCS study. Transplantation 2000;69:1414–19.
16. Kohaut EC, Whelchel J, Waldo FB, Diethelm AG. Aggressive therapy of infants with renal failure. Pediatr Nephrol 1987;1:150–3.
17. Tejani A, Fine R, Alexander S, Harmon W, Stablein D. Factors predictive of sustained growth in children after renal transplantation. J Pediatr 1993;122:397–402.
18. Harmon W, Alexander S, Tejani A. The effect of donor age on graft survival in pediatric cadaveric renal transplant recipients. Transplantation 1992;54:232–7.
19. Kari J, Romagnoli J, Duffy P, Fernando ON, Rees L, Trompeter RS. Renal transplantation in children under 5 years of age. Pediatr Nephrol 1999;13:730–6.
20. Singh A, Stablein D, Tejani A. Risk factors for vascular thrombosis in pediatric renal transplantation: a special report of the North American Pediatric Renal Transplant Cooperative Study. Transplantation 1997;63:1263–7.
21. Evans E, Ettenger RB. Immune response in pediatric renal transplantation. In: Tejani AH, Fine RN (eds) Pediatric renal transplantation. New York: Wiley–Liss; p. 17–21.
22. Hoyer PF, Brohedl J, Ehrich JHH, Offner G. Practical aspects in the use of cyclosporine in pediatric nephrology. Pediatr Nephrol 1991;5:630–8.
23. Laine J, Holmberg C, Salmeda K, Jalanko H, Sairanen H, Peltola K, Ronnholm K, Eklund B, Wikstrom S, Leijala M. Renal transplantation in children with emphasis on young patients. Pediatr Nephrol 1994;8:313–19.
24. Qvist E, Laine J, Ronnholm K, Jalanko H, Leijala M, Holmberg C. Graft function 5–7 years after renal transplantation in early childhood. Transplantation 1999;67:1043.
25. Najarian JS, Almond S, Gillingham KJ, Mauer M, Chavers B, Nevins TE, Kahtan CE, Matas AJ. Renal transplantation in the first five years of life. Kidney Int [Suppl]1993;44;S40–S44.
26. Tyden G, Berg U, Bohlin AB, Sandberg J. Renal transplantation in children less than two years old. Transplantation 1997;63:554–8.
27. Reinberg Y, Gonzalez R, Fryd D, Mauer SM, Najarian JS. The outcome of renal transplantation in children with posterior urethral valves. J Urol 1988;140:1491–3.
28. Connolly JA, Miller B, Bretan PN. Renal transplantation in patients with posterior urethral valves: favorable long-term outcome. J Urol 1995;154:1153–5.
29. Klare B, Strom TM, Hahn H, Engelsberger I, Meusel E. Remarkable long-term prognosis and excellent growth in kidney transplant children under cyclosporin monotherapy. Transplant Proc 1991;23:1013–17.
30. Ingulli E, Sharma V, Singh A, Suthanthiran M, Tejani A. Steroid withdrawal, rejection and the mixed lymphocyte reaction in children after renal transplantation. Kidney Int 1993;43(Suppl):S36–S39.
31. Maxwell H, Haffner D, Rees L. Catch up growth following renal transplantation in children of pubertal age. J Pediatr 1998;133:435–40.
32. Wheeler MA, Taylor CM, Williams M, Moghal N. Factor V Leiden: a risk factor for renal vein thrombosis in renal transplantation. Pediatr Nephrol 2000;4:525–6.
33. Broyer M, Gagnadoux MF, Sierro A, Fischer AM, Niaudet P. Preventative treatment of vascular thrombosis after kidney transplantation in children with low molecular weight heparin. Transplant Proc 1991;23:1384–5.
34. Palleschi J, Novick AC, Braun WE. Vascular complications of renal transplantation. Urology 1990;16:61.
35. Bunchman TE, Fryd DS, Sibley RK, Mauer M. Manifestations of renal allograft rejection in small children receiving adult kidneys. Pediatr Nephrol 1990;4:255–8.
36. Shapiro R, Scantlebury VP, Jordan ML, et al. FK506 in pediatric kidney transplantation—primary and rescue experience. Pediatr Nephrol 1995;9:43–8.
37. Broyer M, Selwood N, Brunner F. Recurrence of primary renal disease in kidney grafts: a European pediatric experience. J Am Soc Nephrol 1992;2:S255–S257.
38. Senggutuvan P, Cameron JS, Hartley RB, Rigden S, Chantler C, Haycock G, Williams DG, Koffman G. Recurrence of focal segmental glomerulosclerosis in transplanted kidneys: analysis of incidence and risk factors in 59 allografts. Pediatr Nephrol 1990;4:21-8.
39. Cameron JS. Recurrent primary disease and de novo nephritis following renal transplantation. Pediatr Nephrol 1991;5:412–21.
40. Stephanian E, Matas AJ, Mauer SM, Chavers B, Nevins T, Kashtan C, Sutherland DE, Gores P, Najarian JS. Recurrence of disease in patients transplanted for focal segmental glomerulosclerosis. Transplantation 1992;53:755–7.
41. Cochat P, Kassir A, Colon S, Glastre C, Tourniaire B, Parchoux B, Martin X, David L. Recurrent nephrotic syndrome after transplantation: early treatment with plasmapheresis and cyclophosphamide. Pediatr Nephrol 1993;7:50–4.
42. Niaudet P, Fuchshuber A, Gagnadoux MF, Habib R, Broyer M. Cyclosporin in the therapy of steroid-resistant idiopathic nephrotic syndrome. Kidney Int [Suppl] 1997;58:S85–S90.
43. Hebert D, Kim E, Sibley R, Mauer MS. Post-transplantation outcome of patients with hemolytic–uremic syndrome: update. Pediatr Nephrol 1991;5:162–7.
44. West C. Childhood membranoproliferative glomerulonephritis: an approach to management. Kidney Int 1986;29:1077–93.
45. Tarshish P, Bernstein J, Tobin JN, Edelmann CM Jr. Treatment of mesangiocapillary glomerulonephritis with alternate-day prednisone—a report of the International Study of Kidney Disease in Children. Pediatr Nephrol 1992;6:123–30.
46. Gagnadoux MF, Niaudet P, Broyer M. Non-immunological risk factors in paediatric renal transplantation. Pediatr Nephrol 1993;7:89–95.
47. Scheinman JI. Transplantation in primary hyperoxaluria. In: Tejani AH, Fine RN, editors. Pediatric renal transplantation. New York: Wiley–Liss; 1994. p. 349–78.
48. Watts RWE, Mansell MA. Oxalate livers and kidneys. Combined renal and hepatic transplants transform the outlook in primary hyperoxaluria type I. BMJ 1990;301:772–3.
49. Schurmann G, Scharer K, Wingen A-M, Otto G, Herfarth C. Early liver transplantation for primary hyperoxaluria type I in an infant with chronic renal failure. Nephrol Dial Transplant 1990;5:825–7.
50. Sharifian M, Rees L, Trompeter R. High incidence of bacteriuria following renal transplantation in children. Nephrol Dial Transplant 1998;13:432–5.
51. Patel R, Paya CV. Cytomegalovirus infection and disease in solid organ transplant recipients. In: Bowden RA, Ljungman, Paya CV, editors. Transplant infections. Philadelphia: Lippincott–Raven; 1998. p. 229–244.
52. Ellis D, Jaffe R, Green M, et al. Epstein–Barr virus-related disorders in children undergoing renal transplantation with tacrolimus-based immunosuppression. Transplantation 1999;68:997–1003.
53. Srivastava T, Zwick DL, Rothberg PG, Warady BA. Posttransplant lymphoproliferative disorder in pediatric renal transplantation. Pediatr Nephrol 1999;13:748–54.
54. Broyer M, Tete MJ, Guest G, et al. Varicella and zoster after kidney transplantation: long-term results of vaccination. Pediatrics 1997;99:35.
55. Penn I. Malignancy in children. In: Tejani AH, Fine RN, editors. Pediatric renal transplantation. New York: Wiley–Liss; 1994. p. 461–70.

56. Broyer M, Guest G, Gagnadoux MF et al. Hypertension following renal transplantation in children. Pediatr Nephrol 1987;1:16–21.
57. Baluarte HJ, Grushkin AB, Ingelfinger JR, Stablein D, Tejani A. Analysis of hypertension in children post renal transplantation—a report of the North American Pediatric Renal Transplant Cooperative Study. Pediatr Nephrol 1994;8:570–3.
58. Niaudet P, Dudley J, Charbit M, Gagnadoux M-F, Macleay K, Broyer M. Pretransplant blood transfusions with cyclosporine in pediatric renal transplantation. Pediatr Nephrol 2000;14:451–6.
59. Paul LC. Pathophysiology of chronic renal allograft rejection. Transplant Proc 1999;31:2715–6.
60. Gellert S, Devaux S, Schonberger B, May G. Donor age and graft function. Pediatr Nephrol 1996;10:716–19.
61. Potter DE. Long-term outcome in kidney transplantation in children. In: Tejani AH, Fine RN, editors. Pediatric renal transplantation. New York: Wiley-Liss; 1994. p. 525–33.

Interventional Radiology and the Transplant Kidney

J. G. Moss and R. Edwards

Renal transplant complications have traditionally been managed by open surgical techniques. There have been many advances in minimally invasive techniques over the last 10–20 years, which include endourology, laparoscopy, and interventional radiology. This chapter will focus on the role and contribution of interventional radiological techniques.

Renal transplants are more challenging than native kidneys in several respects, and transplant patients requiring interventional radiology should be referred to a transplant center where they can benefit from a team approach and the appropriate expertise. A transplant is a precious commodity, and often the most effective management is reached after discussion between the nephrologist, the transplant surgeon, and the interventional radiologist.

■ *Summary points:*

The main interventional radiology techniques for renal transplants are:

- Biopsy
- Drainage and sclerosis
- Renal angioplasty and stenting
- Nephrostomy
- Ureteric dilatation and stenting
- Embolization

Patient Preparation

Informed consent is essential; the risks and benefits should be openly discussed with the patient before embarking on an interventional procedure. Many of the procedures described in this chapter are best performed with the patient under conscious sedation; this will allay the patient's anxiety and pain and generally make the whole procedure less of an ordeal for all concerned. The present authors' preferred medication is diamorphine 2–5 mg and midazolam 1–10 mg given intravenously. It is essential that all patients are appropriately monitored with pulse oximetry, blood pressure measurement, and ECG. It is equally important that a dedicated member of staff in the interventional room is responsible for monitoring these vital signs. This person should not be the radiologist, scrub nurse, or radiographer.[1] Drugs which reverse the effect of diamorphine and midazolam, i.e., flumazenil 200–600 µg (Roche, UK) and naloxone 0.8–2 mg (Dupont, UK), must always be available in the room. Any coagulopathy should be corrected to ensure the international normalized ratio (INR) is below 1.5 and the platelet count above $50{,}000 \times 10^9$/l. Prophylactic antibiotics should be administered for most procedures (excluding biopsy and angioplasty), including the relief of an obstructed urinary tract and drainage of collections, which are often infected or can become infected as a result of catheter manipulation. Fatal septicemia following simple procedures such as nephrostomy have been reported. The present authors prefer a broad-spectrum antibiotic such as cefuroxime 750 mg given intravenously immediately prior to the procedure.

■ *Summary points:*

Preprocedural preparation:

- Informed consent
- Fast for six hours (fluids permitted)
- Check and correct coagulopathy
- Periprocedural antibiotics (except for percutaneous transluminal angioplasty and biopsy)

Requirements for conscious sedation:

- Pulse oximetry
- Pulse and blood pressure monitoring
- ECG monitoring
- Dedicated personnel
- Midazolam 1–10 mg (reversal agent flumenazil)
- Diamorphine 2.5–5 mg (reversal agent naloxone)
- Antibiotic (cefuroxime 750 mg)

Biopsy

Percutaneous biopsy of a renal transplant is normally straightforward as the kidney occupies a relatively superficial anterior position. Ultrasonography should be used to guide the marking of the skin and measure the target depth or, better, to guide needle placement under real-time guidance. The needle should avoid any major vascular structures and the collecting system and provide a suitable core of cortex and medulla. If an uncorrectable coagulopathy is present, a plugged biopsy or transvenous approach should be used.

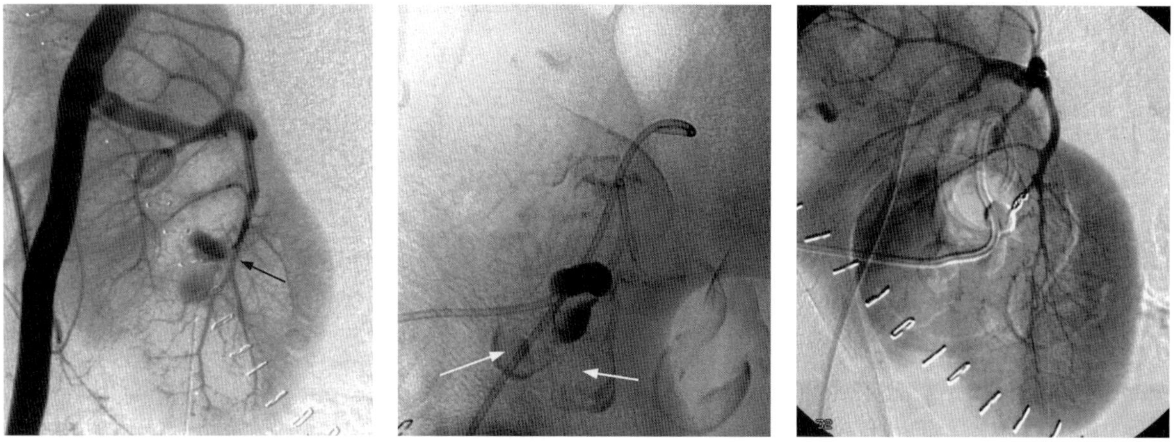

a b c

Fig. 6.**1** **a** Angiogram showing an arteriocalyceal fistula complicating a percutaneous nephrostomy (arrow). **b** A delayed film shows hematoma in a distended collecting system (arrows). **c** Following embolization with 0.018-in. coils the branch vessel and fistula have been occluded (compare with **a**)

Complications of Biopsy

Although percutaneous biopsy is very safe, arteriovenous fistulae, arteriocalyceal fistulae, and pseudoaneurysms are recognized complications. Arteriovenous fistulae (AVFs) are common, occurring in up to 10 % of biopsies, but are usually small; the majority close spontaneously. Persistent AVFs are much less common; again, the majority do not cause any adverse clinical sequelae. Treatment is only indicated if an AVF persists and causes complications such as significant hypertension or deteriorating renal function. Transcatheter embolization is a highly effective technique and should be performed as selectively as possible to minimize the loss of normal renal tissue (Fig. 6.**1**). The use of 2- to 3-Fr coaxial catheters, such as the Tracker system (Boston Scientific, UK), allows the AVF to be precisely catheterized and 1- to 3-mm microcoils can be placed until the AVF is closed. A microcatheter has the additional advantage of minimizing arterial spasm, which can be problematic and can even prevent successful embolization. A color Doppler ultrasound scan the following day should confirm successful occlusion.

Arteriocalyceal fistulae are less common but are more likely to produce symptoms such as persistent hematuria (Fig. 6.**1**). Although they can close spontaneously, more urgent intervention may be required if the hemorrhage is severe.

A pseudoaneurysm caused by biopsy trauma to a peripheral branch of the transplant artery may rupture into the subcapsular or perirenal space and requires urgent embolization.

Calculus Disease

Calculi occur in approximately 1.5 % of renal transplants.[2] The range of techniques used to treat renal transplant calculi are similar to the range used in the native kidney; however, difficulties in retrograde instrumentation of the transplant ureter limit this method of stone retrieval and also preclude the option of opacifying and distending the collecting system prior to percutaneous nephrolithotomy. When percutaneous nephrolithotomy is required, a combined approach utilizing the skills of both the radiologist and the urologist is preferable. Despite its superficial position, the presence of surgical scarring and adhesions around the transplant can make dilatation of the tract difficult. A stiff guide wire such as a Meier wire (Boston Scientific, UK) and a 30-Fr balloon/sheath access system (Tractmaster system, Boston Scientific, UK) is probably superior to Amplatz (Microvena, UK) dilators, where there is an increased risk of losing access. Once the tract has been dilated and the working sheath inserted, the urologist removes the calculus under direct vision using fragmentation techniques when necessary.

Fluid Collections and Abscesses

Fluid collections include lymphoceles (the commonest, occurring in up to 18 % of renal transplant patients), urinomas, hematomas, and abscesses.[3] A small collection of fluid surrounding a transplant during the immediate postoperative period does not necessarily require treatment and will often resolve spontaneously. Inserting a drain risks the introduction of infection, so a "wait and see" policy with follow-up ultrasonography is best for asymptomatic collections. An enlarging collection which is either infected or causing compression of the graft, collecting system, or surrounding structures, requires percutaneous drainage.

Most fluid collections can be drained with an appropriately sized pigtail catheter (8–16 Fr) under imaging guidance. The catheter can be placed directly using the

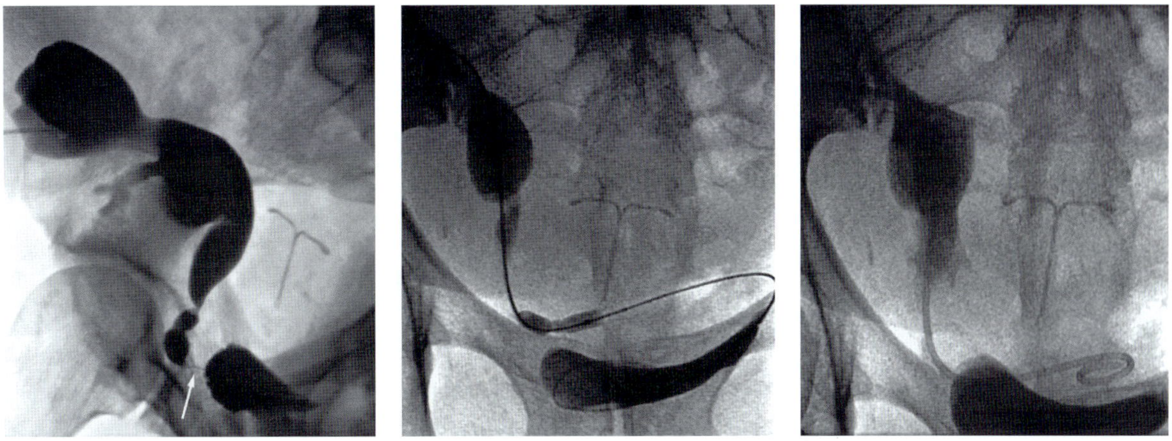

a b c

Fig. 6.2 **a** A distal ureteric stricture (arrow) causing proximal hydronephrosis and impaired renal function. Following passage of an antegrade wire the stricture is balloon-dilated (**b**) and a double pigtail stent placed (**c**). An intrauterine contraceptive device is coincidentally seen

trocar or Seldinger technique under ultrasound and fluoroscopic control. Most unsuccessful drainages fail either because of poor selection (e.g., trying to drain a predominantly solid collection) or because the drainage catheter is of insufficient caliber. Collections of thick pus require a large-bore drain (12–16 Fr), and if adequate drainage is not achieved a second drain may be required. A locking pigtail catheter affords some protection against inadvertent removal. Catheter aftercare is important; the catheter should be flushed with 5 ml saline six-hourly to prevent blockage of the side holes. A contrast study should be carried out weekly to ensure resolution of the cavity and exclude any communication with a viscus. If there is any doubt as when to remove the drain, it should be clamped and an ultrasound scan performed after 24 hours. Reaccumulation of the collection indicates the need for a further period of drainage.

Lymphoceles can be difficult to manage, and if drained percutaneously often require prolonged catheter drainage and sclerosis using one of a variety of agents (absolute alcohol, doxycycline, or povidone iodine). Serious consideration should be given to laparoscopic marsupialization of lymphoceles, which has the advantage of involving a single treatment episode with a very low recurrence rate.[4]

Renal Obstruction

Obstruction is the commonest complication to befall a renal transplant, occurring in 2–10% of patients in the first five postoperative years.[5] Obstruction in the early transplant period may be caused by edema or extrinsic compression from an adjacent fluid collection, but late obstruction is usually due to an ischemic stricture at the ureterovesical anastomosis. The blood supply to this area of the transplant ureter is precarious, as it arises solely from branches of the transplant renal artery, making it potentially vulnerable to ischemia and stricture formation. In addition, if an accessory lower pole artery is inadvertently damaged during transplantation, the ureterovesical anastomosis may be exposed to ischemic damage, which can result in an early postoperative urinary leak or a delayed stricture. Reoperation is difficult in these circumstances, and the benefits of taking a minimally invasive approach and placing a stent percutaneously include the avoidance of a general anesthetic and a prolonged postoperative recovery period. A simple leak can often be managed with a nephrostomy and stent, whereas a stricture will usually require balloon dilatation prior to stenting (Fig. 6.**2**). The results of balloon dilatation and stenting of ureteric strictures varies, with successful outcomes reported in 40–78% of cases. The best results occur in those patients who present with early obstruction (< three months of transplantation) and short distal ureteric strictures.[4,5] Failure of percutaneous treatment will require a surgical revision or, if this is not an option, a permanent ureteric stent.

Nephrostomy

The indications for an urgent nephrostomy are urinary sepsis, a dangerously elevated serum potassium level, and acute rupture of the renal collecting system. In the absence of the above, a nephrostomy can normally be performed electively and need not be performed as an out-of-hours procedure. Although a nephrostomy can be performed at the bedside using ultrasound guidance alone, there is much to commend transferring the patient to the radiology department where the procedure can be performed with a combination of ultrasound and fluoroscopy in an interventional suite under aseptic conditions. A C-arm fluoroscopy unit is

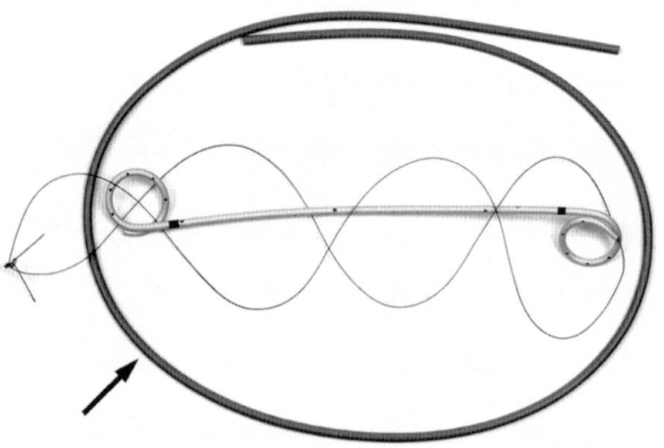

Fig. 6.**3** A modified ureteric stent using an Ethilon loop. The pusher catheter is also shown (arrow)

not essential, but desirable, as it permits the best radiographic projection to be used and minimizes the radiation dose to patient and operator. Careful choice of a suitable calyx is important to minimize radiation to the operator's hand, avoid any scar tissue, and facilitate ureteric stenting should that be required. A direct pelvic puncture must be avoided because of the risk of damaging large vascular structures, with the risk of hemorrhage and loss of the graft.

A 22G Chiba needle is placed into a suitable calyx under ultrasound guidance and a few milliliters of urine aspirated and sent for bacteriological analysis. A small volume of contrast medium is then injected to confirm satisfactory position. The injection of large volumes of contrast should be avoided as this can precipitate endotoxemia. If the needle position is satisfactory, one of the proprietary access systems (Acustix, Boston Scientific, UK; or a Neff Set, Cook, UK) is then used to deliver an 0.018-in. wire followed by a transitional dilator with stiffener. Following removal of the stiffener and inner dilator, a standard 0.035-in. wire is placed and the outer access dilator removed. The original 0.018-in. wire should be left in situ as a safety wire should access be lost at any time. The tract is then dilated to 8 Fr and a locking pigtail catheter placed over the 0.035-in. wire. A small amount of contrast is injected to confirm position and the safety wire is finally removed. It is not necessary to perform a complete nephrostogram in an acute obstruction, and it is safer to defer this until the following day.

Ureteric Balloon Dilatation and Stenting

Although ureteric stenting can be undertaken as a single-stage procedure, a nephrostomy will usually have been established a few days earlier. Once the collecting system has been opacified and the presence of a stricture confirmed, a wire is carefully manipulated across the stricture into the bladder. A useful catheter and wire combination is the biliary manipulation catheter (Cook, UK) and a stiff angled hydrophilic wire (Terumo, UK). Placement of a 9-Fr peel-away sheath provides secure access and support across invariably scarred tissues. A dedicated transplant ureteric stent (Cook Urological, UK) is required. It is useful to modify the stent by placing an Ethilon suture through the trailing end (Fig. 6.**3**), which allows the stent to be pulled proximally if placement is too distal. The stent is then advanced over the wire using the pusher, ensuring that the end of the Ethilon loop protrudes from the sheath. As the guide wire is partially removed, the pigtail must be seen to reform in the bladder, as failure to do so indicates that the distal end of the stent still lies within the ureter. As the wire is removed completely, the trailing pigtail is seen to form in the renal pelvis, and if the stent lies too distal it may be repositioned by traction on the Ethilon loop. It is important to buttress the peel-away sheath against the stent to maintain proximal stent position during removal of the suture, which is simply cut and pulled.

If the stent cannot be advanced across the stricture, it should be removed and a 5- to 6-mm angioplasty balloon placed to dilate the stenosis. Following this, it is usually possible to advance the stent, but occasionally it may be difficult to do so because of tortuous ureteric anatomy. In this situation it may be helpful to establish a "through-and-through" wire by capturing the distal end of the wire within the bladder using an Amplatz Goose Neck snare (Microvena, UK). Excessive tension on the wire should be avoided to minimize damage to the transplant ureter. A temporary nephrostomy should be left in place if there is a significant amount of procedure-related blood clot within the collecting system or if antegrade drainage appears inadequate. The ureteric stent should be removed after six to eight weeks; this can be done either cystoscopically or by snaring under fluoroscopic guidance (Fig 6.**4**).

Renal Artery Stenosis

Renal artery stenosis may be detected in up to 30% of transplant patients. The precise etiology is often unknown, but possible causes include surgical clamp injury, cyclosporine toxicity, donor atherosclerosis, and vessel tortuosity or kinking causing turbulence. Occasionally the stenosis lies in the proximal aortoiliac system, and the presence of claudication in the affected limb is often a clinical clue (Fig. 6.**5**).

The appropriate management of renal transplant artery stenosis is controversial; opinions vary widely between those who advocate revascularization and others who adopt a more conservative approach. The clinical sequelae, i.e., hypertension and impaired renal function, are multifactorial and are not uncommon in the absence of renal artery stenosis. Although the natural history of transplant renal artery stenosis is unknown, there is little evidence to support the assump-

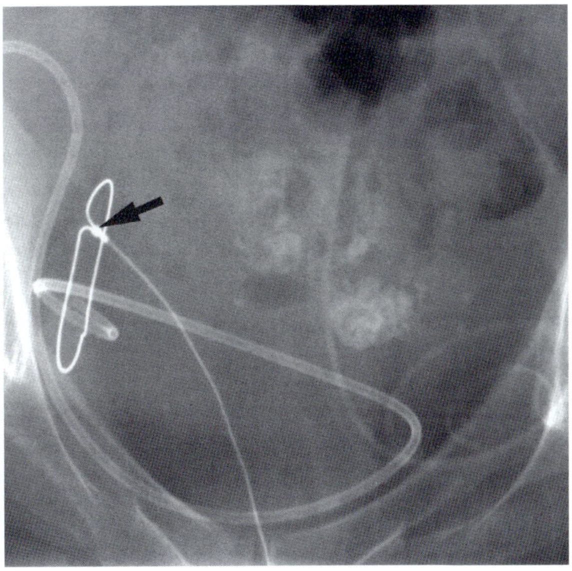

a

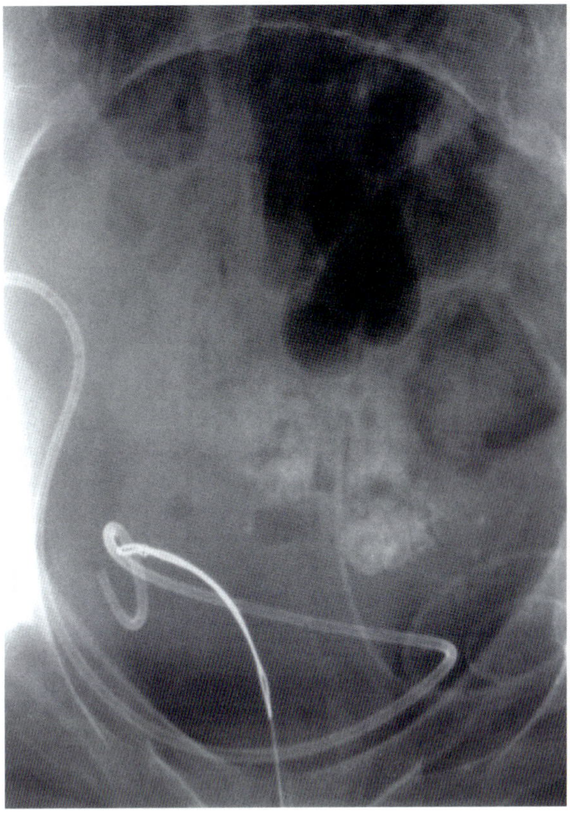

b

Fig. 6.4 **a** An Amplatz gooseneck snare (arrow) is passed via the urethra and guided over the stent using fluoroscopic guidance. Once tightened, the snare and stent are removed together via the urethra (**b**)

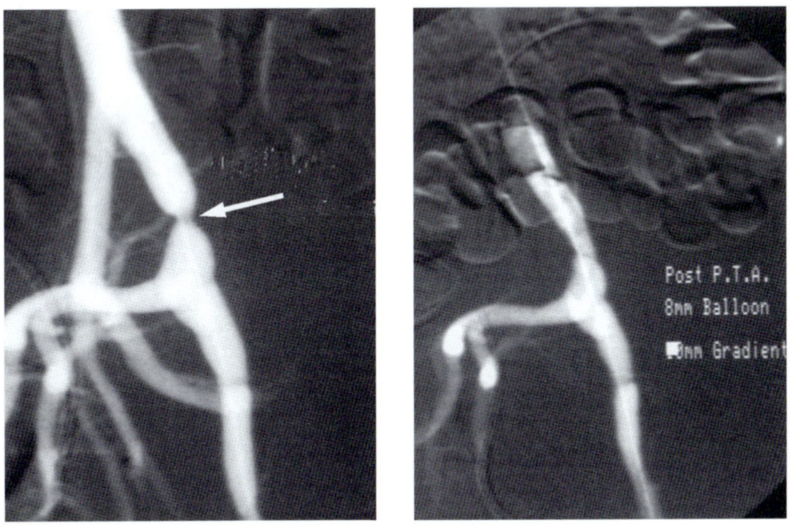

a b

Fig. 6.5 **a** Angiogram of a patient with claudication and impaired renal function showing an external left iliac artery stenosis proximal to the transplant anastomosis (arrow). **b** Satisfactory result following angioplasty. The claudication resolved and the renal function improved

tion of a progressive process similar to that seen in the native kidneys with atheromatous lesions. The restenosis rate following percutaneous transluminal angioplasty is in the region of 20–30%, and stents have been advocated in these cases. Small series have been published reporting the use of stents in postangioplasty restenosis, and although results are encouraging, the long-term outcome is unknown.[6]

Endovascular treatment of transplant renal artery stenosis is preferable to a conventional surgical approach as it is much less invasive. The choice of access will depend upon the surgical anatomy, but generally a cadaveric graft (external iliac anastomosis) is best accessed from an ipsilateral femoral approach and a live donor graft (internal iliac anastomosis) from a contralateral femoral approach.

During a cadaveric organ harvest a small cuff of aortic wall (Carrel patch) is removed with the transplant artery and this is used to fashion a wide vascular anastomosis with the recipient's external iliac artery. For this reason, the site of the arterial stenosis is almost always distal to the anastomosis in a cadaveric transplant, but is very variable in a live donor organ.

Renal Artery Angioplasty

A 6-Fr sheath is placed in the appropriate access vessel and the transplant artery catheterized with an appropriately shaped catheter. The stenosis is crossed with a TAD11 wire (Boston Scientific, UK). This wire is tapered and particularly useful as it has a floppy 0.018-in. tip but a reasonably stiff 0.035-in. shaft for balloon support. Heparin (3000–5000 units) and an antispasmodic, e.g., glycerol trinitrate 200 μg (intra-arterially) should be given routinely once the renal artery has been selected. A short-tip, short-length (2 cm) angioplasty balloon 5–7 mm in diameter is used to dilate the stenosis. The balloon diameter should match the normal artery size. Endovascular stents are rarely indicated unless there is either total vessel collapse or flow-limiting dissection immediately following angioplasty. If a stent is used, one of the small platform systems (Cordis, UK; Medtronic, UK; or Guidant, UK) is recommended, which, when placed through an appropriate guiding catheter, will track around the often tortuous renal artery. The present authors administer an antibiotic (cefuroxime 750 mg i. v.) given as a single dose when the stent is placed.

In conclusion, the role of percutaneous transluminal angioplasty and stenting in transplant renal artery stenosis remains controversial. Although it may bring clinical benefit, it is not without risk, and occasionally the graft can be lost due to vessel occlusion or dissection. In no area is fully informed patient consent more important.

References

1. Callum KG, Whimster F. National CEPOD: A report of the National Confidential Enquiry into Perioperative Deaths. London: NCEPOD, 2000.
2. Hayes JM, Streem SB, Graneto D, et al. Renal transplant calculi: a re-evaluation of risks and management. Transplantation 1984;47:949–52.
3. Lange V, Schardey HM, Meyer G, et al. Laparoscopic deroofing of post-transplant lymphocoeles. Transpl Int 1994;7:140–3.
4. Hobart MG, Streem SB, Gill IS. Renal transplant complications. Minimally invasive management. Urol Clin North Am 2000;27:787–98.
5. Soltes GD, Rainwater GD, Middlebrook MR, et al. Interventional uroradiology. World J Urol 1998;16:52–61.
6. Sierre SD, Raynaud AC, Carreres T, Sapoval MR, Beyssen BM, Gaux JC. Treatment of recurrent transplant renal artery stenosis with metallic stents. J Vasc Interv Radiol 1998;9:639–44.

Indications and Assessment for Liver Transplantation

S. Norris

Introduction

Liver transplantation is now widely accepted as an effective therapeutic modality for a variety of irreversible acute and chronic liver diseases for which there was formerly no other effective therapy. With advances in perioperative techniques, immunosuppressive agents, postoperative care, and a greater understanding of the prognosis of many liver diseases, the results of liver transplantation have improved, with one-year survival figures in excess of 85 % for a number of liver diseases. As a result, the procedure is now being offered for a wider range of diseases and to older patients.

The main goals of liver transplantation are to prolong life and improve the quality of life. To achieve these goals, the timing of transplantation is crucial, but in the absence of international or nationally agreed criteria the selection of patients can be difficult and inexact. Ideally, liver transplantation should be performed at a sufficiently late stage of the disease to allow for spontaneous stabilization or recovery, but before the onset of complications of end-stage liver disease that could potentially increase the risk of liver transplantation. In order to optimize the timing of transplantation to increase survival and decrease postoperative morbidity, a number of survival models have been applied to specific liver diseases, and these will be discussed in subsequent sections.

The indications for liver transplantation broadly fall into four main categories: advanced chronic liver disease, acute liver failure, malignancy, and inherited metabolic disorders (Table 7.**1**). End-stage chronic liver disease accounts for approximately 70% of all liver transplant activity in Europe and America, but the indications for transplantation have changed over the past ten years, with alcohol-related and viral-related cirrhosis presenting an expanding indication (Fig. 7.**1**). In the setting of donor shortages and constriction in healthcare budgets, the timing of transplantation becomes even more important.

■ ***Summary points:***

- The results of liver transplantation have improved, with one-year survival figures in excess of 85 % for a number of liver diseases
- Liver transplantation should be performed at a sufficiently late stage of the disease to allow for spontaneous stabilization or recovery but before the onset of complications of end-stage liver disease that could potentially increase the risk of liver transplantation
- End-stage chronic liver disease accounts for approximately 70% of all liver transplants in Europe and America

Table 7.**1** Indications for liver transplantation in adults

Chronic liver disease:
Primary biliary cirrhosis
Primary sclerosing cholangitis
Secondary biliary cirrhosis
Alcohol
Autoimmune hepatitis
Viral hepatitis (HCV, HBV, HDV)
Budd–Chiari syndrome
Metabolic:
Wilson disease
Hemochromatosis
Alpha$_1$-antitrypsin deficiency
Familial hypercholesterolemia
Familial amyloid polyneuropathy
Primary hyperoxaluria
Cystic fibrosis
Neoplastic:
Hepatocellular carcinoma
Apudomas
Epithelioid hemangioendothelioma
Acute liver failure:
Drugs/toxins
Viral (HAV, HBV)
Wilson disease
Congenital:
Polycystic disease
Caroli disease

HAV, HBV, HBC, HBD, hepatitis A, B, C, and D viruses

Chronic Liver Diseases

Primary Biliary Cirrhosis

Primary biliary cirrhosis (PBC) is a chronic progressive cholestatic disease characterized by inflammatory destruction of the interlobular bile ducts, affecting predominantly females between 40 and 60 years. The disease is thought to be autoimmune in nature and is

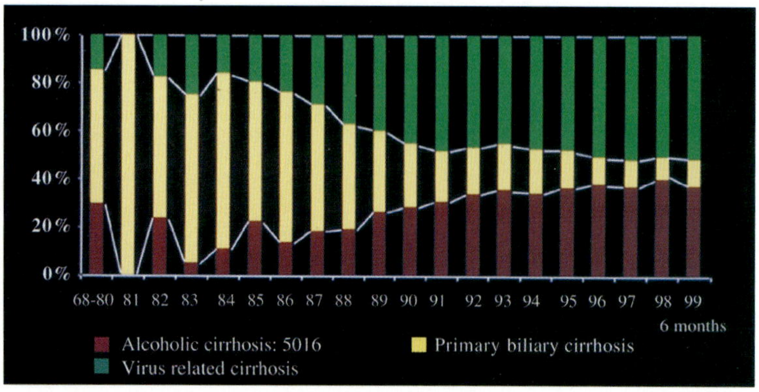

Fig. 7.**1** Indications for liver transplantation from 1968 to 1999 have changed, with alcohol-related and viral-related cirrhosis presenting an expanding indication

Table 7.**2** Clinical indications for liver transplantation

Serum bilirubin 6 mg/dl (170 μmol/l)[a]
Refractory ascites
Recurring encephalopathy
Deteriorating synthetic function (serum albumin <30 g/l, unrelated to active infection)
Recurrent spontaneous bacterial peritonitis
Recurrent bacterial cholangitis[b]
Hepatopulmonary syndrome
Poor quality of life (intractable pruritus, extreme fatigue)
Hepatic osteodystrophy[a,b]

[a]Primary biliary cirrhosis
[b]Primary sclerosing cholangitis

serologically characterized by raised IgM titers in association with positive antimitochondrial antibodies (AMA). Radiology has no role to play in the diagnosis or management of PBC until the onset of complications relating to portal hypertension. The disease progresses through three phases: an asymptomatic phase with normal serum bilirubin, lasting up to 20 years, a symptomatic phase marked by pruritus, jaundice, and fatigue, and a third phase characterized by severe jaundice and complications of portal hypertension. Treatment with ursodeoxycholic acid (UDCA) is the most commonly used therapy. It reduces cholestasis but its effects on survival are less certain, although some studies suggest a delay in the need for transplantation.[1]

In contrast to most other liver diseases that require transplantation, the natural history of PBC is well characterized and this facilitates the timing of transplantation. A number of prognostic models have been developed to determine independent risk factors to estimate survival and therefore facilitate patient selection. The most widely used model was developed at the Mayo Clinic[2] and identified five independent variables which indicated poor prognosis: age, serum albumin, serum bilirubin, prothrombin time (PT), and edema. The European model identified serum bilirubin and albumin, the presence of ascites, history of gastrointestinal bleeding, and age as independent variables indicating poor prognosis. The most useful variable, common to several prognostic models, is the serum bilirubin,[3] and the major indication for transplantation for PBC is a serum bilirubin concentration greater than 6.0 mg/dl (102 μmol/l). At this level of jaundice, the median survival is 25 months, which falls to 17 months when the bilirubin rises above 10 mg/dl (170 μmol/l). Other indications for liver transplantation are listed in Table 7.**2**.

These models have also been used to assess the efficacy of the transplant procedure. Using the Mayo model, estimated survival of patients who underwent transplantation was superior to the simulated survival of these patients if they had been managed conservatively without transplantation, and the benefit was greatest in patients with the highest risk scores. The five-year survival for PBC following transplantation is 70–80 %, and the risk of recurrence at five years seems to be less than 10 %.[4]

Summary points:

- Radiology has no role to play in the diagnosis or management of PBC until the onset of complications relating to portal hypertension
- Five independent variables indicate poor prognosis in PBC: age, serum albumin, serum bilirubin, prothrombin time, and edema
- The five-year survival for PBC following transplantation is 70–80 %, and the risk of recurrence at five years seems to be less than 10 %

Primary Sclerosing Cholangitis

Primary sclerosing cholangitis (PSC) is a chronic progressive obliterative process involving the intra- and extrahepatic biliary tree, which ultimately leads to cirrhosis. The etiology of the disease is unknown, but immunologic mechanisms, genetic predisposition, and bacterial and viral infections have all been postulated.[5] It occurs predominantly in younger men (mean age at diagnosis 39 years), and is commonly associated with inflammatory bowel disease (more than 75 % of cases). Median survival from time of diagnosis is 11.9 years.[6] Many patients are asymptomatic at the time of diagnosis and the disease progresses insidiously, marked by periods of jaundice and pruritus associated with bacterial cholangitis secondary to stricture formation. Other symptoms relate to chronic cholestasis and portal hypertension. A major concern in PSC patients is the risk of developing cholangiocarcinoma, and long-term studies indicate that 8–30% of patients develop this malignancy over 10 years. Most centers consider cholangiocarcinoma to be a contraindication to liver transplantation.

Unlike PBC, radiology has a major role in the diagnosis and management of this condition, and endoscopic retrograde cholangiopancreatography is the method of choice for visualizing the biliary tree. Balloon dilatation and stenting of strictures may be required intermittently, and brushings and biopsies from the bile duct should be obtained for assessment of neoplastic change at each procedure. Treatment with UDCA does not seem to modify the course of the disease.

Several models have been developed on the basis of clinical variables in which a survival risk score can be calculated and translated into a survival function for estimating survival for individual patients with PSC. In the Mayo model, age, serum bilirubin level, hemoglobin, presence or absence of inflammatory bowel disease, and histologic stage were identified as independent predictors of survival. As with PBC, this model indicates that liver transplantation significantly improves the survival rate at all risk stratifications compared with simulated survival in the absence of transplantation.[7] Five-year survival rates between 73% and 85% have been reported following transplantation for PSC, based on studies from three transplant centers. However, the major challenge for clinicians is selecting the appropriate time for transplantation, before the onset of significant muscle loss and the development of cholangiocarcinoma. Latent cholangiocarcinoma remains a risk in PSC as its progression is usually silent, and despite routine ultrasound and computed tomographic scanning prior to transplantation, 10% of PSC patients have an unsuspected tumor at surgery. In patients where tumors are suspected despite negative computed tomography (CT) and magnetic resonance imaging (MRI) imaging, positron emission tomography (PET) may have a role to play.

■ *Summary points:*

- In PSC the risk of developing cholangiocarcinoma is 8–30% over 10 years; most centers consider cholangiocarcinoma to be a contraindication to liver transplantation
- Five-year survival rates of 73–85% have been reported following liver transplantation for PSC
- Latent cholangiocarcinoma is found in 10% of PSC patients at surgery

Alcohol-Related Liver Disease

Alcohol is one of the most significant causes of liver disease in the Western world. While the relationship between alcohol intake and the development of alcohol-related cirrhosis is not simply one of dose-related toxicity, there is a clear relationship between overall alcohol consumption and death from cirrhosis. Recent estimates indicate that the risk of developing cirrhosis with a consumption of 28–41 units per week is 3–4% at 12 years. This risk increases to 6–7% when more than 42 units are consumed per week.[8]

An increasing number of patients with alcohol-related cirrhosis are now undergoing transplantation (Fig. 7.**1**), and alcohol-related disease is the second commonest indication for transplantation in both Europe and America. Long-term survival following transplantation is similar to that for cirrhosis of other causes.[9] Despite this, the percentage of patients undergoing transplantation for alcohol-related cirrhosis is extremely low compared to the incidence of alcohol-related cirrhosis in the community. Reluctance to transplant or refer for transplantation may be explained by concern regarding the risk of recidivism (estimated at between 15–40%) and lack of compliance following transplantation, and the ethics of transplantation for this condition. Most centers have established guidelines for assessing patients with alcohol-related cirrhosis, which usually include a six-month period of abstinence from alcohol ingestion. This allows time to reassess the need for transplantation and to allow assessment of the patient's ability to refrain from consumption (i.e., the patient's alcohol dependency). Assessment of alcohol-induced disease in extrahepatic organs is also mandatory, and careful evaluation for non-alcohol-related liver disease is necessary even when alcohol-related liver disease is the initial diagnosis, as hepatitis C virus (HCV) infection is a frequent co-morbid condition in this patient group. Indications for transplantation are similar to those for other causes of cirrhosis.

■ *Summary point:*

- Alcohol is the second commonest indication for transplantation in both Europe and America

Autoimmune Hepatitis

Autoimmune hepatitis (AIH) is a chronic inflammatory disease of the liver, associated with hypergammaglobulinemia and serum autoantibodies, and responds to immunosuppressive therapy in most cases. It has a strong female preponderance and is associated with HLA-DR3 and HLA-DR4. The diagnosis requires absence of chronic viral hepatitis and metabolic liver diseases such as Wilson disease. AIH can be subclassified into types 1, 2, and 3 depending on the pattern of autoantibodies: type 1 with antinuclear antibodies (ANA) and/or smooth muscle antibodies (SMA); type 2 with anti-liver–kidney microsomal antibodies (LKM); type 3 with anti-soluble liver antigen (SLA). Type 1 AIH is the commonest from of AIH, while type 2 occurs in younger patients and is associated with more severe disease which progresses more rapidly. The condition is confirmed by liver biopsy, which in untreated patients shows portal and lobular hepatitis with lymphocytic and plasma cell infiltration and interface hepatitis. Radiology has no role in the diagnosis of AIH. Therapy consists of steroids alone or in combination with azathioprine used as a steroid-sparing agent. A minority of patients achieve complete remission, but most patients require long-term drug therapy. Alternative strategies include cyclosporine, tacrolimus, cyclophosphamide, UDCA, and rapamycin (sirolimus), but their efficacy remains to be fully evaluated in controlled trials.

Transplantation of the liver is the definitive therapy for AIH, not only for chronic disease resulting in cirrhosis but also for acute liver failure secondary to AIH. There are no specific markers that predict lack of response to conservative therapy, and again the timing of transplantation can be difficult. Symptoms are similar to those of other end-stage liver diseases, mainly fatigue, refractory ascites, and encephalopathy, and deteriorating synthetic function should prompt referral for transplant assessment. The five-year survival rates following transplantation are in excess of 80 %. Patients with AIH are reported to have a higher rate of rejection following transplantation, and many centers continue steroid therapy long-term in this group.

Viral Hepatitis: HCV

Chronic viral hepatitis is one of the commonest causes of end-stage liver disease worldwide, with an estimated 150 million HCV-infected individuals globally. Following exposure to HCV, up to 85 % of infected individuals fail to clear the virus and progress to chronic disease. Progression is variable, but an estimated 20–30 % develop cirrhosis over 20–30 years, 20 % of whom progress to decompensated liver disease.[10] Between 8 % and 40 % of patients have been reported to develop hepatocellular carcinoma (HCC), invariably on a background of cirrhosis. The rate of disease progression is variable and unpredictable, but an accelerated rate of progression is associated with older age at time of infection, increased alcohol consumption, and coinfection with hepatitis B virus (HBV) or the human immunodeficiency virus (HIV). Six genotypes and more than 80 subtypes of hepatitis C have been identified. Blood donors and patients in Western Europe and the USA are frequently infected with genotypes 1a, 1b, 2a, 2b, and 3a, while genotype 4 is commonly found in north and central Africa and the Middle East. Genotype variation has an important bearing on the management of hepatitis C as genotype 1 is less responsive to therapy than genotypes 2 and 3 and a longer duration of therapy is required.

Diagnosis requires detection of antibodies to expressed proteins of HCV, which confirm exposure to the virus. Determination of ongoing viremia requires detection of HCV RNA in serum by polymerase chain reaction. However, as there is poor correlation between serum alanine transaminase (ALT) or viral load and histologic disease, a liver biopsy is essential to determine the degree of inflammation and fibrosis, particularly in assessing the need for antiviral therapy. In cirrhotic patients, six-monthly alpha-fetoprotein and ultrasound assessment are performed for HCC screening, and detection of a suspicious lesion prompts further imaging with CT and angiography to determine the precise size, location, and number of tumors.

HCV cirrhosis has become the leading indication for liver transplantation in the past ten years, and the number of patients undergoing transplantation continues to grow. Indications for liver transplantation are similar to those in cirrhosis of other causes. In addition, the discovery of HCC in a cirrhotic HCV-infected patient also prompts referral for liver transplantation assessment. Five- and ten-year survival rates of 70 % and 60 % respectively have been reported in Europe, similar to rates for other nonmalignant disease. Unfortunately, HCV recurrence following transplantation is almost universal, and although the majority of patients experience mild disease, cirrhosis following transplantation has been reported in 10–28 % of patients at five years.[11,12] Studies using prophylactic antiviral agents to prevent and antiviral drugs to treat graft reinfection are currently under assessment.

Summary points:

- Chronic viral hepatitis is one of the commonest causes of end-stage liver disease worldwide, with an estimated 150 million HCV-infected individuals globally
- HCV-related cirrhosis has become the leading indication for liver transplantation in the past ten years
- Cirrhosis following liver transplantation for HCV infection has been reported in 10–28 % of patients at five years

Viral Hepatitis: HBV

HBV infection is a worldwide problem, with 300 million HBV carriers globally. Unlike HCV, the rate of progression to chronic viral illness following acute infection is less than 5 % in adults, but it is 90 % for perinatally acquired infection. Thus, perinatal infection is the predominant mode of transmission in high-prevalence areas. Unprotected sexual intercourse and intravenous drug use are the major modes of transmission in low endemic regions.

The course of chronic HBV infection is determined by the interaction between the virus and the individual's immune system, and consists of three phases. The first phase is characterized by a very high level of HBV replication without liver disease and is therefore referred to as the "immunotolerant phase." It can last for up to 30 years, and spontaneous HB_eAg clearance is rare. This may be followed by a immune clearance phase, when HB_eAg clearance occurs spontaneously (10–20% of patients per year) but is associated with active liver disease. The third phase is characterized by HB_eAg loss and the development of HB_eAb. HBV replication may have ceased and the liver disease is usually inactive.

Clinical features of HBV-related chronic liver disease may range from fatigue, vague right upper quadrant discomfort, and intermittent jaundice, to cirrhosis and the sequelae of portal hypertension. As with chronic HCV infection, cirrhotic patients require regular screening for HCC. Indications for liver transplantation are similar to those in other nonviral end-stage liver diseases.

Chronic HBV-related liver disease accounts for approximately 10% of all liver transplant indications, although it still remains somewhat controversial due to the risk of graft reinfection following transplantation. In the absence of antiviral therapy, the spontaneous risk of HBV recurrence is 80%; recurrence is characterized by the reappearance of hepatitis B serum antigen (HB_sAg) and HBV DNA in the serum. Reinfection is almost always accompanied by recurrent liver disease. However, the administration of high-dose anti-HB_s immunoglobulin (HBIg) during and immediately following surgery has dramatically reduced the rate of HBV recurrence.[13] With long-term administration of HBIg to maintain hepatitis B serum antibody (HB_sAb) titers above 100 IU/l, five-year survival rates in excess of 80% in those who remain HB_sAg-negative have been reported by the Paris group. The most important predictor of HBV reinfection in the graft is the presence of HB_eAg and/or HBV DNA before transplantation. It is therefore crucial to inhibit HBV replication with antiviral therapy before transplantation. Lamivudine, a nucleoside analogue, is the most effective antiviral drug available to decrease the viral load before transplantation, and it is well tolerated in those with decompensated cirrhosis.

Summary points:

- HBV infection is a worldwide problem, with 300 million HBV carriers globally. The rate of progression to chronic viral illness following acute infection is less than 5% in adults but 90% in patients with perinatally acquired infection
- Chronic HBV-related liver disease accounts for approximately 10% of all transplant indications but remains controversial due to the risk of graft reinfection following transplantation
- The most important predictor of HBV reinfection in the graft is the presence of HB_eAg and/or HBV DNA before transplantation

Acute Liver Failure

Acute liver failure (ALF) is defined as the development of encephalopathy within 12 weeks of the onset of jaundice, and has the subclassifications "hyper-ALF" for patients in whom this interval is less than 7 days and "sub-ALF" for those in whom it is 5–12 weeks. These terms have now superseded the older terms fulminant liver failure and late-onset liver failure. Patients who develop hyper-ALF have the highest chance of recovery with appropriate management, despite the high incidence of cerebral edema and characteristic rapid deterioration. ALF and sub-ALF, by contrast, are associated with a significantly higher mortality rate, around 80–85%.

The main causes of ALF in the United Kingdom are viruses and drugs, but in a proportion of patients no cause can be identified, and in these patients the disease is termed seronegative or non-A-E hepatitis. ALF due to acetaminophen poisoning is commonest in the United Kingdom (54% of cases), followed by seronegative hepatitis (17%), while in France acute HBV infection is the commonest cause of ALF (45%). In the USA, seronegative hepatitis is predominant (39%), followed by ALF due to acute HBV infection (18%). Other causes of ALF include acute liver failure associated with pregnancy, Wilson disease, and mushroom poisoning.

The clinical manifestation of ALF involves all the major organ systems but is characterized by encephalopathy, cerebral edema, renal failure, hypoglycemia, hyperlactatemia, and metabolic acidosis. Hemodynamic changes include profound vasodilatation, and progressive disease leads to circulatory failure. Other potential complications include bacterial and fungal infections.

The prognosis of ALF varies significantly according to the underlying diagnosis, the age of the patient, and the duration of time over which the disease evolves. Since some patients recover spontaneously without the need for transplantation, criteria have evolved to try and identify those patients in most need of liver transplantation (Table **7.3**). In France, coma associated with a significant reduction in the factor V level correlates with a mortality rate of more than 90% irrespective of the cause, and prompts scheduling for transplantation.[14] Factor V levels are not used widely in clinical practice outside France, but their prognostic value has been validated in non-acetaminophen-induced ALF in the UK. The King's College criteria (see Table 7.**3**) are early indicators of prognosis and can be applied quickly before progression to the late stages of encephalopathy.[15] A small or rapidly shrinking liver is also an indicator of poor prognosis, particularly for patients with sub-ALF. Serial ultrasound or CT imaging has been used in Japan to assess the size of the liver and the functional reserve, and to determine prognosis.

Liver transplantation for ALF accounts for 11% of all liver transplant activity in Europe and 5% in the USA. Survival rates range from 59% to 79% in different series.

Table 7.3 Criteria for liver transplantation in acute liver failure

King's College criteria:
- Acetaminophen-related:
  - pH < 7.3, or all three of the following:
  - PT > 100 seconds or INR > 6.5, serum creatinine > 2.3 mg/dl (300 μmol/l), and grade 3–4 encephalopathy
- Non-acetaminophen-related:
  - PT > 100 seconds or INR > 6.5, or any three of the following variables:
    - Age < 10 or > 40 years
    - PT > 50 seconds or INR > 3.5
    - Serum bilirubin > 17.6 mg/dl (300 μmol/l)
    - Duration of jaundice before encephalopathy > 7 days
    - Etiology (drug-induced, seronegative hepatitis)

Clichy criteria
- Factor V < 30 % of normal if age > 30 years, or < 20 % if age < 30 years, and
- Grade 3–4 encephalopathy

Table 7.4 Indications for liver transplantation in children

Metabolic:
- Alpha$_1$-antitrypsin deficiency
- Hereditary tyrosinemia
- Crigler–Najjar type 1 disease
- Glycogen storage disease
- Wilson disease
- Urea cycle defects

Neoplastic:
- Hepatocellular carcinoma
- Hepatoblastoma

Cholestatic diseases:
- Biliary atresia
- Familial intrahepatic cholestasis (Byler disease)
- Alagille syndrome (syndromic bile duct paucity)
- Nonsyndromic bile duct paucity
- Neonatal hepatitis

Acute liver failure:
- Wilson disease
- Budd–Chiari syndrome
- Viral hepatitis
- Toxin/drug

Summary points:

- Patients who develop hyper-ALF have the highest chance of recovery
- Liver transplantation for ALF accounts for 11 % of all liver transplant activity in Europe and 5 % in the USA, with survival rates from 59 % to 79 %

Pediatric Liver Transplantation

Liver transplantation has been widely accepted as a definitive therapy for many end-stage liver diseases in children.[16] Diseases that comprise the common indications for liver transplantation in children are listed in Table 7.**4**. Biliary atresia is the commonest indication, accounting for more than 50 % of cases, and metabolic indications account for a further 20–25 % of pediatric transplants (Fig. 7.**2**). In the USA 4000 liver transplants are performed each year and 15 % of recipients are under 18 years old. The increasing use of liver transplantation for a variety of pediatric liver diseases has placed a huge burden on limited resources, and this has led to a variety of alternative techniques such as reduced-size grafts, split grafts, and living related donor transplantation in an attempt to meet the demand.[17]
The main indications for transplantation are severe jaundice, intractable variceal hemorrhage, encephalopathy, marked deterioration in synthetic function with vitamin-K-resistant coagulopathy, progressive malaise, and failure to grow. Contraindications to liver transplantation are similar to those outlined above for adult liver transplantation. Additional care is needed to determine the presence of irreversible neurologic damage and extrahepatic sepsis, which are further contraindications to surgery.

Survival rates at one year following transplantation are excellent, 85–90 %. The most important factor determining survival is the severity of the child's illness at the time of transplantation. Survival in infants is still less than in older children, and in infants less than one year old or weighing less than 10 kg, survival rates are in the range of 65–88 %. Delaying transplantation until the child is at least one year old and weighs more than 10 kg runs the risk of progressive complications and deterioration in the child's clinical state.

Summary point:

- Biliary atresia accounts for more than 50 % and metabolic indications account for 20–25 % of pediatric transplants

Preoperative Evaluation

Despite drug therapy and support, many patients with chronic liver diseases progress inexorably to end-stage decompensated cirrhosis and become potential recipients for liver transplantation. While many of the models discussed earlier can aid the decision about appropriate timing for transplantation, there are inherent problems with prognostic models. Firstly, they apply to a group of patients rather than to any specific individual with the disease. Secondly, they include no quality-of-life factor, which together with the clinical status of the patient should be taken into account. Finally, certain tables need to be available for these models to calculate the risk scores.
The goals of the pretransplant evaluation process are outlined in Table 7.**5**. The assessment must confirm the diagnosis and assess the severity of the disease, as oc-

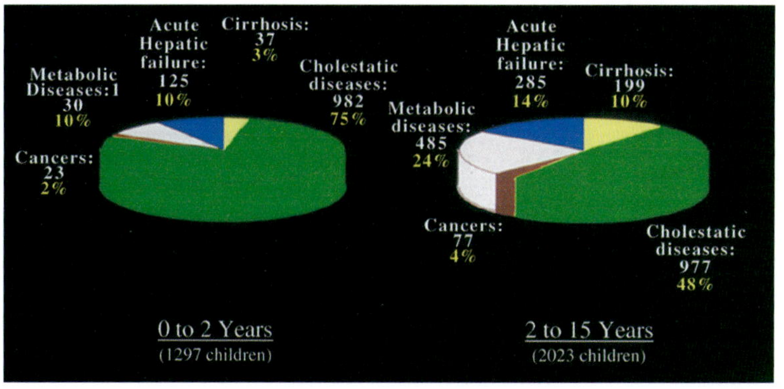

Fig. 7.**2** Indications for liver transplantation in pediatric patients, divided into the 0- to 2-year-old age group and the 2- to 15-year-old age group

casionally patients are referred at an early stage in their disease course when the benefit of transplantation is not so well defined. Occasionally, nontransplant strategies such as transhepatic intrajugular portosystemic shunting may delay the need for transplantation in patients with good synthetic function with refractory ascites or recurrent variceal bleeding. The transplant selection team comprises transplant surgeons, hepatologists, transplant coordinators, anesthesiologists, social workers, and psychologists, with referrals to other specialists including dieticians, cardiologists, radiologists, infectious disease experts, and others. Many patients with end-stage liver disease have poor dental hygiene, and a dental consultation is frequently required to remove potential sources of sepsis.

The preoperative evaluation process is outlined in Table 7.**6**. Ultrasound scanning is routinely performed in all patients to assess portal vein patency and to assess for potential malignant lesions. Where lesions suspicious for HCC are diagnosed, or where HCC is the indication for transplantation, additional imaging is mandatory to determine the precise number, nature, and location of the lesions. Aortoportography and/or magnetic resonance venography may also be required. These investigations are also necessary in the presence of portal vein thrombosis to determine the vascular anatomy. In patients with PSC, colonoscopy is advised to determine the presence or absence of colonic malignancy, and where there is a suspicion of cholangiocarcinoma, PET scanning may aid the diagnosis. In patients with risk factors for cardiac disease, cardiac catheterization is advised. Patients with atypical features of encephalopathy may undergo a CT brain scan to rule out organic causes of confusion, but routine scanning for all patients with hepatic encephalopathy is not cost-effective.

An important component of the transplant assessment is determining the presence of contraindications to surgery. Previous contraindications to liver transplantation, which no longer apply as experience has increased, include an age limit of 55 years, portal vein thrombosis, and HB_sAg positivity. There is now no absolute age limit, and the physiologic age is more im-

Table 7.**5** Goals of pretransplant evaluation

1. Confirm the diagnosis
2. Establish the severity
3. Consider strategic management options:
   Nontransplant options:
      Treatable metabolic disease
      Shunt surgery/TIPPS
   Transplant options:
      Evaluation of living donors (pediatric)
4. Recognize potential contraindications to transplantation
5. Establish plan for interim management
6. Vaccination (pediatric)
7. Maintain nutrition
8. Maximize developmental progression (pediatric)
9. Educate patient and family

Table 7.**6** Preoperative evaluation of the liver transplant candidate

Routine laboratory tests:
Full blood count, INR, blood group, HLA type
Serum electrolytes, urea, creatinine, liver function tests, glucose, Ca^{2+}, Mg^{2+}
Hepatitis screen (HCV, HBV, cytomegalovirus, Epstein–Barr virus), HIV test
Tumor markers (alpha-fetoprotein, CEA)
TSH

Routine radiologic tests:
Chest X-ray
Abdominal ultrasound with Doppler studies

Other routine tests:
ECG
Pulmonary function tests
Arterial blood gas
Echocardiography (if candidate > 40 years)
24-hour creatinine clearance

Additional tests where indicated:
Abdominal CT, MR venography
Celiac/superior mesenteric angiography
Aortoportogram
CT brain
PET scan
Cardiac catheterization
Colonoscopy

Table 7.**7** Contraindications to liver transplantation

Extrahepatic organ failure (heart, lungs)
Uncontrolled systemic sepsis
Extrahepatic malignancy (possible exception: neuroendocrine disease)
AIDS
Portomesenteric thrombosis (portal, splenic, and superior mesenteric veins)
Active substance abuse
Cholangiocarcinoma

portant than the chronologic age. As a result, the number of recipients over the age of 60 years has increased. HIV-positive patients who are HIV RNA-negative on highly active antiretroviral therapy (HAART) with a CD4 count above 200 are undergoing transplantation at some centers. As more HIV-positive patients live longer as a result of HAART, it is likely that the number of coinfected patients referred for transplant assessment as a consequence of HBV- or HCV-related end-stage cirrhosis will increase. Absolute contraindications to liver transplantation are listed in Table 7.**7**. The general criterion for establishing an absolute contraindication to liver transplantation is the extremely poor outcome following transplantation, when it has been performed.

References

1. Poupon RE, Lindor K, Cauch-Dudeck K, Dickson ER, Poupon R, Heathcote EJ. Combined analysis of randomised controlled trials of ursodeoxycholic acid in primary biliary cirrhosis. Gastroenterology 1997;113:884–90.
2. Dickson ER, Grambsch PM, Fleming TR, Fisher LD, Langworthy A. Prognosis in primary biliary cirrhosis: model for decision-making. Hepatology 1989;10:1–7.
3. Shapiro JM, Smith H, Schaffner F. Serum bilirubin: a prognostic factor for primary biliary cirrhosis. Gut 1979;20:137–40.
4. Garcia RFG, Garcia CE, McMaster P, Neuberger J. Transplantation for primary biliary cirrhosis: retrospective analysis of 400 patients in a single centre. Hepatology 2001;33:22–27.
5. Lee YM, Kaplan MM. Primary sclerosing cholangitis. N Engl J Med 1995;332:924–33.
6. Broome U, Olsson R, Loof L, Bodemar G, Hultrantz R, Danielsson A, et al. Natural history and prognostic factors in 305 Swedish patients with primary sclerosing cholangitis. Gut 1996;38:610–15.
7. Wiesner RH, Porayko MK, Dickson ER, Gores GJ, LaRusso NF, Hay JE, et al. Selection and timing of liver transplantation in primary biliary cirrhosis and primary sclerosing cholangitis. Hepatology 1992;16:1290–9.
8. Becker U, Deis A, Thorkild I, Sorensen A, Gronbaek M, Borch-Johnsen K, et al. Prediction of risk of liver disease by alcohol intake, sex and age: a prospective population study. Hepatology 1996;23:1025–9.
9. Poynard T, Barthelemy P, Fratte S, Boudjema K, Doffoel M, Vanlemmens C, et al. Evaluation of efficacy of liver transplantation in alcoholic cirrhosis by a case control study and simulated controls. Lancet 1994;344:502–7.
10. Alberti A, Chemelo L, Benvegnu L. Natural history of hepatitis C. J Hepatol 1999;31(S1):17–24.
11. Gane EJ, Portmann BC, Naoumov NV, Smith HM, Underhill JA, Donaldson PT, et al. Longterm outcome of hepatitis C infection after liver transplantation. N Engl J Med 1996;334:815–20.
12. Prieto M, Berenguer M, Rayon JM, Cordoba J, Arguello L, Carrosco D, et al. High incidence of allograft cirrhosis in hepatitis C virus genotype 1b infection following transplantation: relationship with rejection episodes. Hepatology 1999;29:250–6.
13. Samuel D, Muller R, Alexander G, Fassati L, Ducot B, Benhamou JP, et al. Liver transplantation in European patients with the hepatitis B surface antigen. N Engl J Med 1993;329:1842–7.
14. Bernuau J, Gondeau A, Poynard T. Dubois F, Lesage, G, Yvonnet B, et al. Multivariate analysis of prognostic factors in fulminant hepatitis B. Hepatology 1986;6:648–51
15. O'Grady JG, Alexander GJM, Hayllar KM, Williams R. Early indicators of prognosis in fulminant hepatic failure. Gastroenterology 1989;97:439–45.
16. Whitington PF, Baliestreri WF. Living transplantation in pediatrics: indications, contraindications and pre-transplant management. J Pediatr 1991;119:169–77.
17. Broelsch CE, Emond JC, Whitington PT, Thistlewaite JR, Baker AL, Lichtor JL. Application of reduced-size liver transplantation as split grafts, auxillary orthotopic grafts, and living related segmental transplantation. Ann Surg 1990;212:368.

Liver Transplantation: Surgical Techniques

M. Bowles and M. Rela

Introduction

In order to understand the techniques of liver transplantation a clear appreciation of the segmental anatomy of the liver is essential. Classification according to the Couinaud nomenclature[1,2] is now generally accepted and it is possible to define the segments on both ultrasound[3] and CT examination.[3] This chapter begins with an introduction to liver anatomy relevant to surgical and radiological practice, including the common variants of hepatic vascular anatomy. The standard technique of liver transplantation and its various modifications are then described.

Liver Anatomy

An imaginary plane, the principal plane of the liver, which runs between the inferior vena cava (IVC) posteriorly and the gallbladder anteroinferiorly, separates the right and left lobes of the liver. The two lobes are defined by their blood supplies, which are the right and left branches of the hepatic artery and portal vein.[4] The segmental anatomy of the liver can be appreciated by consideration of the hepatic venous drainage. The major part of the venous drainage of the liver is via the right, middle, and left hepatic veins, which emerge from the posterosuperior aspect of the liver and drain into the IVC, the middle and left veins often having a confluent orifice.[5] The posterior part of the liver that is in contact with the IVC (segment 1, the caudate lobe) drains via short caudate tributaries directly into the IVC.

The middle hepatic vein lies between the right and left lobes in the principal plane. The left hepatic vein lies along the line of the falciform ligament in a plane that separates the left lateral segment (segments 2 and 3) from the remainder of the left lobe (segment 1 and segment 4, the quadrate lobe). The right hepatic vein lies in a plane that divides the right lobe into segments 5 and 8 anteriorly and segments 6 and 7 posteriorly. The numbering of the segments runs roughly clockwise when the liver is viewed in the anatomical position (Fig. 8.**1**).

The portal vein lies in front of the IVC on the inferior surface of the liver.[6] The portal vein is formed by the confluence of the superior mesenteric vein and the splenic vein behind the pancreas and divides into its main right and left branches at the hilum of the liver.

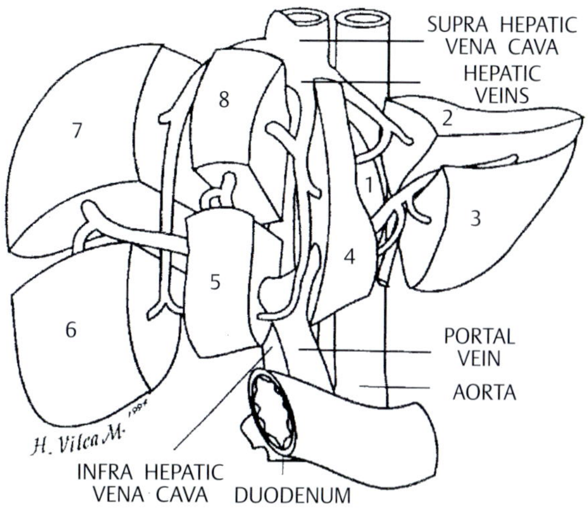

Fig. 8.**1** Segmental liver anatomy based on the Couinaud classification (segments 1–8). The description is based on portal segments, with each segment having its own blood supply (arterial, portal, hepatic venous), lymphatics, and biliary drainage, allowing surgical resection of each segment. (From Couinaud 1957[1])

The arterial blood supply of the liver is via the celiac trunk and the common hepatic artery, which becomes the hepatic artery proper after giving off the gastroduodenal and right gastric arteries (Fig. 8.**2a**). The hepatic artery lies anterior to the left side of the portal vein and divides into right and left branches at the hilum.

Variations in the hepatic arterial anatomy are common (Fig. 8.**2**).[7] There may be an accessory left hepatic artery arising from the left gastric artery and entering the liver through the lesser omentum (14% of individuals, Fig. 8.**2b**); in some cases this may completely replace the conventional left hepatic artery. There may be an accessory right hepatic artery arising from the superior mesenteric artery and entering the liver by passing behind the superior mesenteric vein and to the right of the portal vein (10%, Fig. 8.**2c**); again, in some cases this may replace the conventional right hepatic artery. Both accessory/replaced left and right arteries may be present in the same individual (4%, Fig. 8.**2d**).

Biliary radicals drain into the right and left hepatic ducts which then form the common hepatic duct.[8-10]

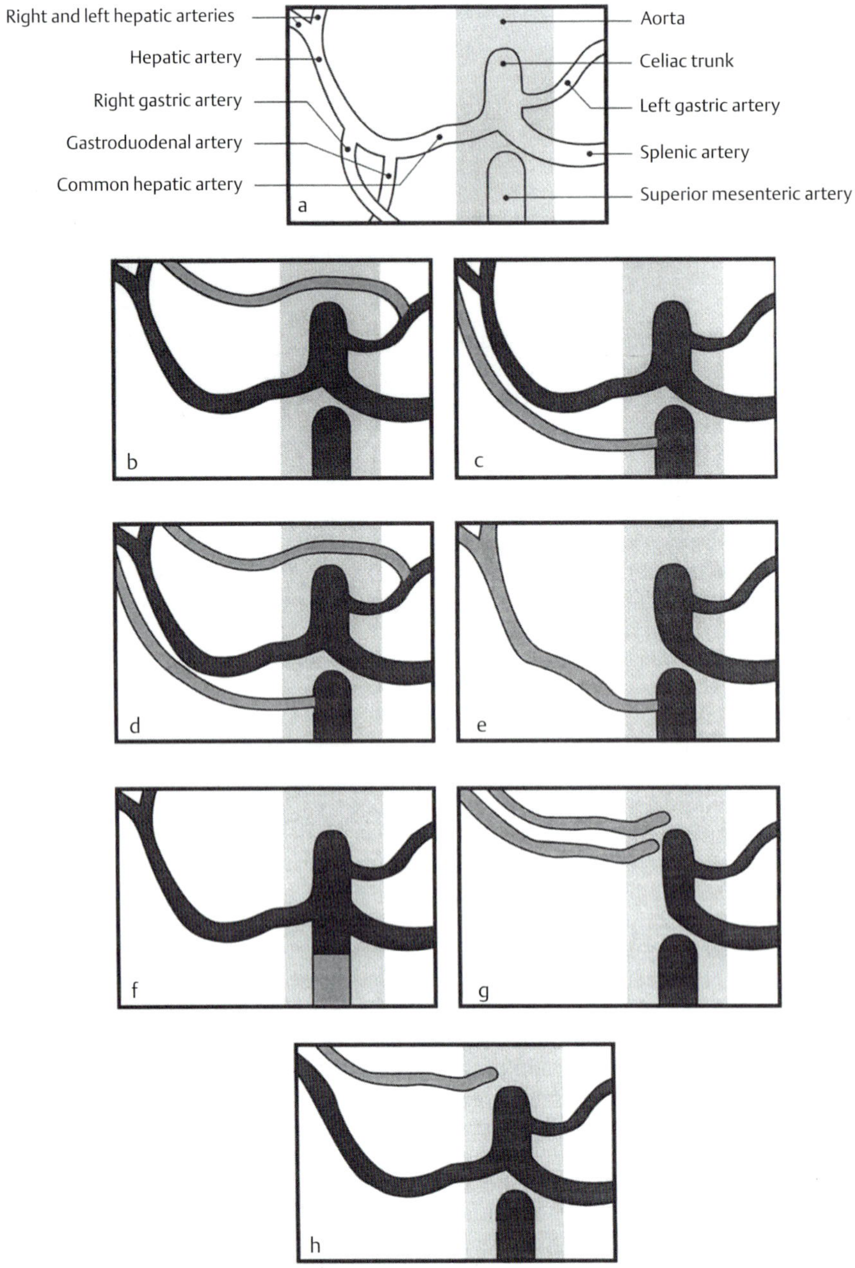

Fig. 8.2 **a** Conventional anatomy of the hepatic arterial system and commonly encountered variations: **b** Accessory left hepatic artery (LHA) arising from the left gastric artery (LGA). **c** Accessory right hepatic artery (RHA) arising from the superior mesenteric artery (SMA). **d** Accessory RHA and accessory LHA. **e** Total replacement of the common hepatic artery from the SMA. **f** Common celiac axis and SMA trunk. **g** The RHA and LHA arising directly from the aorta. **h** The RHA arising from the celiac axis and the LHA from the aorta

This becomes the common bile duct after the entry, at a variable level, of the cystic duct from the gallbladder. The common hepatic and common bile ducts lie anterior to the portal vein and to the right of the hepatic artery.

Summary points:

- The principal plane of the liver, which runs between the inferior vena cava posteriorly and the gallbladder anteroinferiorly, separates the right and left lobes of the liver.
- Variations in the hepatic arterial anatomy are common.

Standard Orthotopic Cadaveric Liver Transplantation

The liver, unlike the kidney, is almost always transplanted in an orthotopic position, i.e., in its usual anatomical site: the diseased liver is removed and the transplanted organ takes its place.[11] The firm attachment of the retrohepatic IVC to the liver by the caudate veins means that the most straightforward way to remove the liver is to take the retrohepatic IVC with it, having already divided the common bile duct, hepatic artery, and portal vein. A very similar operation will have previously been performed in the cadaveric organ donor.

There are therefore five structures which require anastomosis between the recipient and the graft: the suprahepatic IVC, the infrahepatic IVC, the portal vein, the hepatic artery, and the common bile duct[12] (Fig. 8.**3**). The above vessels are clamped from the time that the diseased liver is removed until the vascular anastomoses to the graft are completed. Clamping of the infrahepatic (suprarenal) IVC results in congestion in the lower half of the body and the kidneys. Patients in poor condition may not tolerate the resultant diminished venous return to the heart, and venous congestion of the kidneys may also result in renal dysfunction in the early postoperative period.[13] Similarly, clamping of the portal vein may result in worsening of portal hypertension, congestion of the bowel, and increased blood loss during the procedure. In order to minimize these problems, it is common practice to perform veno-venous bypass: cannulae are inserted into the portal vein and a common iliac vein (via the femoral vein), and blood is returned to the heart via a bypass pump connected to a cannula in the left axillary or internal jugular vein.

All anastomoses are performed in an end-to-end fashion (Fig. 8.**3**). A modification of end-to-end anastomosis is frequently used for the hepatic arterial anastomosis, which often has a small caliber.[14] The diameter of the cut end of an artery can be increased if the vessel is divided at the origin of a branch. This produces a "branch patch", the most commonly used being a gastroduodenal branch patch of the common hepatic artery. Branch patches may be used on both recipient and graft arteries and result in a slight increase in diameter of the arterial lumen at the point of anastomosis.[15]

The gallbladder is removed from the transplanted liver after implantation. This is in order to avoid potential post-transplantation gallbladder complications due to stasis in a denervated gallbladder. The common bile duct of the donor liver is usually anastomosed to the common bile duct of the recipient. This is referred to as a "duct-to-duct anastomosis." A T tube may be placed across the anastomosis when there is a significant size discrepancy between the donor and the recipient ducts. As caliber differences are fairly common, the postoperative appearance of a graft bile duct larger in caliber than the recipient duct does not necessarily imply biliary obstruction.

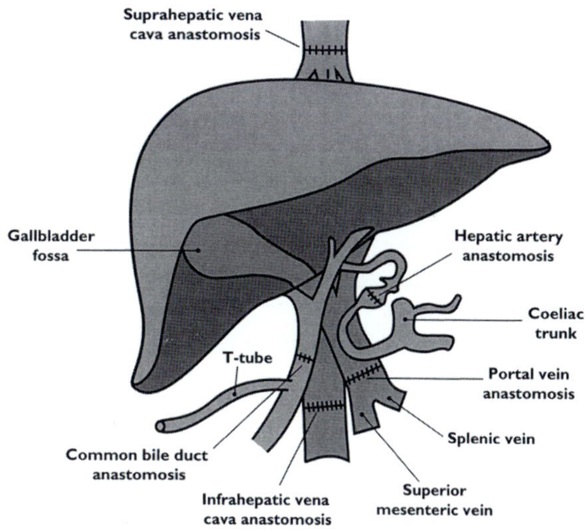

Fig. 8.**3** Donor/recipient sites for vascular and biliary anastomoses

Summary points:

- The liver, unlike the kidney, is almost always transplanted in an orthotopic position, i.e., in its usual anatomical site: the diseased liver is removed and the transplanted organ takes its place.
- There are five structures which require anastomosis between the recipient and the graft: the suprahepatic IVC, the infrahepatic IVC, the portal vein, the hepatic artery and the common bile duct.
- The gallbladder is removed from the transplanted liver after implantation in order to avoid potential post-transplant gallbladder complications due to stasis in a denervated gallbladder.

Variations in Standard Technique

Inferior Vena Caval Anastomosis: The "Piggy-Back" Technique

The standard technique of liver implantation described in the preceding paragraph is referred to as "caval replacement."[16,17] A common variation of this is the "piggy-back" technique. In the transplant recipient, instead of removing the retrohepatic IVC with the liver, the liver is "filleted" off the IVC by division of all the short caudate tributaries. The three hepatic veins are then clamped and the liver is removed without interrupting blood flow within the IVC. With the clamp flush with the anterior surface of the IVC, the three hepatic venous orifices are joined together to form a single large orifice.

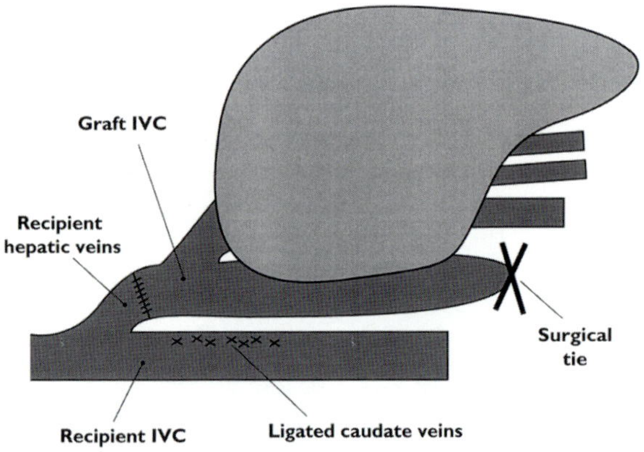

Fig. 8.**4** "Piggy-back" implantation in liver transplantation (sagittal section)

The graft's suprahepatic IVC is then anastomosed to the recipient's hepatic venous confluence and the graft's infrahepatic IVC is tied off (Fig. 8.**4**). The new liver therefore lies in a piggy-back position on the recipient IVC, with the graft and recipient IVCs lying in parallel. The advantage of the piggy-back technique over caval replacement is that flow in the IVC is not interrupted and therefore veno-venous bypass is not required. The disadvantage is that filleting the liver off the IVC can be difficult and time-consuming.

On occasions the recipient's right hepatic venous orifice may be significantly separated from the middle and left orifice(s) and it may not be feasible to form a common orifice for anastomosis to the suprahepatic IVC of the graft. In this situation the right hepatic venous orifice is usually closed and the graft's suprahepatic IVC is anastomosed to the confluence of the recipient's middle and left hepatic veins only. This technique therefore carries a slightly higher risk of venous outflow obstruction to the graft.

■ ***Summary point:***

- The advantage of the "piggy-back" liver transplant technique over "caval replacement" is that flow in the IVC is not interrupted and therefore veno-venous bypass is not required.

Hepatic Arterial Anastomosis

The common hepatic artery of the graft is usually anastomosed to that of the recipient. However, there are circumstances in which this does not provide optimal arterial flow. In this case an arterial conduit is constructed between the anterior wall of the aorta below the level of the origins of the renal arteries and the graft common hepatic artery or celiac trunk. Iliac artery, taken from the donor at the time of organ retrieval, is used for the conduit. The course of the conduit is usually through the transverse mesocolon and between the pancreas and stomach.[11,18]

Various techniques are used to re-establish the entire arterial inflow to the graft, which may therefore have more than one principal arterial trunk. An accessory or replaced right hepatic artery is generally reconstructed anterior rather than posterior to the portal vein.

Biliary Anastomosis

There are some circumstances in which it may not be possible or desirable to drain the graft's biliary system into the recipient bile duct. In this case the graft common hepatic duct is anastomosed directly to the small bowel. This is accomplished by dividing the proximal jejunum and forming a Roux-en-Y jejunal loop. A hepaticojejunostomy is then fashioned between the common hepatic duct of the graft and the blind end of the Roux loop. This is routine practice when the indication for transplantation is primary sclerosing cholangitis, because the recipient common bile duct may be diseased and unsuitable for end-to-end anastomosis.[11]

An alternative method of biliary drainage is anastomosis of the graft gallbladder to the recipient common bile duct. This gallbladder conduit technique was used in the early years of liver transplantation but was susceptible to bile stasis within the gallbladder with subsequent stone formation and cholangitis. The gallbladder conduit has therefore been abandoned, but there are some patients at long-term follow-up who have this type of biliary reconstruction.

■ ***Summary point:***

- A hepaticojejunostomy is fashioned between the common hepatic duct of the graft and the blind end of the Roux loop when the indication for transplantation is primary sclerosing cholangitis, because the recipient common bile duct may be diseased and unsuitable for end-to-end anastomosis.

Pediatric Liver Transplantation

If a liver becomes available from a pediatric organ donor and is implanted into a similar-sized recipient, the technical principles of the transplant operation are very similar to those of the adult operation. However, the majority of biliary anastomoses in children are hepaticojejunostomies rather than duct-to-duct anastomoses, because the recipient duct is usually either absent (in extrahepatic biliary atresia) or very small.[18]

Pediatric organ donors are much less common than adult donors. The inevitable consequence of this is that children have to wait longer for a suitable liver to become available for transplantation. Various techniques have been developed to provide suitable organs for pediatric recipients; these are reduced, split, and living related donor liver transplantation.[19] These techniques have the potential to overcome discrepancies between donor and recipient weights in a ratio of up to 10:1.

Reduced Liver Transplantation

The liver can be reduced to provide one of a variety of different implantable parts, depending on the size of the recipient. This is done under sterile conditions on a back table in the operating theatre with the liver surrounded by ice to prevent it from rewarming.[20] The term "liver reduction" is used when a liver is cut down to the required size for the recipient and the remaining segments are discarded.[21] The left lobe (segments 1–4) can be removed, leaving the right lobe (segments 5–8) for transplantation, or the right lobe can be removed and the left lobe transplanted. In both these cases the IVC is retained with the transplanted lobe, so either caval replacement or "piggy-back" techniques can be used (Fig. 8.**5** shows a left lobe graft with caval replacement).

A liver can also be reduced to a left lateral segment (segments 2 and 3) by removing the extended right lobe (segments 1 and 4–8); this allows an adult liver to be used for a small pediatric recipient.[22] In this case, the IVC of the donor liver cannot be retained with the left lateral segment and the "piggy-back" technique has to be used, anastomosing the left hepatic vein of the donor liver to the confluence of the hepatic veins on the anterior wall of the IVC of the recipient (Fig. 8.**6**). A left lateral segment reduction is rarely performed these days as the right lobe can be used for another recipient, resulting in what is described as a split liver transplant (see below), in which one organ is used for two recipients.[23]

A reduced right lobe is used when the donor-to-recipient weight ratio is approximately 3:2, a left lobe when the ratio is 3:1 and a left lateral segment when this ratio is 10:1. Following transplantation, the principal difference between a reduced graft and a whole organ is that there is a relatively flat cut surface (representing the plane of back table hepatic parenchymal division) which has the potential to bleed or leak bile (Figs. 8.**5**, 8.**6**).

■ ***Summary point:***

- The term "liver reduction" is used when a liver is cut down to the required size for the recipient and the remaining segments are discarded.

Split Liver Transplantation

The technique of liver splitting is an extension of liver reduction and enables a donor liver to be used to transplant two recipients rather than just one.[24] The liver is usually split into an extended right lobe and the left lateral segment. Segment 4 is sometimes excised from

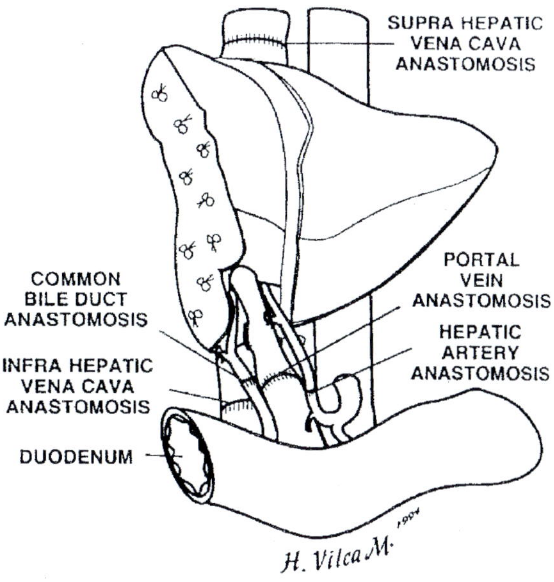

Fig. 8.**5** Left lobe liver transplantation

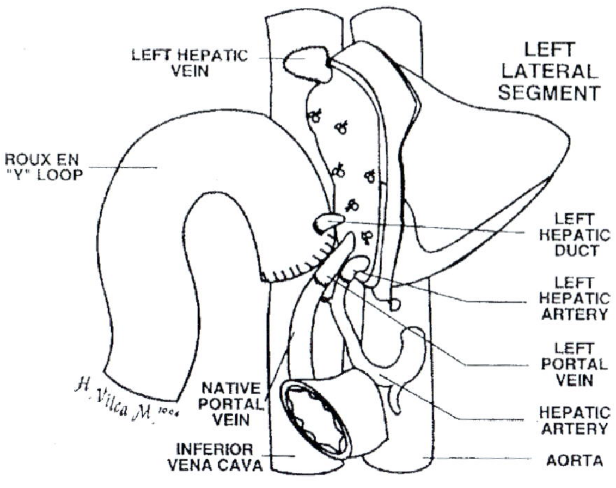

Fig. 8.**6** Left lateral segment liver transplantation

the right lobe and discarded. The IVC is retained with the right lobe. The main portal trunk and hepatic artery are assigned to one or other side of the split (not necessarily the same side). This inevitably results in anastomoses closer to the hilum than usual on the grafts with a short portal vein or hepatic artery. An exception to this arises if there is a replaced right or left hepatic artery, in which case both sides of the split liver graft can have a good length of artery.[25]

■ ***Summary point:***

- The technique of "liver splitting" is an extension of "liver reduction" and enables a donor liver to be used to transplant two recipients rather than just one, the liver usually being split into an extended right lobe and the left lateral segment.

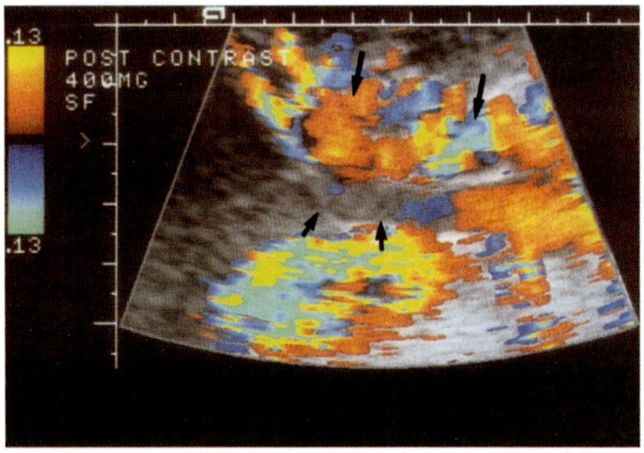

a

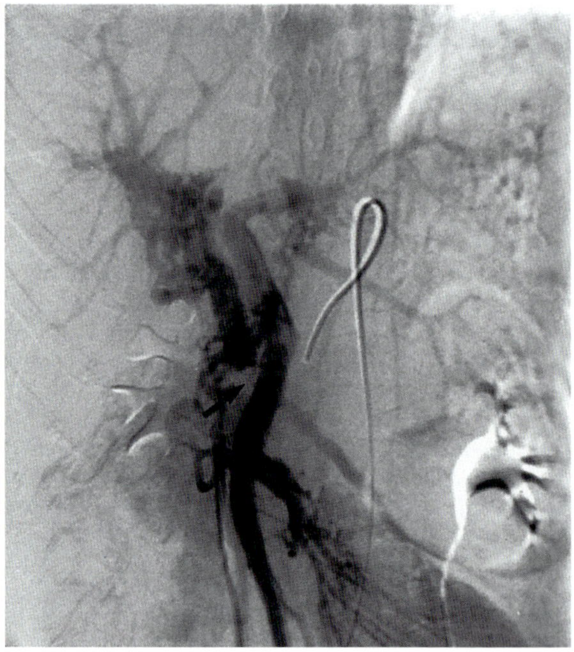

b

Fig. 8.**7** **a** Ultrasound image of a left auxiliary transplant in Crigler–Najjar syndrome, demonstrating an occluded native portal vein (short arrows) with surrounding cavernous transformation (arrows) maintaining portal venous blood flow to the native liver, albeit reduced. **b** The ultrasound findings confirmed at the portal venous phase of a selective superior mesenteric arteriogram, where a short segmental occlusion of the native portal vein is demonstrated (arrow). (Reproduced from *European Radiology*,[28] by permission of the editor)

Living Related Liver Transplantation

In the majority of countries, and particularly in those without well-developed and coordinated transplantation and organ donation programs, there is a relative excess of organ demand over supply. Living related organ donation provides a means of transplanting patients who might otherwise not be found a suitable cadaveric organ.[26] Adult-to-child living related liver transplantation (LRLT) usually involves the resection of the left lateral segment from the healthy living donor and its implantation into the pediatric recipient. Adult-to-adult LRLT has become more popular recently and involves the use of the right lobe for transplanting an adult patient. This is a much bigger procedure for the donor, with higher risk of donor morbidity. In LRLT the vessels to the graft are short, making the operation technically demanding with an increased risk of technical complications in the recipient.

■ *Summary point:*

- Adult-to-child living related liver transplantation usually involves resection of the left lateral segment from the healthy living donor and its implantation into the pediatric recipient.

Auxiliary Liver Transplantation

The final type of liver transplantation to consider is auxiliary liver transplantation.[18] In this situation, instead of removing the whole of the diseased liver, only part of it is resected. A donor reduced or split lobe is used to replace the resected lobe. This form of transplantation may be used in two circumstances: (1) when the liver failure is acute (e.g., acute viral hepatitis or drug toxicity) and there is potential for recovery of the native liver, thus allowing removal of the auxiliary liver and withdrawal of immunosuppressive treatment at some time in the future; (2) when the indication for transplantation is a single metabolic enzyme defect (e.g., Crigler–Najjar syndrome) in an otherwise normal liver, when the metabolic defect can be cured by a small segmental transplant.[27] In this situation, therefore, in addition to the vascular and biliary connections of the transplant, those of the native liver remnant remain intact.

Any dysfunction of the transplanted liver, such as rejection, cholestasis, or ischemia, results in an increase in the graft's resistance to portal venous inflow. This may be beneficial in auxiliary liver transplantation performed for acute liver failure because portal inflow will be relatively increased to the native liver, aiding regeneration. However, in auxiliary transplantation for single enzyme defects, the hemodynamics of the native liver are entirely normal and the graft is therefore relatively deprived of portal venous inflow, which is detrimental to graft function. In the latter situation, therefore, the native portal vein is narrowed with a tie at the time of transplantation in order to encourage preferential portal flow to the graft. This obviously has implications for the interpretation of post-transplantation ultrasound appearances (Fig. 8.**7**).[28]

Summary point:

- In auxiliary liver transplantation, instead of removing the whole of the diseased liver, only part of it is resected, and a donor reduced or split lobe is used to replace the resected lobe.

References

1. Couinaud C. Le foie. Etudes anatomiques et chirurgicales. 1st ed. Paris: Masson et Cie, 1957;
2. Sugarbaker PH. Toward a standard nomenclature for surgical anatomy of the liver. Neth J Surg 1988;P0:100
3. Lafortune M, Madore F, Patriquin H. Segmental anatomy of the liver: a sonographic approach to the Couinaud nomenclature. Radiology 1991;181:443.
4. Marks WM, Filly RA, Callen PW. Ultrasonic anatomy of the liver: a review with new applications. J Clin Ultrasound 1979;7:137–46.
5. Cosgrove DO, Arger PH, Coleman BG. Ultrasonic anatomy of the hepatic veins. J Clin Ultrasound 1987;15:231–5.
6. Fraser-Hill MA, Atri M, Bret PM, Aldis AE, Illescas FF, Herschorn SD. Intrahepatic portal venous system: variations demonstrated with duplex and color US. Radiology 1990;177:523–6.
7. Winter TC, Nghiem HV, Freeny PC, Hommeyer SC, Mack LA. Hepatic artery anatomy: demonstration of normal supply and vascular variants with three-dimensional CT angiography. Radiographics 1995;15:771–80.
8. Mittelstaedt CA. Ultrasound of the bile ducts. Semin Roentgenol 1997;32:161–71.
9. Wittich GR, Steiner E, Baxter RB. Segemental anatomy of the intrahepatic bile ducts: relevance to biliary interventions. Semin Interv Radiol 1995;12:173.
10. Taourel PG, Bret PM, Reinhold C, Barkun AN, Atri M. Anatomic variants of the biliary tree with MR cholangiopancreatography. Radiology 1996;199:521–7.
11. Corbally MT, Rela M, Heaton ND, Tan KC. Standard orthotopic operation, retransplantation and piggybacking. In: Williams R, Portmann B, Tan KC, editors. The practice of liver transplantation. 1st ed. London: Churchill Livingstone; 1995. p. 135–42.
12. Starzl TE, Iwatsuki S, Shaw BW. Transplantation of the human liver. In: Swarts SI, editor. Maingot's abdominal operations. 8th ed. Connecticut: Appleton-Century-Crofts; 1985. p. 1681–722.
13. Klintmalm G, Busuttil R. The recipient hepatectomy and grafting. In: Busuttil RW, Klintmalm GBG, editors. Transplantation of the liver. 1st ed. Philadelphia: Saunders; 1996. p. 405–18.
14. Kalayoglu M, Belzer O. A new technique for arterialisation of the hepatic graft. Surg Gynaecol Obstet 1987;164:564–7.
15. Quinones-Baldrich WJ, Memsic L, Ramming K, Hiatt J, Busuttil RW. Branch patch for arterialisation of hepatic grafts. Surg Gynaecol Obstet 1986;162:489–91.
16. Calne RY, Williams R. Liver transplantation in man. I. Observations on technique and organisation in 5 cases. BMJ 1968;4:535–40.
17. Bismuth H, Castaing D, Sherlock DJ. Liver transplantation by "face-a-face" venacavaplasty. Surgery 1990;111:151–5.
18. Heaton ND, Corbally MT, Rela M, Tan KC. Surgical techniques of segmental reduction. Split and auxiliary liver transplantation. In: Williams R, Portmann B, Tan KC, editors. The practice of liver transplantation. 1st ed. London: Churchill Livingstone; 1995. p. 143–51.
19. Bismuth H, Houssin D. Reduced-sized orthotopic liver graft in hepatic transplantation in children. Surgery 1984;95:367–70.
20. Starzl TE, Miller C, Bronznick B, Makowka L. An improved technique for multiple organ harvesting. Surg Gynaecol Obstet 1987;165:343–8.
21. de Hemptinne B, Salizzoni M, Tan KC, Otte JB. The technique of liver reduction in orthotopic liver transplantation. Transplant Proc 1988;20:508–11.
22. Strong RW, Ong TH, Pillay P, Baldeson G, Lynch S. A new method of segmental orthotopic liver transplantation in children. Surgery 1988;104:104–7.
23. Bismuth H, Morino M, Castaing D, et al. Emergency orthotopic liver transplantation in two patients using one donor. Br J Surg 1989;76:722–4.
24. Rela M, Vougas V, Muiesan P, et al. Split liver transplantation. Kings College Hospital experience. Ann Surg 1998;227:282–8.
25. Shaw BW, Wood RP, Stratta RJ, et al. Management of arterial anomalies encountered in split-liver transplantation. Transplant Proc 1990;22:420–2.
26. Broelsch CE, Whitington PF, Edmond JC, et al. Liver transplantation in children from living related donors. Surgical techniques and results. Ann Surg 1991;214:428–38.
27. Rela M, Muiesan P, Vilca-Melendez H, et al. Auxiliary partial orthotopic liver transplantation for Crigler–Najjar syndrome type 1. Ann Surg 1999;229:565–9.
28. Sidhu PS, Marshall MM, Ryan SM, Ellis SM. Clinical use of Levovist, an ultrasound contrast agent, in the imaging of liver transplantation: assessment of the pre and post transplant patient. Eur Radiol 2000;10:1114–26.

Ultrasound Assessment of the Liver Transplant Candidate

A. Shaw and P. S. Sidhu

Introduction

Ultrasonography is frequently the initial investigation in patients with hepatobiliary disease, and the same is true of the evaluation of candidates for transplantation, with its advantages of being readily available, relatively inexpensive, and involving no ionizing radiation. The majority of patients referred for assessment have chronic liver disease, the cause of which has already been established. Therefore, the emphasis in investigating these patients is on recognizing the sequelae of chronic disease and excluding any contraindications to transplantation.

A smaller, but significant, population will present with acute liver failure having had no antecedent hepatic dysfunction. The role of the radiologist in this group is more limited, but will be considered later in the chapter. Finally, the role of ultrasound within the neonatal and pediatric transplant assessment will be reviewed, as this group has a different spectrum of disease and requires the use of novel surgical techniques.

Chronic Liver Disease

Parenchymal Imaging

The sonographic techniques used in imaging the liver are well described.[1] In imaging the patient with chronic liver disease, they remain essentially unchanged, but may require the use of a lower-frequency transducer (2–3 MHz) than usual in order to compensate for both the increased attenuation seen in the cirrhotic liver and for the presence of ascites. This will, of course, reduce the resolution of the image, so a balance should be found.

The cirrhotic liver has a coarse, heterogeneous echotexture with increased reflectivity (Fig. 9.**1**). There is often relative atrophy of segments 4–8, with hypertrophy of the caudate (segment 1) and left lateral lobes (segments 2 and 3) (Fig. 9.**2**). Although several authors have described the use of various ratios in the diagnosis of cirrhosis,[2–6] these are not in common clinical use and are of no relevance in the transplant patient group. Nodularity may be a feature, particularly where histological analysis shows the patient to have a macronodular cirrhosis (nodules 3 mm), more commonly seen in chronic viral hepatitis, Wilson's disease, and alpha$_1$-antitrypsin deficiency.[2] Alcohol, biliary obstruction, hemochromatosis, and Budd–Chiari syndrome more commonly give a micronodular cirrhosis, although there is considerable overlap between the two groups (Fig. 9.**3**).

Nodules within the liver are classified as regenerative, cirrhotic, dysplastic, or hepatocellular carcinoma (HCC), in accordance with agreed nomenclature.[7] It is thought that HCC develops from cirrhotic and sub-

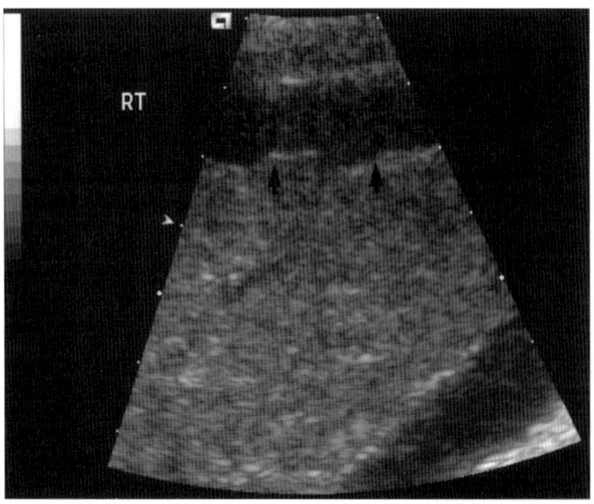

Fig. 9.**1** Ascites surrounding a contracted and cirrhotic liver. The liver surface is irregular (arrows) in keeping with macronodular change

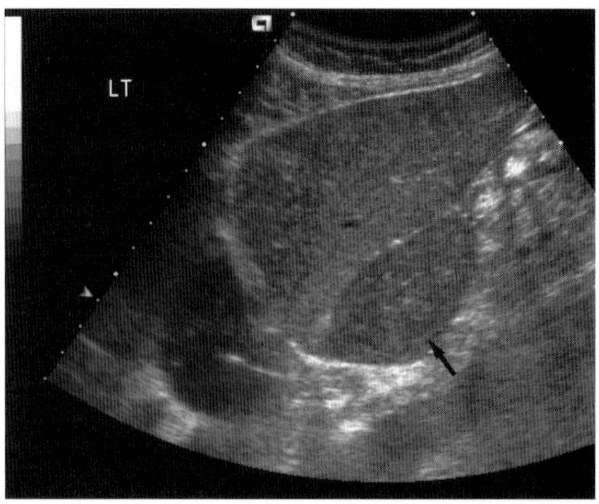

Fig. 9.**2** Hypertrophy of the caudate lobe. A hyporeflective enlarged caudate lobe (arrow) in a patient with biopsy-proven liver cirrhosis

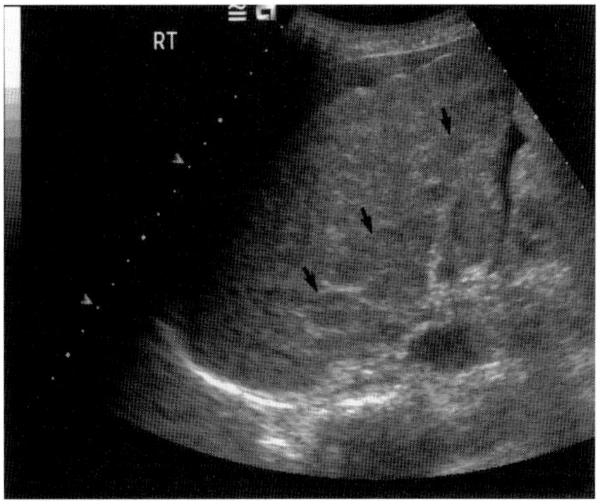

Fig. 9.**3** Multiple areas of low reflectivity representing regenerating nodules (arrows) in a patient with advanced primary biliary cirrhosis

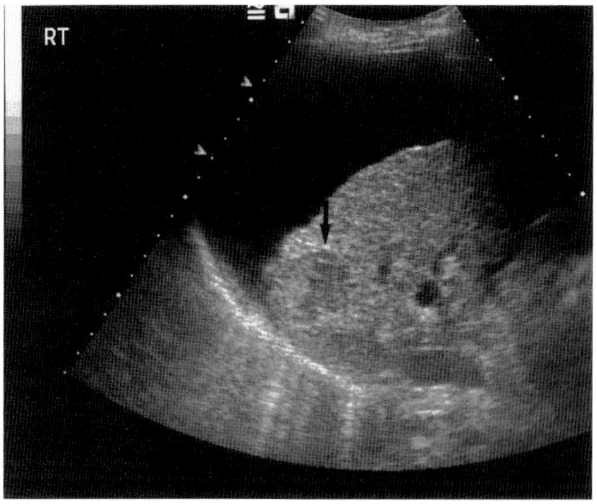

Fig. 9.**4** Advanced liver cirrhosis complicated by the development of a hepatocellular carcinoma (HCC) in the right lobe of liver (arrow)

sequently dysplastic nodules, and hence it is of prime importance to try and differentiate these wherever possible. An observational study from Denmark has shown that patients with cirrhosis have an approximately 60-fold risk of developing HCC and a 10-fold risk of cholangiocarcinoma, in addition to variably increased incidence of other alcohol-related and, to a lesser extent, tobacco-related tumors.[8]

The sonographic appearances of HCC are variable, depending on the size and constitution of the tumor (Fig. 9.**4**). Small tumors are commonly hypoechoic and well defined, but may be hyperechoic, resembling hemangiomata. As tumors grow, they tend to become more ill defined, with central necrosis giving rise to a more heterogeneous echogenicity. HCC may be solitary, or may be in the form of multifocal nodules. Occasionally, there may be infiltrative disease, giving a diffuse change easily missed on ultrasound.

It is of vital importance that the size and number of tumor nodules are established before the planning of treatment. In patients with a single dominant lesion less than 4 cm in size, transplantation offers potential cure, with one series documenting no recurrence in 14 patients.[9] Patients who undergo partial hepatectomy have a poorer prognosis, with more frequent recurrence and 5-year survival rates as low as 25%.[10] This is compared with higher disease-free survival at 5 years in transplant recipients (60% versus 14%).[11] Recurrence may be due to either undiagnosed "daughter" nodules or de novo malignancy in a susceptible liver. Patients with a tumor larger than 4 cm or multifocal disease are known to do poorly in the postoperative period, with a high incidence of disease recurrence.[9] Indeed, transplantation is not recommended in patients with tumor exceeding 5 cm or more than three in number, and is contraindicated in patients with local or systemic extrahepatic spread.[12]

The detection of malignant nodules within the liver with ultrasound has been extensively investigated. Although some authors claim 100% detection of dominant nodules,[13] few others have had such success, and a figure of 80% is more common.[10,14] One series showed a malignant nodule detection rate of 50% in patients with cirrhotic liver disease.[15] It is thought that variation in study populations may account for much of this discrepancy, as not all patients studied had cirrhotic liver disease. By comparison, computed tomography (CT) detects malignancy in 86–100% of cases[10,13,14] and hepatic angiography in 90–100%.[13,14]

The detection of smaller tumors representative of either intrahepatic spread or multifocal primary lesions is much more problematic, with studies showing a detection range from 16%[14] to 45%.[15] Indeed, all modalities have been shown to be poor in this respect, perhaps the most successful techniques being hepatic angiography and CT aortoportography, although these detect at most 40% of lesions.[13]

Recent studies with ultrasound microbubble contrast agents have demonstrated a late liver-specific phase three to five minutes after injection. The use of nonlinear methods such as pulse or phase inversion harmonic imaging and stimulated acoustic emission techniques (SAE)[16] at this late stage leads to increased conspicuity of focal lesions,[17–19] enabling the detection of subcentimeter metastases not detected by conventional ultrasound techniques or CT[20,21] (Fig. 9.**5**). In SAE imaging, HCC and metastases exhibit reduced emission from within the lesions, thought to be due to the absence of Kupffer cells, whereas the presence of high late-phase microbubble contrast uptake is taken as evidence of a benign lesion[22] (Fig. 9.**6**).

Differentiation of focal nodular lesions in distinct types or categories by ultrasound has been reported as accurate in 98% of patients on the basis of B mode features

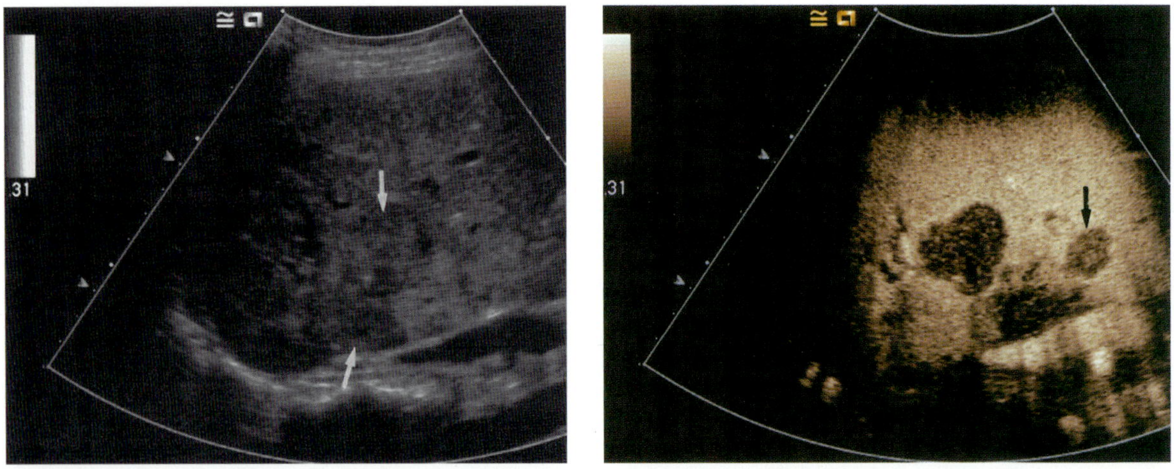

a b

Fig. 9.**5** **a** Multiple secondary lesions from a primary colon carcinoma seen on B mode imaging (arrows). **b** Tumors demonstrated in the late phase after administration of microbubble contrast (Levovist) using agent detection imaging (ADI), showing absence of microbubble uptake in the tumors and a further lesion not seen on the baseline image (arrow)

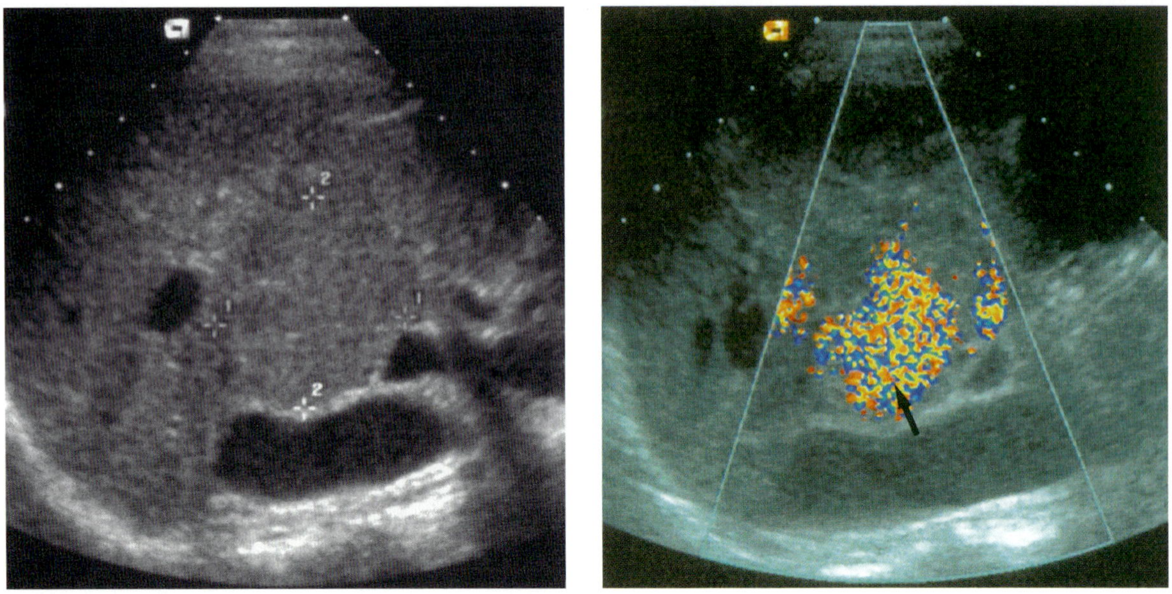

a b

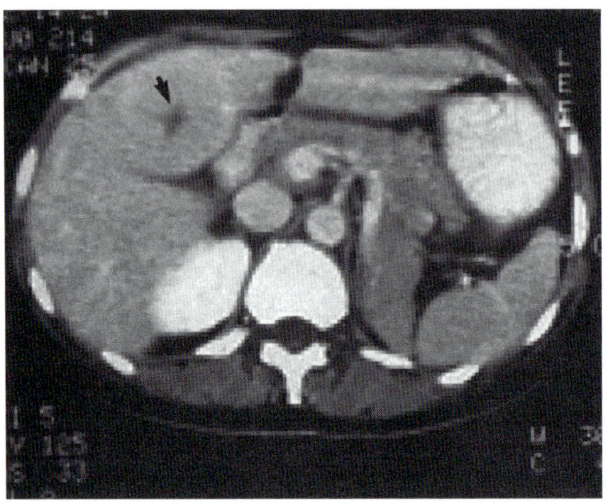

c

Fig. 9.**6** **a** A low-reflective, well-circumscribed mass (cursors) in the right lobe of the liver in keeping with an area of focal nodular hyperplasia. **b** Following administration of microbubble contrast (Levovist), imaging in the late phase using stimulated acoustic emission (SAE). Normal functioning tissue shows uptake of the contrast (arrow). **c** CT (after contrast enhancement) demonstrates uniform enhancement of a focal nodular hyperplaisia except for the "central scar" (arrow)

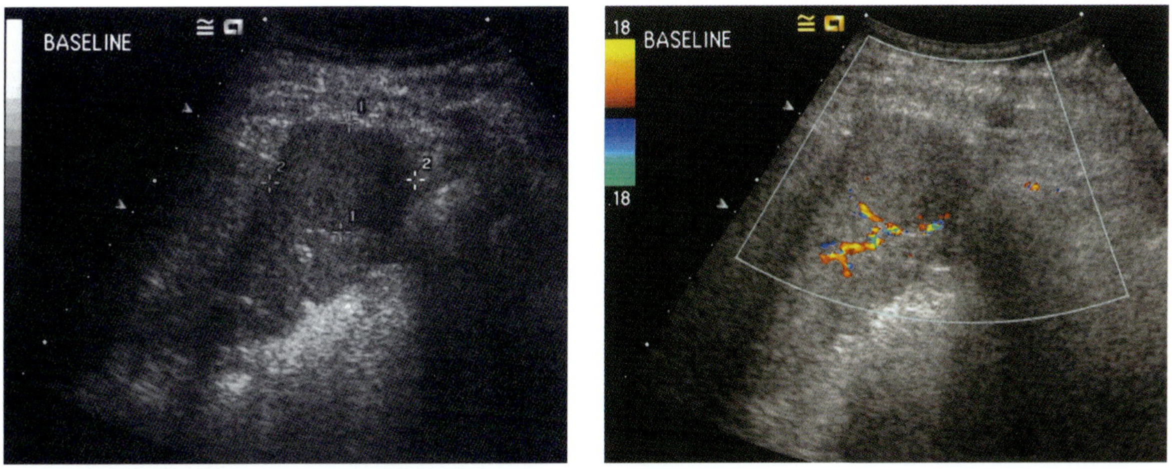

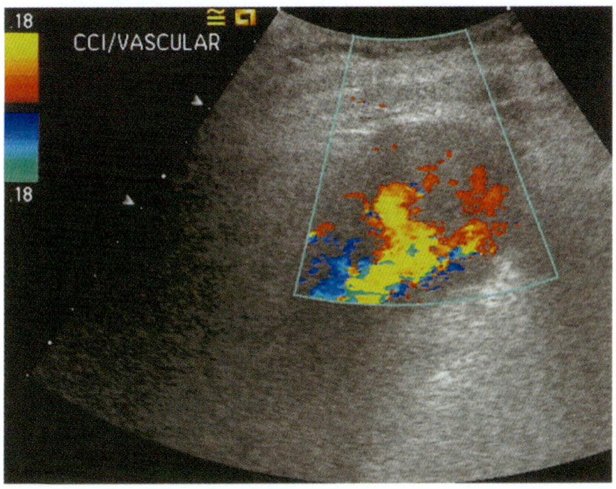

Fig. 9.**7** **a** HCC on B mode ultrasound imaging (cursors). **b** Color Doppler image showing surrounding vascularity but no vascular supply to the central aspect of the tumor. **c** Following the administration of microbubble contrast (Levovist), vascular enhancement is seen both surrounding the tumor and within the tumor itself

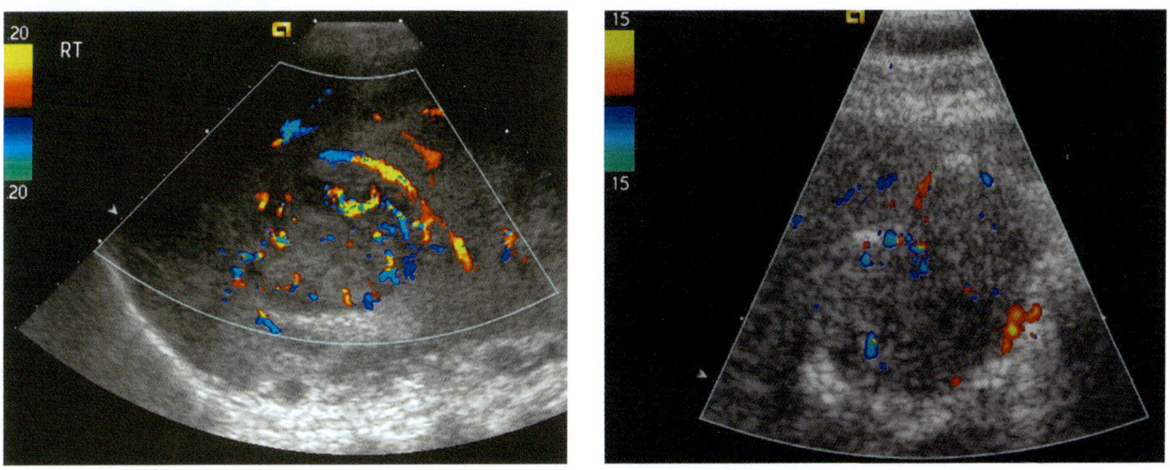

Fig. 9.**8** **a** HCC demonstrating a "basket pattern" of abnormal tumor vascularity on color Doppler imaging. **b** A metastasis from a primary lung tumor demonstrating a "vessel-within-the-tumor" pattern of vascularity on color Doppler imaging

alone.[15] However, other studies have failed to replicate these results. Further attempts at characterizing the lesions by means of tumor vascularity have been reported, but only 76% of lesions known to be HCC demonstrated internal abnormal vascularity in one study.[23] Improvements in imaging techniques have resulted in increased flow detection using both power Doppler[24] and contrast-enhanced studies,[25,26] making assessment of tumor vascularity a potential marker of malignancy[23,25,27,28] (Fig. 9.**7**).

There are two documented "typical" patterns of vascularity of HCC (Fig. 9.**8**). The first is a "basket pattern,"

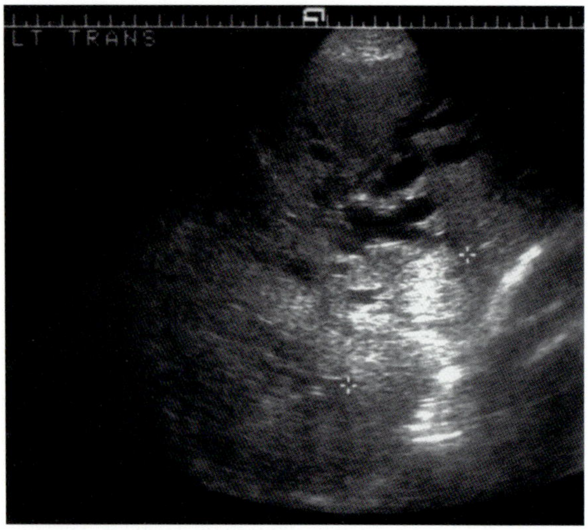

Fig. 9.**9** Hyper-reflective hilar cholangiocarcinoma (cursors) causing marked dilatation of the intrahepatic bile ducts

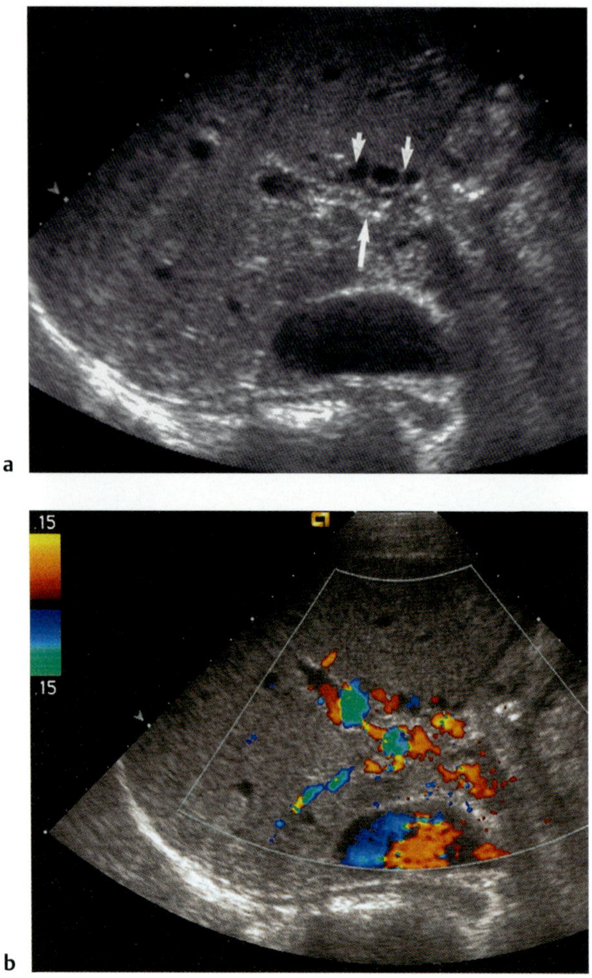

Fig. 9.**10** **a** Attenuated echogenic portal vein (arrow) surrounded by low-reflective areas (short arrow). **b** Color Doppler ultrasound imaging demonstrates cavernous transformation around a long-standing portal vein occlusion

where there is encasement of tumor by a feeding artery and portal vein, with both pulsatile and continuous Doppler spectra present. Alternatively, there is the "vessel-within-the-tumor" pattern, characterized by branches of the feeding artery seen within the lesion and displaying a pulsatile Doppler waveform.[27] Unfortunately, while these may be indicators of malignant disease where present, there is considerable overlap between HCC and metastases,[23] with cavernous hemangiomata also having been reported with abnormal arterial Doppler traces.[29]

The presence of a spontaneous arterioportal fistula should suggest the possibility of HCC in patients with cirrhosis, since such fistulae are reported in over 60% of cases. Although shunts may be seen in patients with nontumoral cirrhosis, these are usually subcapsular or peripheral,[30] in contrast to the random distribution of HCC-associated shunts.

Cholangiocarcinoma, seen most commonly as a consequence of primary sclerosing cholangitis, may be seen on ultrasound as a hyper- to hypoechoic ill-defined mass, usually in the region of the liver hilum, giving rise to dilated intrahepatic ducts (Fig. 9.**9**). Further imaging of suspect lesions with endoscopic retrograde cholangiopancreatography allows more accurate assessment of the biliary anatomy and gives the opportunity for diagnostic brushings and palliative stenting of strictures. Proven cholangiocarcinoma is a contraindication to transplantation,[12] though patients may be considered for radical resective surgery.

Summary points:

- The cirrhotic liver has a coarse, heterogeneous echotexture with reduced pulsatility of the hepatic venous waveform
- Ultrasound is approximately 80% sensitive in the detection of HCC. This may be improved by the use of contrast agents
- Differentiation of focal liver nodules by ultrasound is enhanced by the evaluation of the vascular pattern and postcontrast appearances

Imaging the Vasculature

Portal Vein

Portal venous thrombosis is a common complication of chronic liver disease, occurring in 5–10% of patients with end-stage cirrhosis[31] (Fig. 9.**10**). Although not an absolute contraindication to transplantation,[12] preoperative detection is vital as the full extent of any thrombus needs be demonstrated so that surgery can be planned and techniques modified accordingly.[32,33] Portal venous Doppler imaging in normal patients should give a continuous, undulating hepatopetal trace, although there is considerable variation in flow velocity (Fig. 9.**11**).

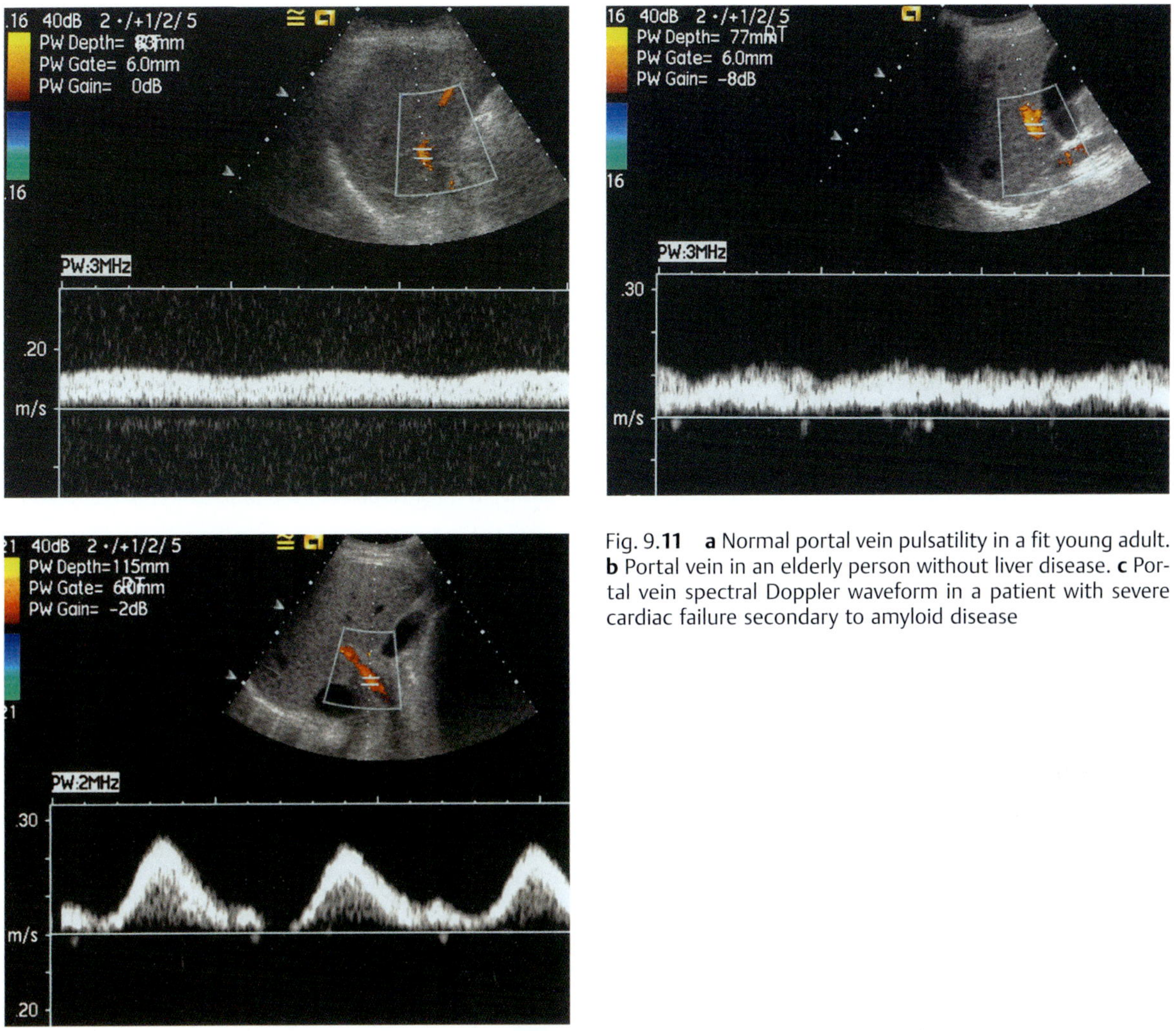

Fig. 9.**11** **a** Normal portal vein pulsatility in a fit young adult. **b** Portal vein in an elderly person without liver disease. **c** Portal vein spectral Doppler waveform in a patient with severe cardiac failure secondary to amyloid disease

In the cirrhotic liver, portal hypertension develops, the increase in pressure accounting for the ensuing complications. Portal velocity and portal venous flow vary inversely with the hepatic venous pressure gradient.[34] Recanalization of the umbilical vein in the ligamentum teres may be seen, allowing patency of the portal vein with antegrade flow to be inferred (Fig. 9.**12**). Reverse flow may also be seen; ultrasound is a reliable indicator of flow direction.[35]

Portal venous flow characteristics do not predict the presence or otherwise of varices.[34] However, among patients in whom variceal bleeding has previously occurred, a 12 % or greater reduction in the maximal portal flow velocity four hours after the administration of 40 mg propranolol has been found to be a significant predictor of which patients are less likely to rebleed.[36]

Portal hypertension may also result in splenomegaly, which may be readily assessed by ultrasound and monitored over time.

B mode imaging of thrombus may show the presence of echogenic material lying within the portal vein, seen as either complete occlusion or a tongue of thrombus with some surrounding flow (Fig. 9.**13**). Ultrasound is both sensitive and specific in the detection of portal venous thrombosis,[37–39] with the small proportion of inaccurate investigations attributed to a diminished flow rate. Demonstration of the portal venous system is enhanced with ultrasound microbubble contrast medium,[32,40] ideally given as an infusion,[41] and this has significant benefits in improving confidence in the diagnosis. Compared to CT angiography,[42,43] ultrasonography is sufficiently accurate in predicting portal venous patency that it has been advocated as the sole means of assessment in patients with no prior surgery.[43] In equivocal cases either magnetic resonance venography, which has been shown to be accurate in demonstrating the portal vein,[44] or, alternatively, indirect portography should be performed.[33] In patients with HCC, which has a tendency to invade the portal veins, differentiation between benign and malignant thrombus by ultrasound has been described. The presence of a pulsatile Doppler trace

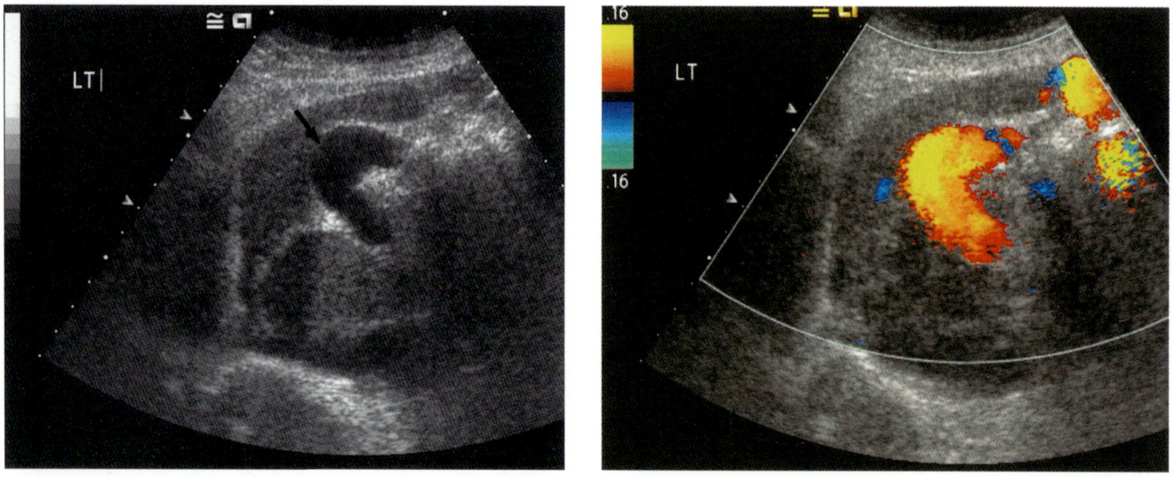

a b

Fig. 9.**12** **a** B mode ultrasound image of a patent umbilical vein (arrow). **b** Color Doppler image of patent umbilical vein

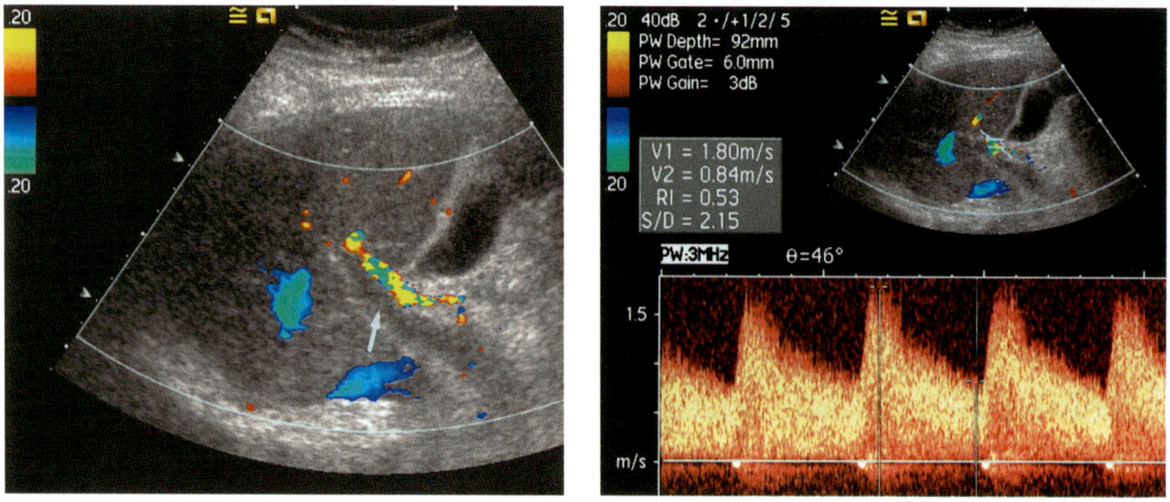

a b

Fig. 9.**13** **a** Portal vein thrombosis (arrow) in a patient without underlying liver disease. No color Doppler signal is seen in the portal vein, but a prominent signal is obtained from the hepatic artery. **b** Spectral Doppler waveform from the hepatic artery demonstrates a "hyperdynamic" waveform with a low resistive index of 0.53

within a thrombus is reported to be 62–89 % sensitive and at least 95 % specific for malignant thrombus,[45,46] whereas a continuous or absent trace was more likely in benign thrombus.

Hepatic Veins

Patency of the hepatic veins should be assessed, particularly in patients with Budd–Chiari syndrome, in order that surgery may be planned accordingly (Figs. 9.**14**, 9.**15**). Particular attention should be paid to whether there is evidence of thrombus extending into the inferior vena cava (IVC). The hepatic vein Doppler waveform may be of value in the diagnosis of cirrhosis, with progressive reduction in pulsatility[47] which has been correlated to histologic findings[48] (Fig. 9.**16**). Detection of early enhancement of the hepatic veins following microbubble contrast injection in patients with cirrhosis has been reported,[49] presumably due to anomalous portovenous shunts, but similar early enhancement is also seen in metastatic disease.[50]

Hepatic Artery

The hepatic artery is not routinely imaged in chronic liver disease as this has little bearing on clinical management. The arterial anatomy does not need to be established since this does not affect the operative pro-

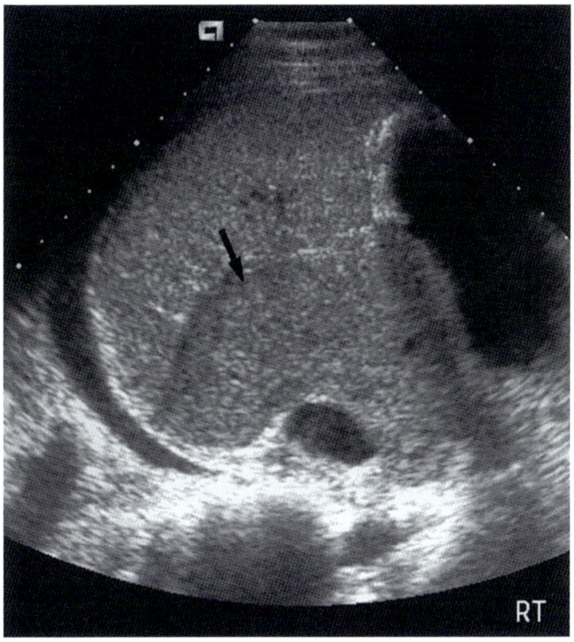

a

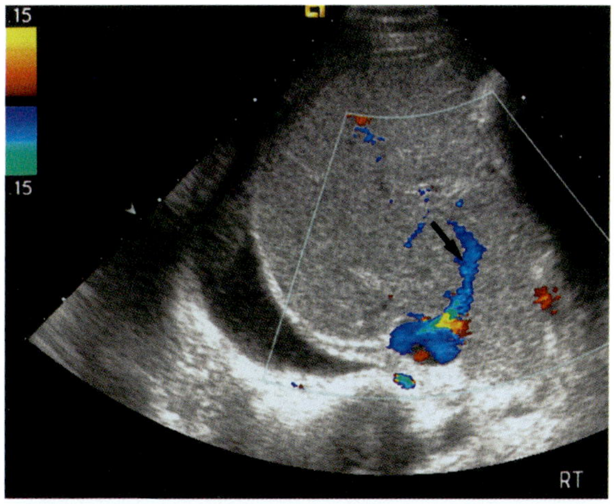

b

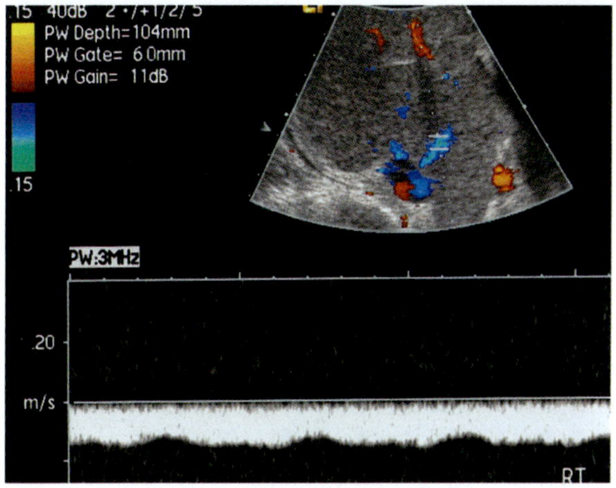

c

Fig. 9.**14** Chronic Budd–Chiari Syndrome. **a** Hypertrophy of the caudate lobe (arrow) in a patient with chronic Budd–Chiari syndrome. A small amount of ascites is present. **b** Direct drainage of vessels (arrow) into the inferior vena cava (IVC) from the caudate lobe. **c** Spectral Doppler waveform demonstrates marked flattening of the caudate lobe vein signal

cedure, whereas that of the donor is of importance. Cirrhosis produces a blunting of hepatic artery pulsatility,[51] with an increase in the resistive index[52] (Fig. 9.**17**). The resistive index will fall, however, if portal vein thrombosis occurs, with a value below 0.5 reported to be 44% sensitive but 100% specific.[53] Ultrasound is not reliable in the delineation of the anatomy.[38]

Shunts

Transjugular intrahepatic portosystemic shunt (TIPSS)—the creation of a shunt between the portal and hepatic venous systems—is a common procedure in the management of variceal hemorrhage and intractable ascites secondary to portal hypertension. Unfortunately, TIPSS stents have a significant rate of stenosis and occlusion[54–59] and require frequent monitoring, usually at one, three, and six months initially and six-monthly thereafter.[60] Clearly, therefore, noninvasive imaging is preferable in this group of patients.

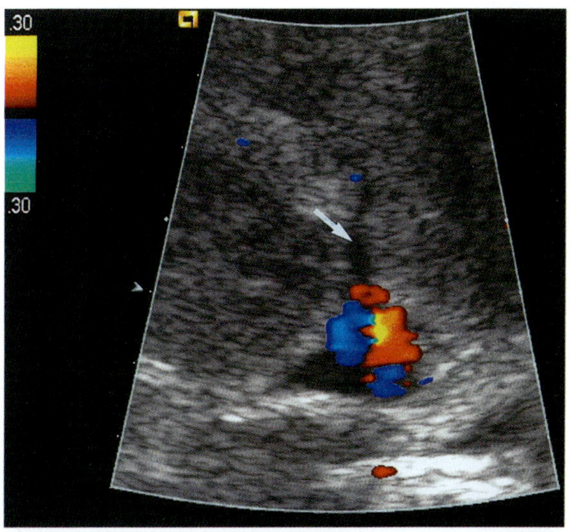

Fig. 9.**15** Acute Budd–Chiari Syndrome. No color Doppler signal is seen in the region of hepatic vein drainage into the IVC (arrow)

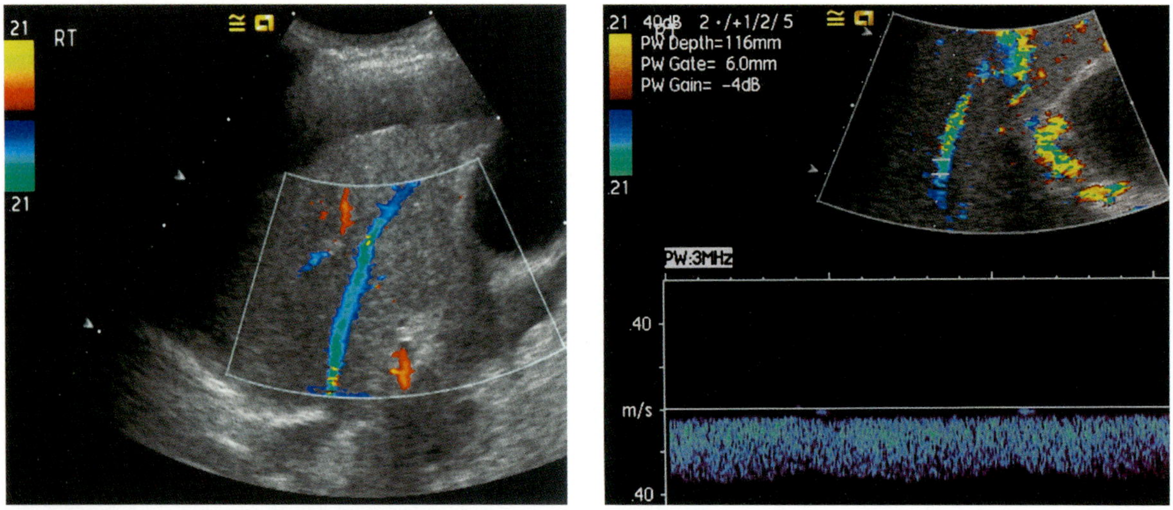

a b

Fig. 9.**16** **a** No reversal of flow on color Doppler US in a hepatic vein in a patient with advanced cirrhosis. **b** Spectral Doppler waveform demonstrates absence of any normal pulsatility

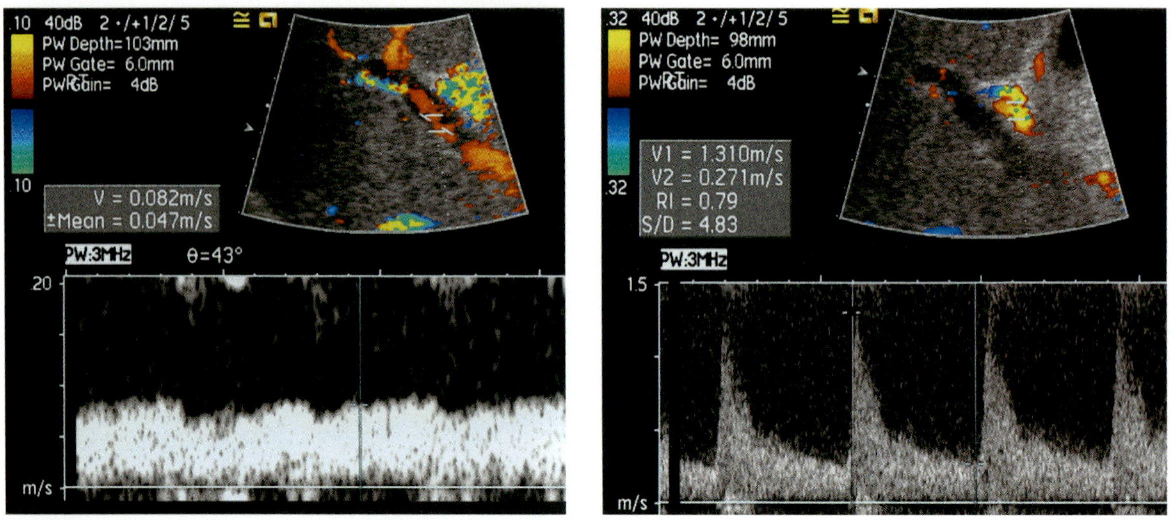

a b

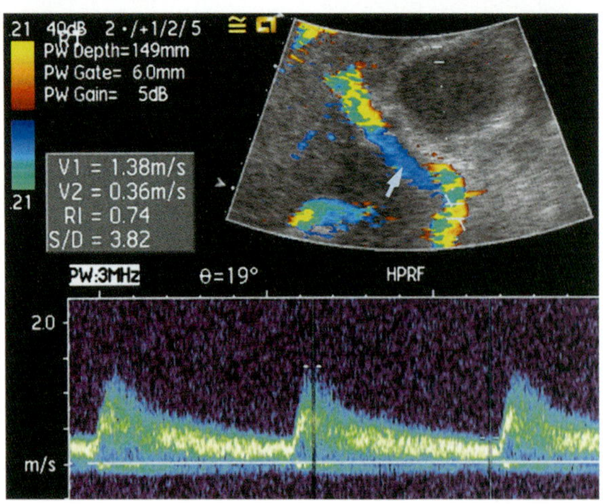

c

Fig. 9.**17** **a** Patient with advanced cirrhosis complicated by the presence of an HCC. There is low-velocity forward flow in the portal vein. **b** Prominent color Doppler signal from the hepatic artery in the same patient demonstrating a hyperdynamic appearance, but with a high resistive index of 0.79. **c** Flow reversal in the portal vein (arrow) also results in a “hyperdynamic” hepatic artery with a high resistive index of 0.74. (Compare with Fig. 9.**13**)

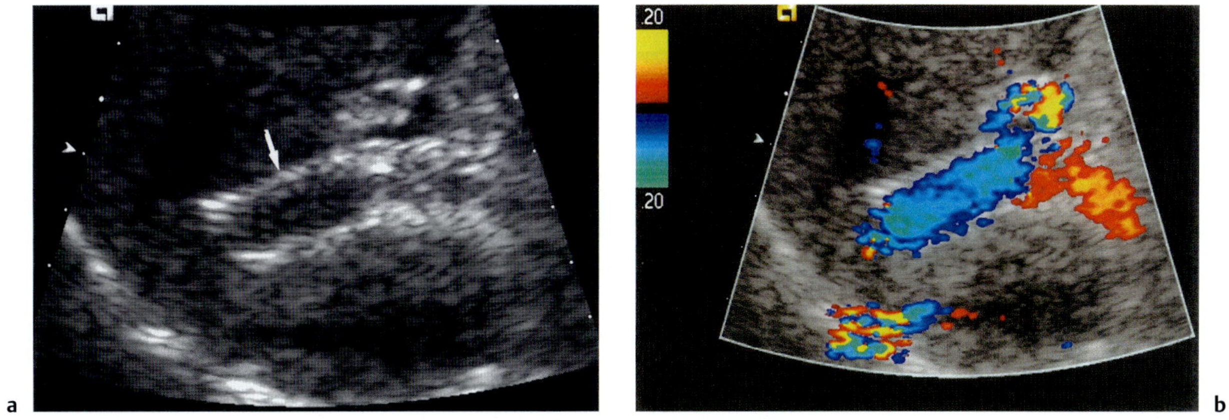

Fig. 9.**18** **a** Transjugular intrahepatic portosystemic shunt (TIPPS) stent on B mode ultrasound imaging demonstrating echogenic walls (arrow). **b** Normal color Doppler signal from a patent TIPPS stent

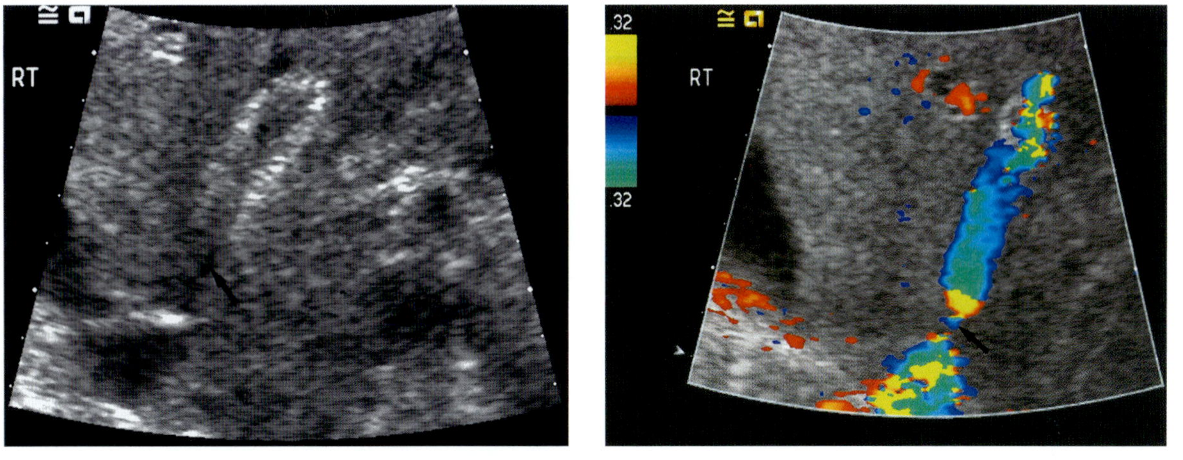

Fig. 9.**19** **a** TIPPS stent with incomplete visualization of terminal aspect in the hepatic vein (arrow). **b** Color Doppler US demonstrates marked narrowing and color turbulence at this point (arrow), suggesting a stenosis

B mode imaging of the TIPSS stent will demonstrate a highly echogenic grid pattern, the wall of the stent, through which the internal lumen often cannot be adequately visualized with ultrasound (Fig. 9.**18**). Several groups have evaluated examination of the flow characteristics of blood through a TIPSS stent. The patient should be examined during gentle respiration, since deep inspiration has been shown to decrease velocity by an average of 0.22 m/s, although the same authors found no significant variation in flow with patient in sitting, supine, or left lateral decubitus positions.[61] The exact range of "normal" flow velocity is disputed. Whereas some authors have found that a flow velocity of 0.90–1.90 m/s yields in excess of 95 % sensitivity and specificity in predicting stent patency[62–64] and a maximum velocity of less than 0.50–0.60 m/s or flow reversal is similarly accurate in predicting occlusion,[62,63] others have found these criteria only 75 % sensitive for detection of occlusion and only 35 % sensitive in detecting stenosed and occluded stents combined.[65] Other series have found ultrasound both sensitive and specific in detecting TIPSS complications, using reversal of flow in the hepatic vein, temporal change in flow velocity greater than 0.50 m/s, or complete absence of flow as criteria, although absolute flow velocity was found to be a poor predictor of occlusion.[66] Flow velocities in excess of 2.00 m/s should be regarded as suggestive of a narrow stenosis.[64] In view of these contradictory data, a suspected TIPSS stenosis by any criteria should be referred for further imaging, either with MRV or transjugular venography (Fig. 9.**19**).

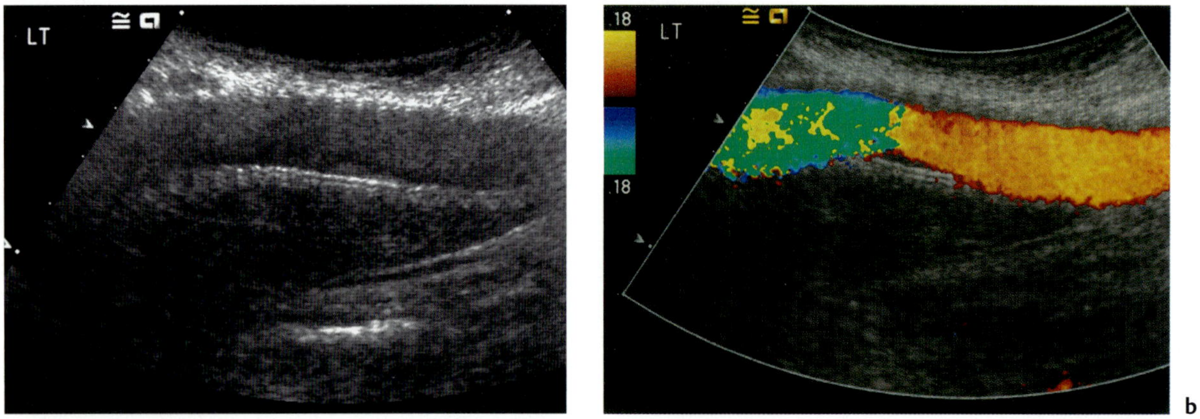

Fig. 9.**20** **a** Shunt on B mode ultrasound imaging a in patient with chronic Budd–Chiari syndrome. **b** Color Doppler imaging demonstrating patency of the shunt

End-to-side portocaval shunts may be demonstrated with some difficulty by ultrasound,[67] but there are no published data regarding the accuracy in comparison with direct venography (Fig. 9.**20**).

■ ***Summary points:***

- Portal vein thrombosis is common in chronic liver disease. Ultrasound provides an accurate assessment of patency and flow direction, although in equivocal cases contrast enhancement may be needed
- Pulsatile flow within a portal vein thrombus is highly suggestive of malignant disease
- In the assessment of a TIPSS, flow characteristics should be assessed and compared with those recorded in previous examinations in order to optimize detection of shunt dysfunction

Fibrolamellar Hepatocellular Carcinoma

Fibrolamellar hepatocellular carcinoma (FLHCC) is a subtype of HCC that occurs in a different population, has distinct radiographic features and a better prognosis (Fig. 9.**21**). FLHCC occurs primarily in young adults of either sex, without any associated cirrhosis or elevation of alpha-fetoprotein[68] and is relatively slow-growing. On ultrasound, FLHCC usually presents as a large (mean diameter 13 cm in one large series[69]), solitary mass within a noncirrhotic liver. The mass is usually of mixed echogenicity, but this is variable. Surface lobulations, punctate calcification, and a central fibrous scar, similar to that seen in focal nodular hyperplasia, are evident in the majority of patients.[70]

All cases should undergo further cross-sectional imaging with CT and magnetic resonance imaging (MRI), which may demonstrate features characteristic enough for a confident diagnosis to be made,[69] and to further assess staging. These patients may be candidates for either resection or transplantation despite large-volume tumors, as the size criteria given above for transplantation in HCC do not apply to FLHCC.[12]

■ ***Summary point:***

- Fibrolamellar HCC occurs in young patients with noncirrhotic livers. The diagnosis is vital as the surgical management and transplant criteria are different

Acute Liver Failure

Acute liver failure, in most cases caused by either drugs (especially paracetamol overdose) or viral hepatitis, is the indication for transplantation in approximately one-sixth of cases.[12] In this group, the role of ultrasound lies in excluding any focal liver lesions and establishing the patency of the vessels prior to surgery.

Serial Doppler ultrasound of patients presenting with acute liver failure has demonstrated that patients with a mean hepatic artery resistance index (HARI) greater than 0.75 or a mean maximum HARI greater than 0.86 were statistically more likely to fulfil transplant criteria, with the possibility that this could be used as an indicator of prognosis.[71] This study also examined portal vein diameter, blood flow, and splenic size, but found no statistically significant differences in these between patient groups.

Pediatric Liver Transplantation

Over the past 15 years liver transplantation in the pediatric population has developed dramatically in the wake of nursing, medical, and surgical advances. In the neonatal period, patients present most commonly with acute hepatic failure, usually from idiopathic hepatitis or iron storage disease.[72] As the age of the population increases, the presentation becomes one of decompensated chronic liver disease. After three months of age, biliary atresia becomes the predominant cause for transplantation, with alpha$_1$-antitrypsin deficiency, Alagille syndrome, and cirrhosis of varying etiology also commonly seen.[73,74] As in the adult population, the role of imaging lies in establishing the anatomy and patency of the hepatic vasculature, to monitor for the sequelae of chronic liver disease, and to exclude where possible any pathology that may contraindicate transplantation. In ultrasonography of the vasculature, it should be borne in mind that portal vein assessment in patients in whom a Kasai portoenterostomy has been performed has been shown to be inaccurate.[43] In addition, biliary atresia is associated with other developmental abnormalities in up to 20% of patients, including situs inversus, portal vein hypoplasia and caval interruption.[75]

Portal hypertension in pediatric patients with chronic liver disease is as for adults, whereas the development of HCC is very rare in the pediatric population. Hepatoblastoma may be treated by transplantation where the tumor remains unresectable following chemotherapy,[76] but there is no published data on the use of ultrasound in staging.

Absolute contraindications to liver transplantation are not well established in this age group, but given that the majority of patients are referred with either metabolic or anatomical congenital abnormalities, a survey of other abdominal organs is prudent in all cases. The majority of pediatric patients will receive a reduced-size graft,[72,73] either from a living related donor or cadaveric, due to the shortage of appropriately sized whole grafts.

Assessment of Living Related Donors

It is important to remember that liver donation is a voluntary undertaking in a healthy individual that is not without risk. Potential donors therefore must undergo a battery of blood tests, radiologic investigations, and independent psychiatric assessment[77] in order that no previously undetected medical problem exists that may preclude donation or unduly increase the risk of surgery.

Ultrasound of the abdomen is routinely performed as part of the radiologic work-up, with visualization of all of the solid organs in order to confirm their normality. The focus of the examination, however, is the hepatic vasculature, with particular attention paid to the anatomy of the hepatic veins, bearing in mind the surgical techniques described in other chapters. In addition to ultrasonography, patients will routinely undergo dual-phase CT of the liver (portal and hepatic venous phases) and aortoportography, giving the surgeon as much information as possible with which to plan surgery.

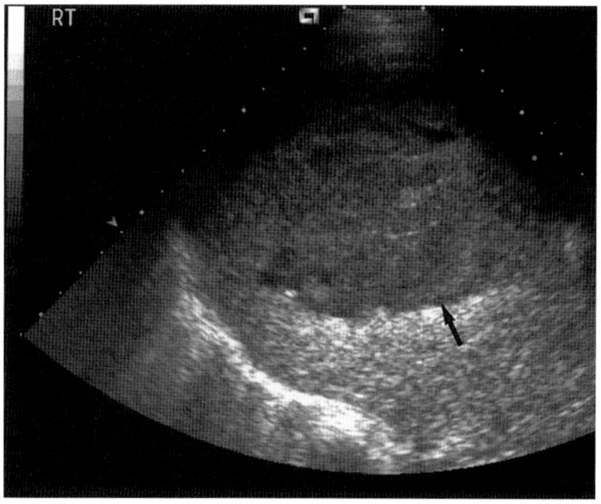

Fig. 9.**21** Fibrolamellar hepatocellular carcinoma (arrow)

Liver Volume Assessment

Of critical importance in determining the successful outcome of transplantation, particularly with the advent of split liver grafts in the fields of pediatric and living related donor transplantation, is the size of the graft used. Small livers should be no less than 50% of the size of the native, since below this there is a risk of hepatic failure postoperatively. Conversely, a graft may be up to 20% larger than the explanted liver. Grafts above this size may cause compression of the adjacent vascular structures and be poorly perfused. In all cases, mismatches lead to problems in performing the anastamoses.[78,79]

Ultrasound determination of volume can be performed by measuring the cross-sectional area of the liver as seen on consecutive scans in the sagittal plane at 1-cm intervals and adding these together, a technique that has been shown to be both accurate and reproducible.[80] However, this is a time-consuming procedure and has now been superseded by CT, which is equally accurate[80,81] and has the additional capability of calculating segmental volumes, but with the inherent risk associated with ionizing radiation exposure.

References

1. Meire HB, Farrant P. The liver. In: Baxter GM, Allan PL, Morley PM, editors. Clinical diagnostic ultrasound. Oxford: Blackwell Science; 1999. p. 369–86.
2. Brown JJ, Naylor MJ, Yagan N. Imaging of hepatic cirrhosis. Radiology 1997;202:1–16.
3. Giorgio A, Amborso P, Lettieri G, Fico P, de Stefano G, Finelli L, et al. Cirrhosis: value of caudate to right lobe ratio in diagnosis with ultrasound. Radiology 1986;161:443–5.
4. Hess CF, Schmiedl UP, Coelbel G, Knecht R, Kurtz B. Diagnosis of liver cirrhosis with US: receiver-operating charac-

teristic analysis of multi-dimensional caudate lobe indexes. Radiology 1989;171:349–51.
5. Goyal AK, Pokhana DS, Sharma SK. Ultrasonic diagnosis of cirrhosis: reference to quantitive measurements of hepatic dimensions. Gastrointest Radiol 1990;15:32–4.
6. Harbin WP, Robert NJ, Ferrucci JT. Diagnosis of cirrhosis based on regional changes in hepatic morphology. Radiology 1980;135:273–83.
7. International Working Party. Terminology of nodular hepatocellular lesions. Hepatology 1995;22:983–93.
8. Sorensen HT, Friis S, Olsen JH, Thulstrup AM, Mellemkjer L, Linet M, et al. Risk of liver and other types of cancer in patients with cirrhosis: a nationwide cohort study in Denmark. Hepatology 1998;28:921–5.
9. McPeake JR, O'Grady J, Zaman S, Portmann B, Wight DGD, Tan KC, et al. Liver transplantation for primary hepatocellular carcinoma: tumor size and number determine outcome. J Hepatol 1993;18:226–34.
10. Miller WJ, Federle MP, Campbell WL. Diagnosis and staging of hepatocellular carcinoma: comparison of CT and sonography in 36 liver transplantation patients. AJR Am J Roentgenol 1991;157:303–6.
11. Michel J, Suc B, Montpeyroux F, Hachemanne S, Blanc P, Domergue J, et al. Liver resection or transplantation for hepatocellular carcinoma? Retrospective analysis of 215 patients with cirrhosis. J Hepatol 1997;26:1274–80.
12. Devlin J, O'Grady J. Indications for referral and assessment in adult liver transplantation: a clinical guideline. Gut 1999;45:VI1.
13. Utsunomiya T, Matsumata T, Adachi E, Honda H, Sugimachi K. Limitations of current preoperative liver imaging techniques for intrahepatic metastatic nodules of hepatocellular carcinoma. Hepatology 1992;16:694–701.
14. Rizzi PM, Kane PA, Ryder SD, Ramage JK, Gane E, Tan KC, et al. Accuracy of radiology in detection of hepatocellular carcinoma before liver transplantation. Gastroenterology 1994;107:1425–9.
15. Dodd GD, Miller WJ, Baron RL, Skolnick ML, Campbell WL. Detection of malignant tumors in end-stage cirrhotic livers: efficacy of sonography as a screening technique. AJR Am J Roentgenol 1992;159:727–33.
16. Powers J, Averkiou M, Hope-Simpson D. Pulse inversion harmonics and other contrast imaging methods. Bothell, Washington: Advanced Technology Laboratories Ultrasound, 1998.
17. Blomley MJK, Albrecht T, Cosgrove DO, Patel N, Jayaram V, Butler-Barnes J, et al. Improved imaging of liver metastases with stimulated acoustic emission in the late phase of enhancement with the US contrast agent SH U 508A: early experience. Radiology 1999;210:409–16.
18. Albrecht T, Hoffmann CW, Schettler S, Overberg A, Ilg M, Von Behren PL, et al. B-mode enhancement at phase-inversion US with air-based microbubble contrast agent: initial experience in humans. Radiology 2000;216:273–8.
19. Forsberg F, Goldberg BB, Liu JB, Merton DA, Rawool NM, Shi WT. Tissue-specific US contrast agent for evaluation of hepatic and splenic parenchyma. Radiology 1999;210:125–32.
20. Harvey CJ, Blomley MJK, Eckersley RJ, Heckemann RA, Butler-Barnes J, Cosgrove DO. Pulse-inversion mode imaging of liver specific microbubbles: improved detection of subcentimetre metastases. Lancet 2000;355:807–8.
21. Blomley MJK, Albrecht T, Wilson SR, Burns PN, Leen E. Improved detection of metastatic liver lesions using pulse inversion harmonic imaging with Levovist: a multicentre study. Radiology 1999;213:491.
22. Blomley MJK, Sidhu PS, Cosgrove DO, Albrecht T, Harvey CJ, Heckemann RA. Do different types of liver lesion differ in their uptake of the microbubble Levovist (SHU508) in its late liver phase, and can this be used to distinguish between them? Radiology 1999;213:489.
23. Nino-Murcia M, Ralls PW, Jeffrey RB, Johnson M. Color flow Doppler characterization of focal hepatic lesions. AJR Am J Roentgenol 1992;159:1195–7.
24. Lencioni R, Pinto F, Armillotta N, Bartolozzi C. Assessment of tumor vascularity in hepatocellular carcinoma: comparison of power Doppler US and color Doppler US. Radiology 1996;201:353–8.
25. Tano S, Ueno N, Tomiyama T, Kimura K. Possibilty of differentiating small hyperechoic liver tumours using contrast-enhanced colour Doppler ultrasonography: a preliminary study. Clin Radiol 1997;52:41–5.
26. Kim AY, Choi BI, Kim TK, Han JK, Yun EJ, Lee KY, et al. Hepatocellular carcinoma: power Doppler US with a contrast agent—preliminary results. Radiology 1998;209:135–40.
27. Hosten N, Puls R, Bechstein WO, Felix R. Focal liver lesions: Doppler ultrasound. Eur Radiol 1999;9:428–35.
28. Yasuhara K, Kimura K, Ohto M, Matsutani S, Ebara M, Tsuchiya Y, et al. Pulsed Doppler in the diagnosis of small liver tumours. Br J Radiol 1988;61:898–902.
29. Wachsberg RH, Jilani M. Duplex Doppler sonography of small (< 3 cm diameter) liver tumours: intralesional arterial flow does not exclude cavernous haemangioma. Clin Radiol 1999;54:103–106.
30. Lane MJ, Jeffrey RB, Katz DS. Spontaneous intrahepatic vascular shunts. AJR Am J Roentgenol 2000;174:125–31.
31. Lamont J, Koff R, Isselbacher K. Cirrhosis. In: Petersdorf R, Adams R, Braunwald E, editors. Harrison's principles of internal medicine. New York: McGraw-Hill, 1983. p. 1811.
32. Sidhu PS, Marshall MM, Ryan SM, Ellis SM. Clinical use of Levovist, an ultrasound contrast agent, in the imaging of liver transplantation: assessment of the pre and post transplant patient. Eur Radiol 2000;10:1114–26.
33. Karani JB, Heaton ND. Imaging in liver transplantation [review]. Clin Radiol 1998;53:317–22.
34. Taourel P, Blanc P, Dauzat M, Chabre M, Pradel J, Gallix B, et al. Doppler study of mesenteric, hepatic, and portal circulation in alcoholic cirrhosis: relationship between quantitative Doppler measurements and the severity of portal hypertension and hepatic failure. Hepatology 1998;28:932–6.
35. Nelson RC, Lovett KE, Chezmar JL, Moyers JH, Torres WE, Murphy FB, et al. Comparison of pulsed Doppler sonography and angiography in patients with portal hypertension. AJR Am J Roentgenol 1987;149:77–81.
36. Cioni G, Turrini F, Ticani E, D'Alimonte P, Cristani A, Boldrini E, et al. Prevention of a first episode of variceal bleeding: role of duplex Doppler sonographic measurement of the acute response to beta-blockers. J Ultrasound Med 1999;18:633–8.
37. Tessler FN, Gehring BJ, Gomes AS, Perrella RR, Ragavendra N, Busuttil R, et al. Diagnosis of portal vein thrombosis: value of color Doppler imaging. AJR Am J Roentgenol 1991;157:293–6.
38. Kolmannskog F, Jakobsen JA, Schrumpf E, Bergan A. Duplex Doppler sonography and angiography in the evaluation for liver transplantation. Acta Radiol 1994;35:1–5.
39. Alpern MB, Rubin JM, Williams DM, Capek P. Porta hepatis: duplex Doppler US with angiographic correlation. Radiology 1987;162:53–6.
40. Marshall MM, Beese RC, Sarma DI, Muiesan P, Kane PA, Karani JB, et al. Demonstration of the portal venous system by Doppler ultrasound is improved by the use of an echo-enhancing agent. Eur Radiol 1999;9:S31.
41. Sellars ME, Sidhu PS, Heneghan M, Blomley MJK, Bauer A. Infusions of microbubbles are more cost effective than bolus injections in Doppler studies of the portal vein: a quantitive comparison of normal volunteers and patients with cirrhosis. Radiology 2000;217:396.
42. Bach AM, Hann LE, Brown KT, Getrajdman GI, Herman SK, Fong Y, et al. Portal vein evaluation with US: comparison to angiography combined with CT arterial portography. Radiology 1996;201:149–54.
43. Raby N, Karani JB, Powell-Jackson P, Meire H, Williams R. Assessment of portal vein patency: comparison of arterial

portography and ultrasound scanning. Clin Radiol 1988;39:381–5.
44. Nghiem HV, Winter TC, Mountford MC, Mack LA, Yuan C, Coldwell DM, et al. Evaluation of the portal venous system before liver transplantation: value of phase-contrast MR angiography. AJR Am J Roentgenol 1995;164:871–8.
45. Dodd GD, Memel DS, Baron RL, Eichner L, Santaguida LA. Portal vein thrombosis in patients with cirrhosis: does sonographic detection of intrathrombus flow allow differentiation of benign and malignant thrombus? AJR Am J Roentgenol 1995;165:573–7.
46. Tanaka K, Numata K, Okazaki H, Nakamura S, Inoue S, Takamura Y. Diagnosis of portal vein thrombosis in patients with hepatocellular carcinoma: efficacy of color Doppler sonography compared with angiography. AJR Am J Roentgenol 1993;160:1279–83.
47. Farrant P, Meire HB. Hepatic vein pulsatility assessment on spectral Doppler ultrasound. Br J Radiol 1997;70:829–32.
48. Colli A, Cocciolo M, Riva C, Martinez E, Prisco A, Pirola M, et al. Abnormalities of Doppler waveform of the hepatic veins in patients with chronic liver disease: correlation with histologic findings. AJR Am J Roentgenol 1994;162:833–7.
49. Albrecht T, Blomley MJK, Cosgrove DO, Taylor-Robinson S, Jayaram V, Eckersley RJ, et al. Non-invasive diagnosis of hepatic cirrhosis by transit-time analysis of an ultrasound contrast agent. Lancet 1999;353:1579–83.
50. Blomley MJK, Albrecht T, Cosgrove DO, Jayaram V, Eckersley RJ, Patel N, et al. Liver vascular transit time analyzed with dynamic hepatic venography with bolus injections of an US contrast agent: early experience in seven patients with metastases. Radiology 1998; 209:862.
51. Iwao T, Toyonaga A, Shigemori H, Oho K, Sakai T, Tayama C, et al. Hepatic artery hemodynamic responsiveness to altered portal blood flow in normal and cirrhotic livers. Radiology 1996;200:793–8.
52. Schneider AW, Kalk JF, Klein CP. Hepatic arterial pulsatility index in cirrhosis: correlation with portal pressure. J Hepatol 1999;30:876–81.
53. Platt JF, Rubin JM, Ellis JH. Hepatic artery resistance changes in portal vein thrombosis. Radiology 1995;196:95–8.
54. LaBerge JM, Somberg KA, Roberts JP, Ascher NL. Creation of transjugular intrahepatic portosystemic shunts with the Wallstent endoprosthesis: results in 100 patients. Radiology 1993;187:413–20.
55. Nazarian GK, Ferral H, Castaneda-Zuniga WR, Bjarnason H, Foshager MC, Rank JM, et al. Development of stenoses in transjugular intrahepatic portosystemic shunts. Radiology 1994;192:231–4.
56. LaBerge JM, Somberg KA, Lake JR, Gordon RL, Kerlan RK, Ascher NL, et al. Two-year outcome following transjugular intrahepatic portosystemic shunt for variceal bleeding: results in 90 patients. Gastroenterology 1995;108:1143–51.
57. Freedman AM, Luketic VA, Purdum PP, Darcy MD, Posner MP. Complications of transjugular intrahepatic portosystemic shunt: a comprehensive review. Radiographics 1993;13:1185–210.
58. Haskal ZJ, Pentecost MJ, Soulen MC, Shalansky-Goldberg RD, Baum RA, Cope C. Transjugular intrahepatic portosystemic shunt stenosis and revision: early and mid term results. AJR Am J Roentgenol 1994;163:439–44.
59. Hausegger KA, Sternthal HM, Klein GE, Karaic R, Stauber R, Zenker G. Transjugular intrahepatic portosystemic shunt: angiographic follow-up and secondary interventions. Radiology 1994;191:177–81.
60. LaBerge JM, Feldstein VA. Ultrasound surveillance of TIPS—why bother ? Hepatology 1998;28:1433–4.
61. Kliewer MA, Hertzberg BS, Heneghan JP, Suhocki PV, Sheafor DH, Gannon PA, et al. Transjugular intrahepatic portosystemic shunts (TIPS): effects of respiratory state and patient position on the measurement of Doppler velocities. AJR Am J Roentgenol 2000;175:149–52.
62. Foshager MC, Ferral H, Nazarian GK, Castaneda-Zuniga WR, Letourneau JG. Duplex sonography after transjugular intrahepatic portosystemic shunts (TIPS): normal hemodynamic findings and efficacy in predicting shunt patency and stenosis. AJR Am J Roentgenol 1995;165:1–7.
63. Feldstein VA, Patel MD, LaBerge JM. Transjugular intrahepatic portosystemic shunts: accuracy of Doppler US in determination of patency and detection of stenoses. Radiology 1996;201:141–7.
64. Ferguson JM, Jalan R, Redhead DN, Hayes PC, Allan PL. The role of duplex and colour Doppler ultrasound in the follow-up evaluation of transjugular intrahepatic portosystemic stent shunt (TIPSS). Br J Radiol 1995;68:587–9.
65. Owens CA, Bartolone C, Warner DL, Aizenstein R, Hibblen J, Yaghmai B, et al. The inaccuracy of duplex ultrasonography in predicting patency of transjugular intrahepatic portosystemic shunts. Gastroenterology 1998;114:1433–4.
66. Dodd GD, Zajko AB, Orons PD, Martin MS, Eichner LS, Santaguida LA. Detection of transjugular intrahepatic portosystemic shunt dysfunction: value of duplex Doppler sonography. AJR Am J Roentgenol 1995;164:1119–24.
67. Ralls PW, Lee KP, Mayekawa DS, Boswell WD, Radin DR, Colletti PM, et al. Color Doppler sonography of portocaval shunts. J Clin Ultrasound 1990;18:379–81.
68. Mahfouz AE, Vogl T, Hamm B. Tumour diagnosis in the adult liver transplant candidate. Eur Radiol 1999;9:841–52.
69. Ichikawa T, Federle MP, Grazioli L, Madariaga J, Nalesnik M, Marsh W. Fibrolamellar hepatocellular carcinoma: imaging and pathologic findings in 31 recent cases. Radiology 1999;213:352–61.
70. Brandt DJ, Johnson CD, Stephens DH, Weiland LH. Imaging of fibrolamellar hepatocellular carcinoma. AJR Am J Roentgenol 1988;151:295–9.
71. Deasy NP, Wendon J, Meire HB, Sidhu PS. The value of serial Doppler ultrasound as a predictor of clinical outcome and the need for transplantation in fulminant and severe acute liver failure. Br J Radiol 1999;72:134–43.
72. Woodle ES, Millis JM, So SKS, McDiarmid SV, Busuttil RW, Esquivel CO, et al. Liver transplantation in the first three months of life. Transplantation 1998;66:606–9.
73. Beath SV, Brook GD, Kelly DA, Cash AJ, McMaster P, Mayer AD, et al. Successful liver transplantations in babies under 1 year. BMJ 1993;307:825–88.
74. Andrews WS, Wanek E, Fyock B, Gray S, Benser M. Pediatric liver transplantation: a 3-year experience. J Pediatr Surg 1989;24:77–82.
75. Howard ER. Biliary atresia; aetiology, management and complications. In: Howard ER, editor. Surgery of liver disease in children. London: Butterworth Heinemann; 1991. p. 39–56.
76. Baker A, Dhawan A, Heaton ND. Who needs a liver transplant ? (new disease specific indications). Arch Dis Child 1998;79:460–4.
77. Baker A, Dhawan A, Devlin J, Mieli-Vergani G, O'Grady J, Williams R, et al. Assessment of potential donors for living related liver transplantation. Br J Surg 1999;86:200–5.
78. Redvanly RD, Nelson RC, Stieber AC, Dodd GD. Imaging in the preoperative evaluation of adult liver-transplant candidates: goals, merits of various procedures, and recommendations. AJR Am J Roentgenol 1995;164:611–7.
79. Kawasaki S, Makuuchi M, Matsunami H, Hashikura Y, Ikegami T, Chisuwa H, et al. Preoperative measurement of segmental liver volume of donors for living related liver transplantation. Hepatology 1993;18:1115–20.
80. Van Thiel DH, Hagler NG, Schade RR, Skolnick ML, Heyl AP, Rosenblum E, et al. In vivo hepatic volume determination using sonography and computed tomography. Validation and a comparison of the two techniques. Gastroenterology 1985;88:1812–17.
81. Schiano TD, Bodian C, Schwartz ME, Glajchen N, Min AD. Accuracy and significance of computed tomographic scan assessment of hepatic volume in patients undergoing liver transplantation. Transplantation 2000;69:545–50.

Early Postoperative Liver Transplant Ultrasound

S. M. Ryan and P. S. Sidhu

Introduction

Patients who have undergone liver transplantation are susceptible to a wide variety of complications that can threaten both allograft and patient survival. Some complications are of the kind seen in any patient who has undergone a major surgical procedure or is receiving immunosuppressive drug therapy, but other complications are unique to the surgical transplantation procedure performed.[1]

The main postoperative complications may be grouped into:

1 Vascular abnormalities
2 Nonvascular abnormalities
   –Graft rejection
   –Biliary tract complications
   –Localized or systemic infection
3 Miscellaneous complications

The clinical diagnosis and management of these complications may be difficult as the clinical and laboratory findings are nonspecific,[1] with imaging, especially ultrasonography, providing the necessary stimulus to further diagnostic or interventional procedures.

Ultrasound is normally the first line of evaluation in the post-transplant phase; used either as an investigative tool, when there is clinical evidence of graft dysfunction, or routinely for the early detection of complications before there is any clinical suspicion of abnormality. A detailed ultrasound examination evaluating the biliary system, hepatic vasculature, hepatic parenchyma, and perihepatic spaces may add information crucial to the patient management.

Prior to performing an ultrasound examination it is imperative to know the type of surgical procedure that has been performed, as numerous variations exist from transplant of the whole liver to transplant of a single liver lobe or segmental liver transplantation. In orthotopic liver transplantation (OLT), revascularization of the allograft requires anastomoses of the hepatic artery, portal vein, and inferior vena cava (IVC), with biliary tract reconstruction performed to establish bile drainage (Fig. 10.**1**). Many different anastomoses may be performed according to the preference of the surgeon, the anatomy of the donor and recipient vessels, as well as the underlying disease.

Vascular Complications

Hepatic Artery

In the first two weeks following liver transplantation, routine color Doppler ultrasonography (CDUS) plays an important role in the detection of both clinically evident and clinically unsuspected vascular complications, particularly hepatic artery thrombosis. There is evidence to suggest that routine CDUS of all the he-

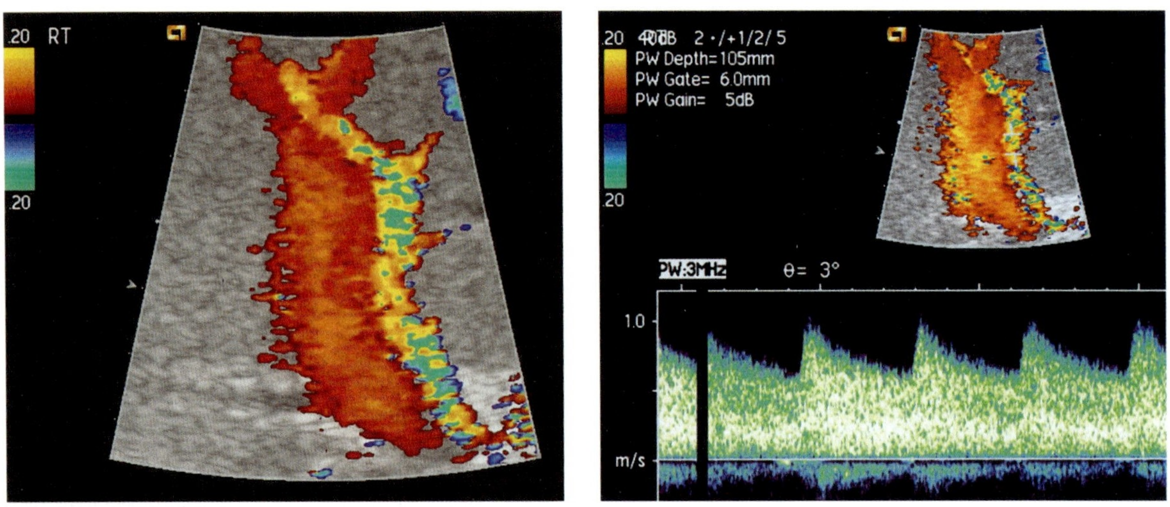

a b

Fig. 10.**1** **a** Normal color Doppler imaging of the portal vein/hepatic artery. **b** Normal spectral Doppler appearances of the post-transplant hepatic artery

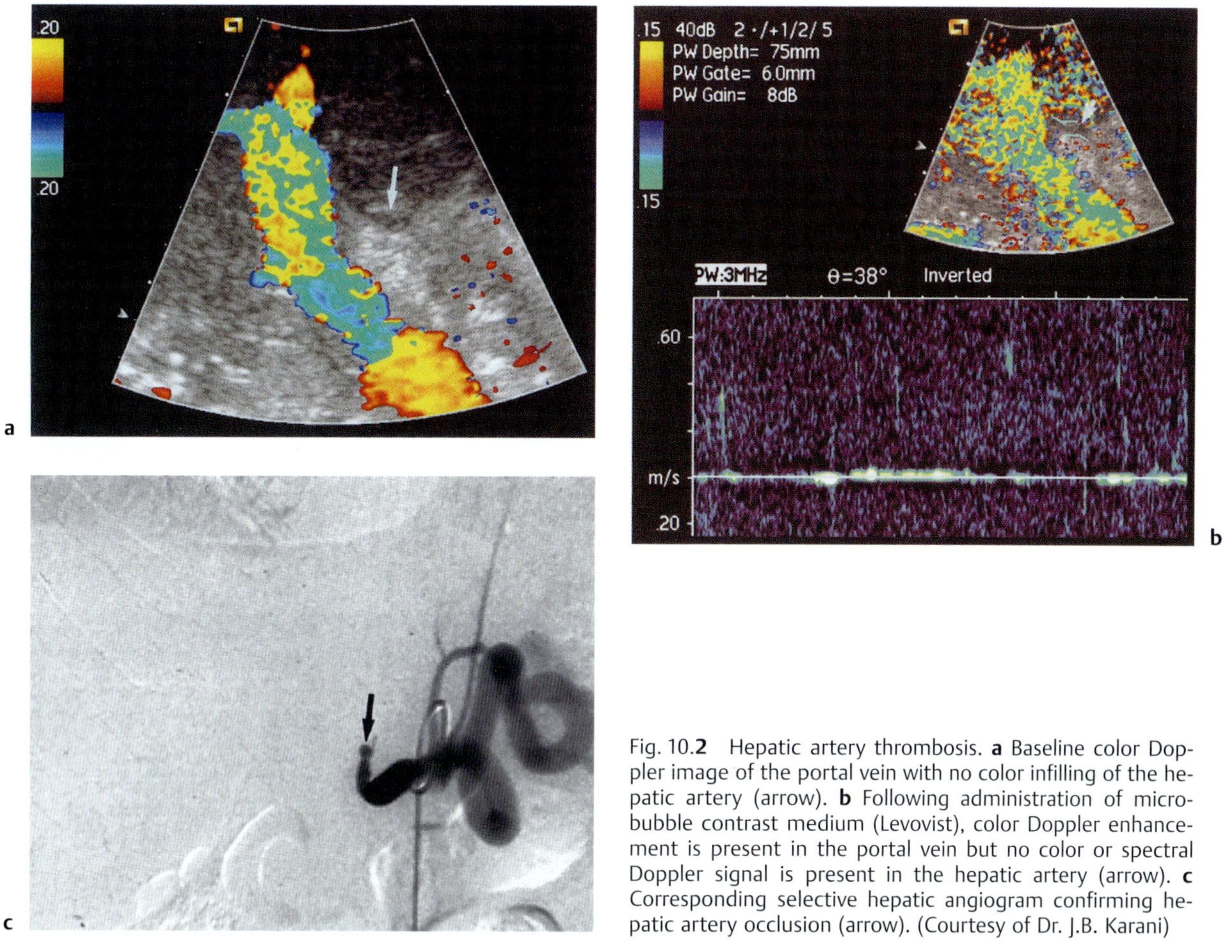

Fig. 10.**2** Hepatic artery thrombosis. **a** Baseline color Doppler image of the portal vein with no color infilling of the hepatic artery (arrow). **b** Following administration of microbubble contrast medium (Levovist), color Doppler enhancement is present in the portal vein but no color or spectral Doppler signal is present in the hepatic artery (arrow). **c** Corresponding selective hepatic angiogram confirming hepatic artery occlusion (arrow). (Courtesy of Dr. J.B. Karani)

patic vessels on the first day following liver transplantation and subsequently every three days in the early postoperative phase is beneficial.[2] Our practice is to perform CDUS in the first 24 hours after liver transplantation, then to perform a repeat ultrasound at day 4 and finally another prior to discharge. Any clinical change would prompt immediate CDUS of the hepatic artery, as after transplantation the donor biliary system is entirely dependent on hepatic arterial blood supply, in particular the right hepatic artery.[3]

Hepatic Artery Thrombosis

The quoted incidence of hepatic artery thrombosis (HAT) is 5 % of adult and 9–18 % of pediatric transplant patients.[4] HAT (Fig. 10.**2**) is a serious complication with a mortality of 50–58 %; retransplantation is often required, and even after retransplantation mortality remains high at 27–30 %.[5]

The ultrasound features of HAT include an absence of color and spectral Doppler flow, with a wall “thump” on Doppler imaging. Ultrasound microbubble contrast medium, by markedly increasing the intensity of the Doppler signal, may help to prevent false-positive diagnosis of HAT.[6] HAT is most common in the first six weeks following transplantation,[7] with CDUS interrogation of the vessels recommended in the first 24 hours after liver transplantation; the highest incidence of vascular complications in patients without symptoms occurs in this period.[2] Collateral formation (Fig. 10.**3**) very rarely occurs in adults, and takes at least three weeks to become apparent, but it is more common in children.

Clinically, impending or complete occlusion of the hepatic artery is often indicated by generalized nonspecific deterioration of the liver function tests, with a characteristic rise in the AST, or with indications of leakage of bile.[8] Tzakis et al.[9] described three clinical presentations of HAT that occur with equal frequency:

- Massive hepatic necrosis, a dramatic clinical emergency, requiring retransplantation for survival
- Delayed biliary leak as a consequence of bile duct ischemia and necrosis
- Intermittent episodes of sepsis without an evident source

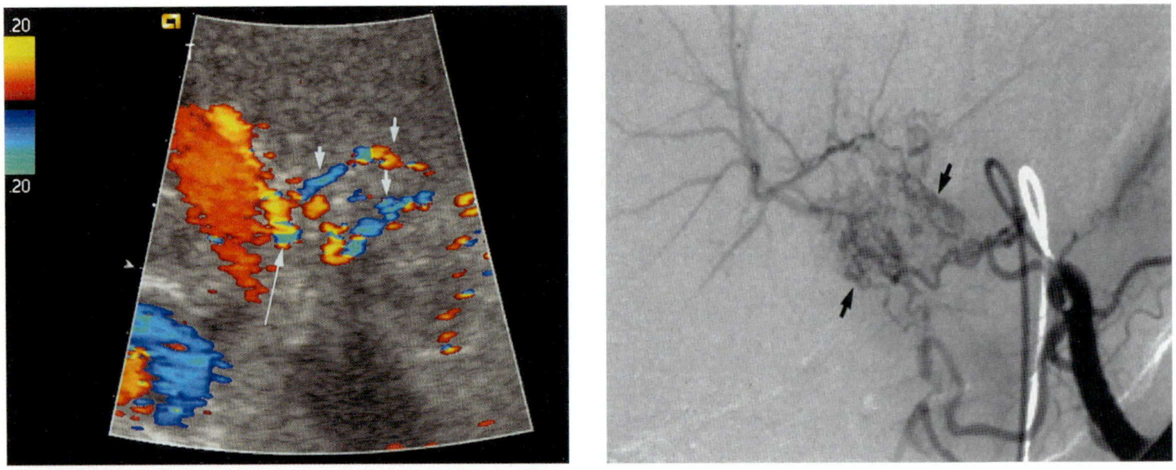

a b

Fig. 10.**3** **a** Color Doppler image of the portal vein and intrahepatic hepatic artery demonstrates collaterals (arrows) forming an intrahepatic hepatic artery branch (long arrow) following long-standing hepatic artery occlusion. **b** Corresponding selective celiac axis angiogram demonstrating collateral formation (arrows) around an occluded hepatic artery. (Reproduced from *Clinical Radiology*[16] by permission of the Editor.)

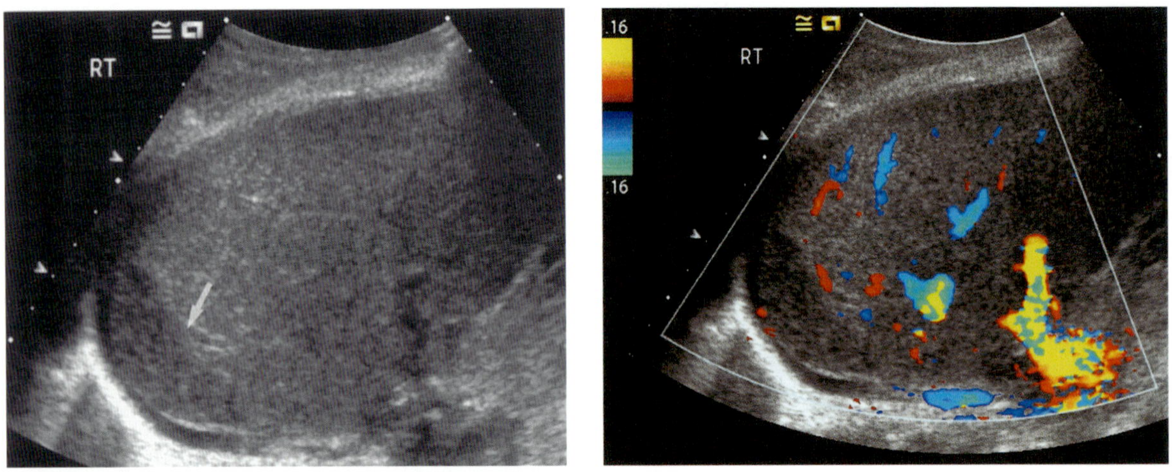

a b

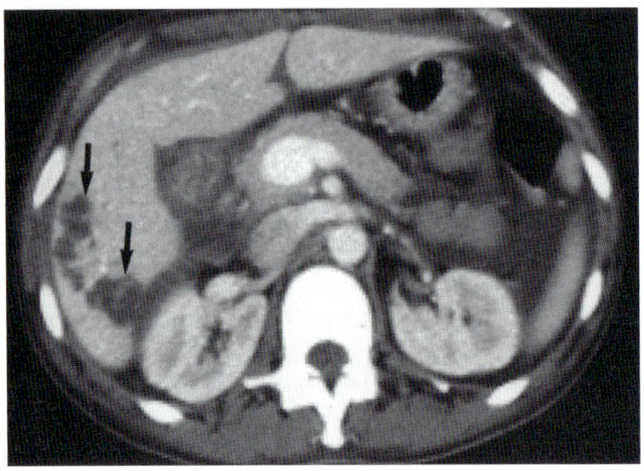

c

Fig. 10.**4** **a** B-mode ultrasound examination of a transplant liver demonstrating an area of low reflectivity corresponding to an area of infarction (arrow). **b** Color Doppler image of same region showing no color signal in the infarcted area. **c** Contrast enhanced CT in a different patient demonstrating focal low-attenuation areas of infarction in a transplant liver (arrows). (Courtesy of Dr. P.A. Kane)

B-mode ultrasonography will demonstrate areas of ischemia as areas of inhomogeneity and decreased echogenicity (Fig. 10.**4**), but this is a late development and revascularization will not save the graft.

In the early postoperative period, the spectral Doppler waveform can be quite variable, from the high forward diastolic flow to absence of flow in diastole (Fig. 10.**5**). Absence or reversal of flow in diastole does not appear to indicate a predisposition to thrombosis in the immediate postoperative period.[7] While absence of any color or spectral Doppler flow in the hepatic artery is suggestive of thrombosis in the immediate post-trans-

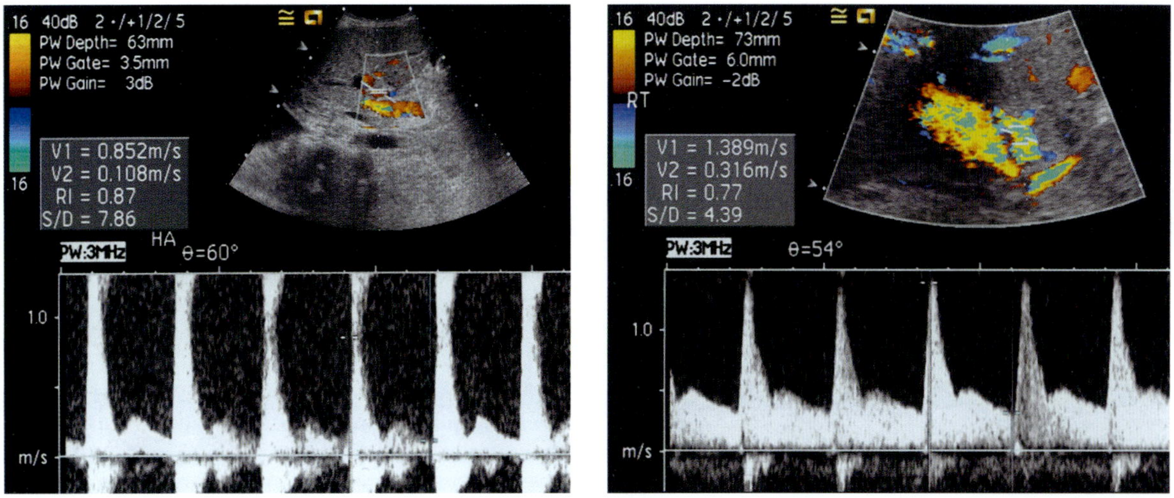

a b

Fig. 10.5 **a** Day 4 after transplantation showing a high-resistance (RI = 0.87) spectral Doppler waveform of the hepatic artery. **b** Day 12 after transplantation in the same patient demonstrating a reduction in the measured resistive index (RI = 0.77) of the transplant artery

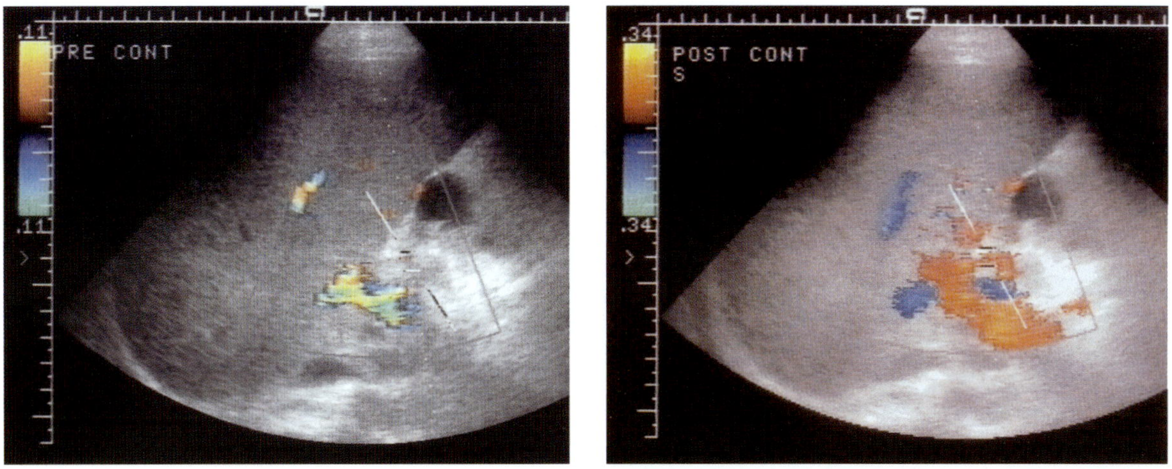

a b

Fig. 10.6 **a** Nonvisualization of any color Doppler signal from the hepatic artery (cursor) despite optimization of machine settings. **b** Following administration of microbubble contrast medium (Levovist), color Doppler signal fills the arterial lumen, allowing confirmation of a patent post-transplant hepatic artery

plant period, other factors may contribute to an undetectable hepatic artery signal.[5] An increased RI occurs, as the newly transplanted liver is relatively ischemic, with reperfusion edema persisting for up to 72 hours. Furthermore, any cause of edema or inflammation in the transplant may produce a similar result; viral hepatitis or rejection can cause severe edema that can markedly damp the hepatic artery waveform.[5] One early study suggested that CDUS has a sensitivity of 92 % in the diagnosis of HAT,[10] but a more recent study suggests a lower value of 82 %, and a positive predictive value of 64–68 %.[5] Our experience suggests that CDUS of the hepatic artery will visualize 96 % of hepatic arteries in the post-transplant period, and further interrogation of the nonvisualized hepatic artery using ultrasound microbubble contrast medium improves detection to 98.7 % (Fig. 10.**6**).[6] Using microbubble contrast has the advantage of reinforcing the signal from the hepatic artery in patients with diminished but present hepatic arterial flow, and precludes the need for more invasive imaging with angiography. Patients who still demonstrate absence of flow following contrast-enhanced CDUS should undergo selective hepatic artery angiography.

The normal Doppler waveform in the hepatic artery is of a broad systolic peak with high diastolic velocity and low RI. Any deviation from this pattern must be carefully watched and followed up with serial CDUS, with a low threshold for proceeding to arteriography, the gold standard in evaluation of hepatic artery patency. Although the hepatic arterial waveform in the immediate postoperative period varies, impending thrombosis

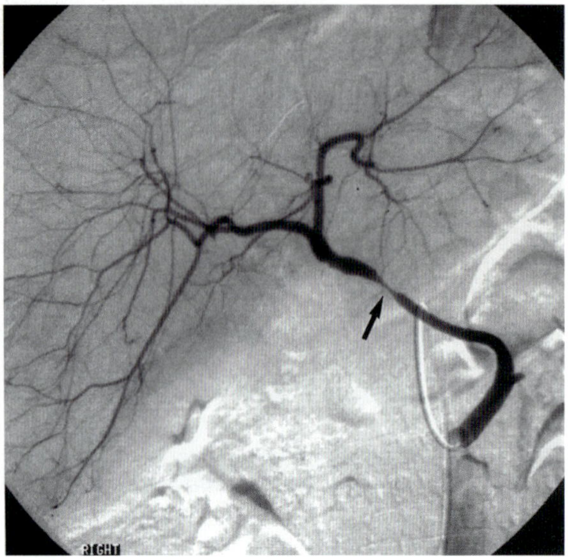

Fig. 10.**7** Arteriography of a transplant hepatic artery demonstrates a narrowing of the artery at the surgical anastomotic site (arrow). (Reproduced from *Clinical Radiology*[16] by permission of the Editor.)

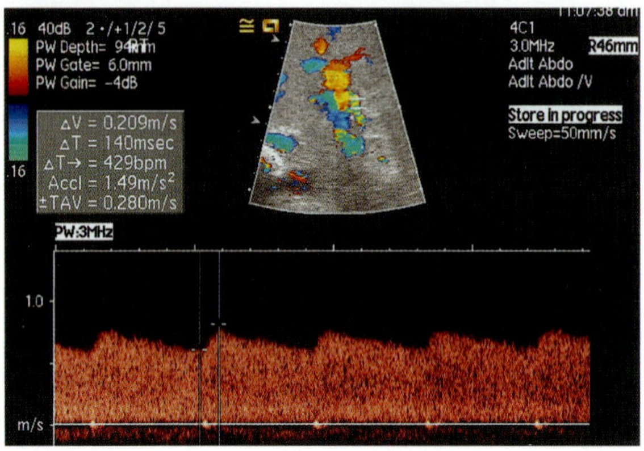

Fig. 10.**8** Spectral Doppler waveform obtained from an intrahepatic section of the hepatic artery demonstrating the tardus parvus waveform (acceleration time 0.14 seconds, RI = 0.23)

is suggested when a previously normal Doppler waveform proceeds to absence of diastolic flow with dampening of the systolic peak. This is thought to occur prior to progression to complete loss of the hepatic arterial signal.[5]

With the advent of multislice capabilities, computed tomographic arteriography (CTA) of the liver is now a practical noninvasive method of detecting hepatic artery complications after liver transplantation. The excellent spatial resolution and fast scan times allow CTA to depict smaller vessels for evaluation of both patency and stenosis and may eventually replace arteriography.[11] In addition, dual-phase contrast-enhanced three-dimensional magnetic resonance angiography (3D MRA) of the hepatic blood supply using fat-saturation techniques, the administration of a high caloric liquid prior to scanning, and digital image subtraction, can give comparable results to arteriography for the evaluation of hepatic arteries.[12–14] Ultrasound will, however. continue to provide first-line imaging assessment of the post-transplant hepatic artery.

Hepatic Artery Stenosis

Stenosis of the hepatic artery has been reported to occur in up to 5 % of hepatic transplant recipients,[15] but in our experience the incidence is close to 3 %.[16] Hepatic artery stenosis (HAS) commonly occurs in the early postoperative period, but may do so several years after transplantation; it occurs most often at the site of the surgical anastomosis (Fig. 10.**7**). If untreated, severe stenosis can lead to allograft rejection and progress further to the development of all the complications associated with HAT.[17]

HAS after liver transplantation may be attributable to inadequate surgical technique, surgical clamp injury, allograft rejection, microvascular injury associated with disrupted vasa vasorum, underlying liver disease, or preservation injury.[15] HAS produces an intrahepatic spectral Doppler tardus parvus waveform, which is defined as a reduced RI of less than 0.5, and a prolonged systolic acceleration time (SAT) greater than or equal to 0.08 seconds (Fig. 10.**8**).[18] Based on the tardus parvus waveform, sensitivity of between 85 % and 97 % for CDUS in detecting the presence of HAS has been quoted.[15,18] However, if only one of the defining parameters—reduced RI or prolonged SAT—is present, the frequency of finding HAS is decreased.[18]

The tardus parvus spectral waveform is nonspecific for stenosis: similar patterns may be seen in severe aortoceliac atherosclerotic disease, arteriovenous fistula, arteriobiliary fistula formation, and long-standing thrombosis with collateral development.[6] Therefore, the primary Doppler ultrasound criterion of arterial stenosis in any location of the body—a marked focal increase in peak systolic velocity (2 m/s) should be sought and is dependent on the direct evaluation of the site of the stenosis. In OLT, poor ultrasound evaluation of the vessels, particularly in the subhepatic space, markedly reduces the possibility of detecting a raised peak systolic velocity.[6] The use of ultrasound microbubble contrast medium may be beneficial in patients with HAS (Fig. 10.**9**). Microbubble contrast enhances the Doppler and color signal by 20 dB, making it easier accurately to identify the exact site of the stenosis, and to identify collateral vessel formation if present.[6]

There are two situations in which the diagnosis of HAS should be made with caution: during surgery, using intraoperative Doppler ultrasonography; and in the early postoperative period (up to 48 hours). Frequently, the postoperative RI will over time return to normal in these patients. Therefore follow-up CDUS is recommended when a low RI is detected in the hepatic artery in the presence of normal hepatic function in the post-

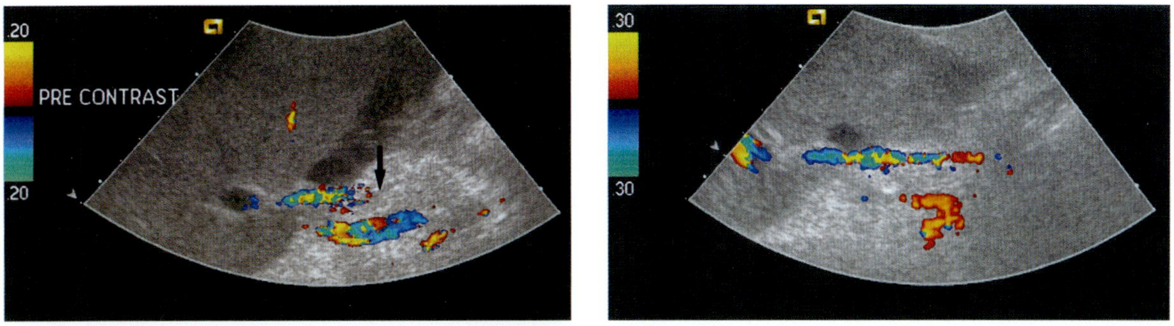

a b

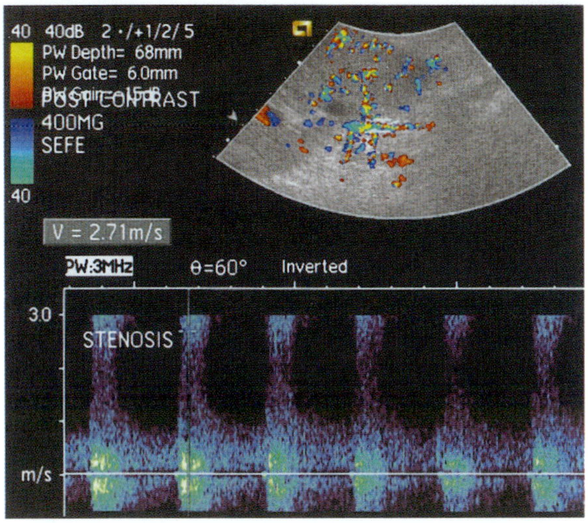

c

Fig. 10.**9** **a** Incomplete color Doppler signal from the hepatic artery in the subhepatic space (arrow) in a post-transplant patient. **b** Following administration of microbubble contrast medium (Levovist) the hepatic artery fills with color Doppler signal. **c** Interrogation of the hepatic artery with spectral Doppler imaging reveals an area of increased velocity corresponding to a focal hepatic artery stenosis. (Reproduced from *Clinical Radiology*[16] by permission of the Editor)

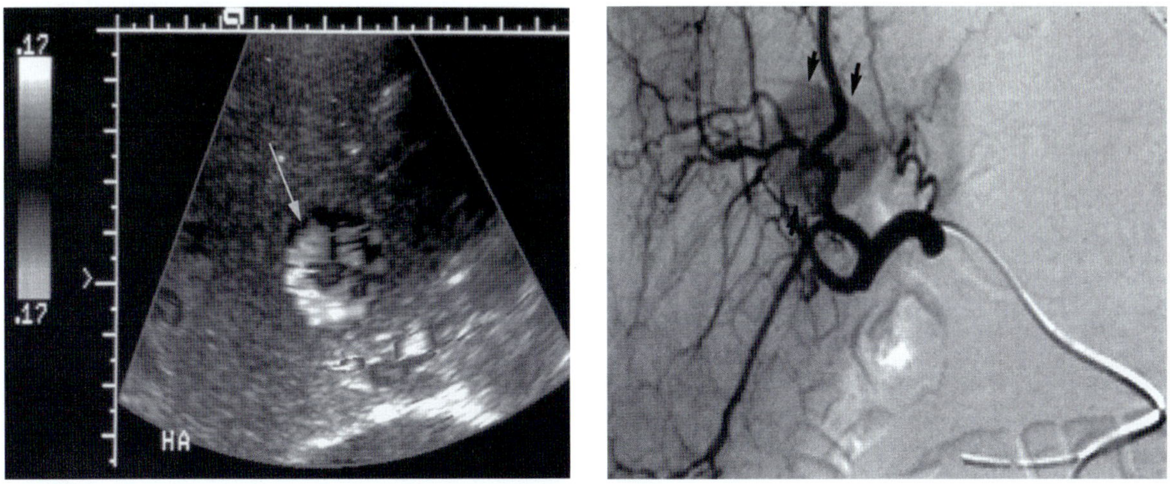

a b

Fig. 10.**10** **a** Ultrasound examination of an extrahepatic pseudoaneurysm (arrow) in a patient with biliary anastomosis breakdown and sepsis. **b** Corresponding selective hepatic artery arteriography demonstrates faint opacification of the pseudoaneurysm (arrows). (Reproduced from *Clinical Radiology*[19] by permission of the Editor)

operative period.[18] If clinical suspicion of HAS remains high, a normal CDUS examination should not prevent follow-up angiography, as HAS may not manifest the tardus parvus Doppler ultrasound abnormality.[18] In the absence of a tardus parvus waveform the HAS is less severe, but nevertheless important to identify, in order that appropriate clinical management is undertaken.

Hepatic Artery Pseudoaneurysm

Pseudoaneurysm formation following OLT is an uncommon vascular complication. The reported incidence following transplantation is 1%[19] (Fig. 10.**10**). Pseudoaneurysms may be caused by defective vascular reconstruction or infection, and usually occurs at the

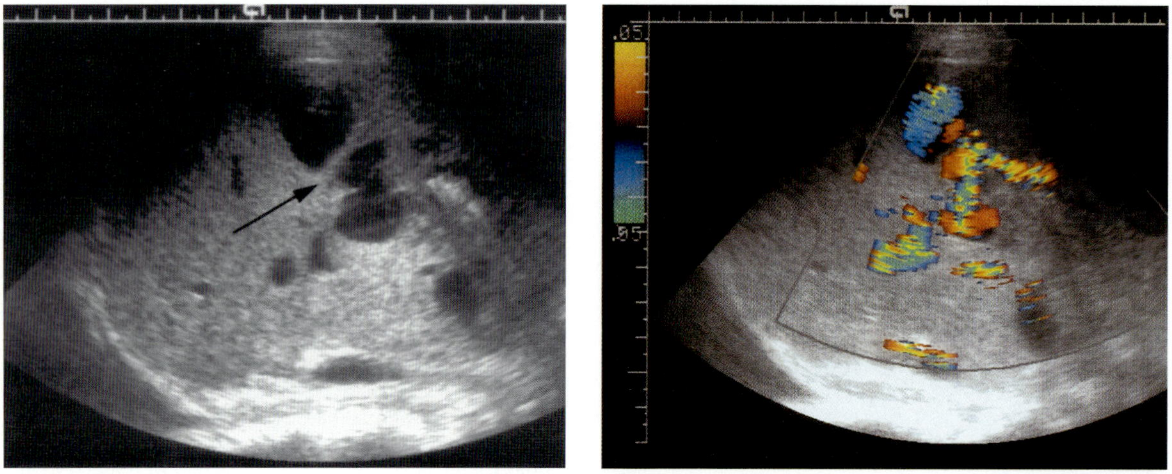

a b

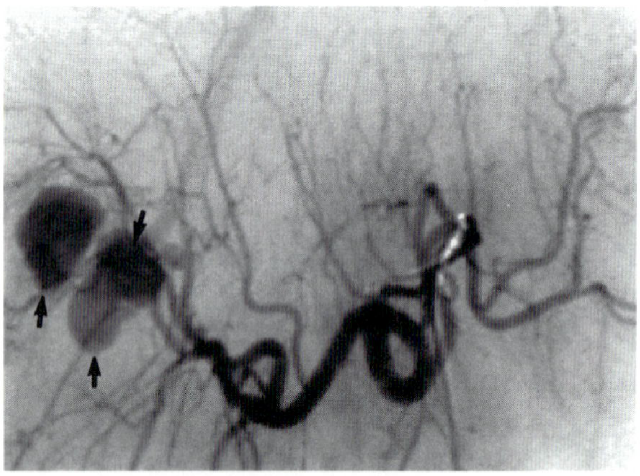

c

Fig. 10.**11** **a** B-mode image of a trilobulated low-reflective area in the right lobe of a transplant liver (arrow). **b** Color Doppler image of the same area demonstrates "ying-yang" color filling of these low-reflective areas, suggesting the presence of pseudoaneurysms. **c** Corresponding selective hepatic artery arteriography confirms the presence of a trilobulated intrahepatic artery pseudoaneurysm (arrows). (Reproduced from *Clinical Radiology*[19] by permission of the Editor)

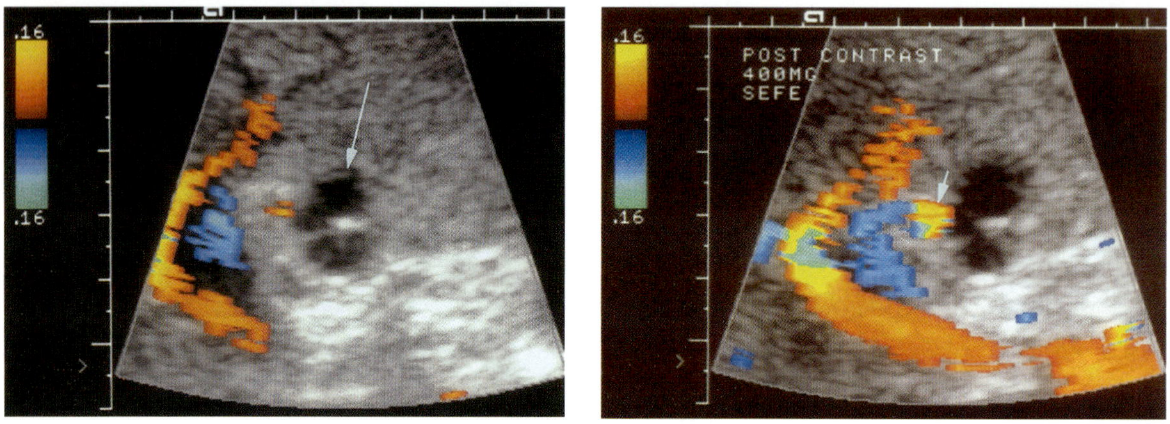

a b

Fig. 10.**12** **a** Hypoechoic area in close proximity to the post-transplant hepatic artery (arrow), suggestive of a hepatic artery pseudoaneurysm. **b** Following administration of microbubble contrast medium (Levovist), the hepatic artery fills with color Doppler signal (arrow), but no filling is seen in the low-reflective area. Subsequent endoscopic retrograde cholangiopancreatography confirmed focal biliary dilatation

site of the anastomosis. When seen in an intrahepatic site, percutaneous needle biopsy is usually responsible (Fig. 10.**11**). The potential for rupture, followed by fatal hemorrhage, makes early diagnosis and treatment important.

Diagnosis of pseudoaneurysm requires a high degree of suspicion, as these entities are often asymptomatic. Any hypoechoic collection in the vicinity of the hepatic artery anastomosis must be evaluated with CDUS (Fig. 10.**12**). Biopsy-related intrahepatic pseudo-

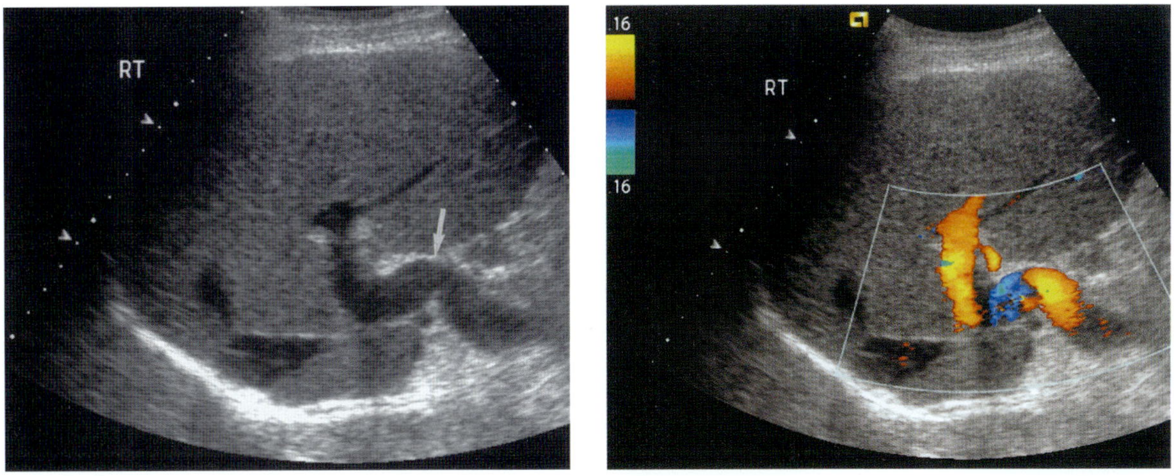

a

b

Fig. 10.**13** **a** Redundant portal vein on B-mode ultrasound (arrow). **b** Color Doppler imaging of the redundant portal vein demonstrating turbulent flow. **c** Confirmation on portal venous phase of selective splenic artery arteriography of the portal vein redundancy (arrow). (Courtesy of Dr. J.B. Karani)

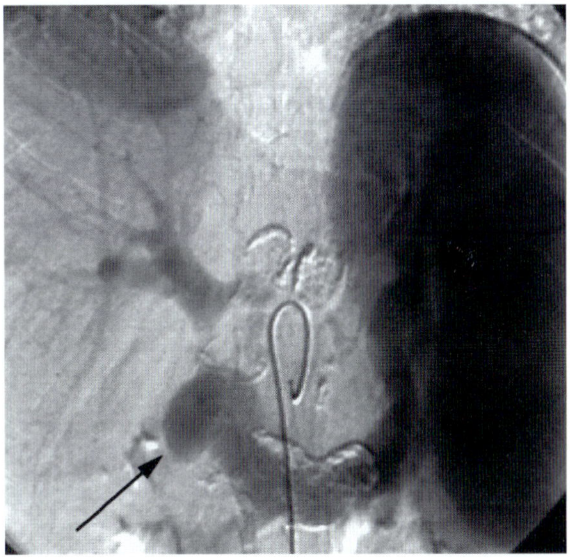

c

aneurysms may be small and may not be seen with ultrasound or CT; arteriography is the gold standard for detection.[20] Pseudoaneurysm formation must be considered in any patient with hemobilia or gastrointestinal bleeding beyond the second part of the duodenum without an endoscopically visible source, and also in those with enlarging intrahepatic hematomas on ultrasound.[1] Mortality from an extrahepatic pseudoaneurysm approaches 70%; retransplantation is often required, with transarterial embolization a temporary holding maneuver.[19]

Portal Vein Stenosis/Occlusion

The flow characteristics in the transplanted portal vein are often abnormal owing to a degree of infolding at the portal anastomosis (Fig. 10.**13**). This leads to flow disturbances beyond the anastomosis, manifest by color turbulence on CDUS. Portal vein occlusion following liver transplantation is uncommon (Fig. 10.**14**), occur-

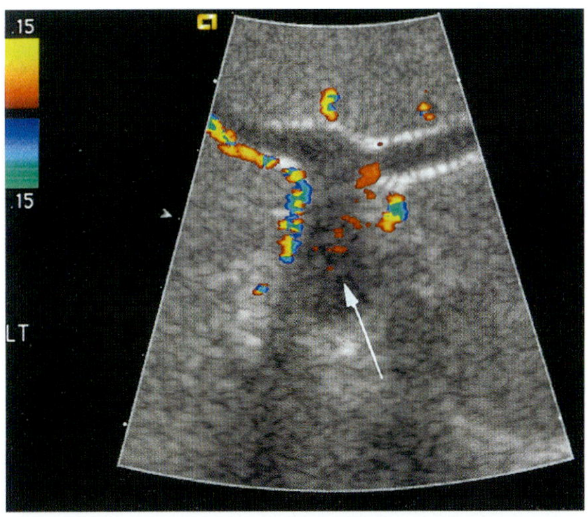

Fig. 10.**14** Absence of color Doppler signal in the portal vein following transplantation indicates the presence of thrombus (arrow)

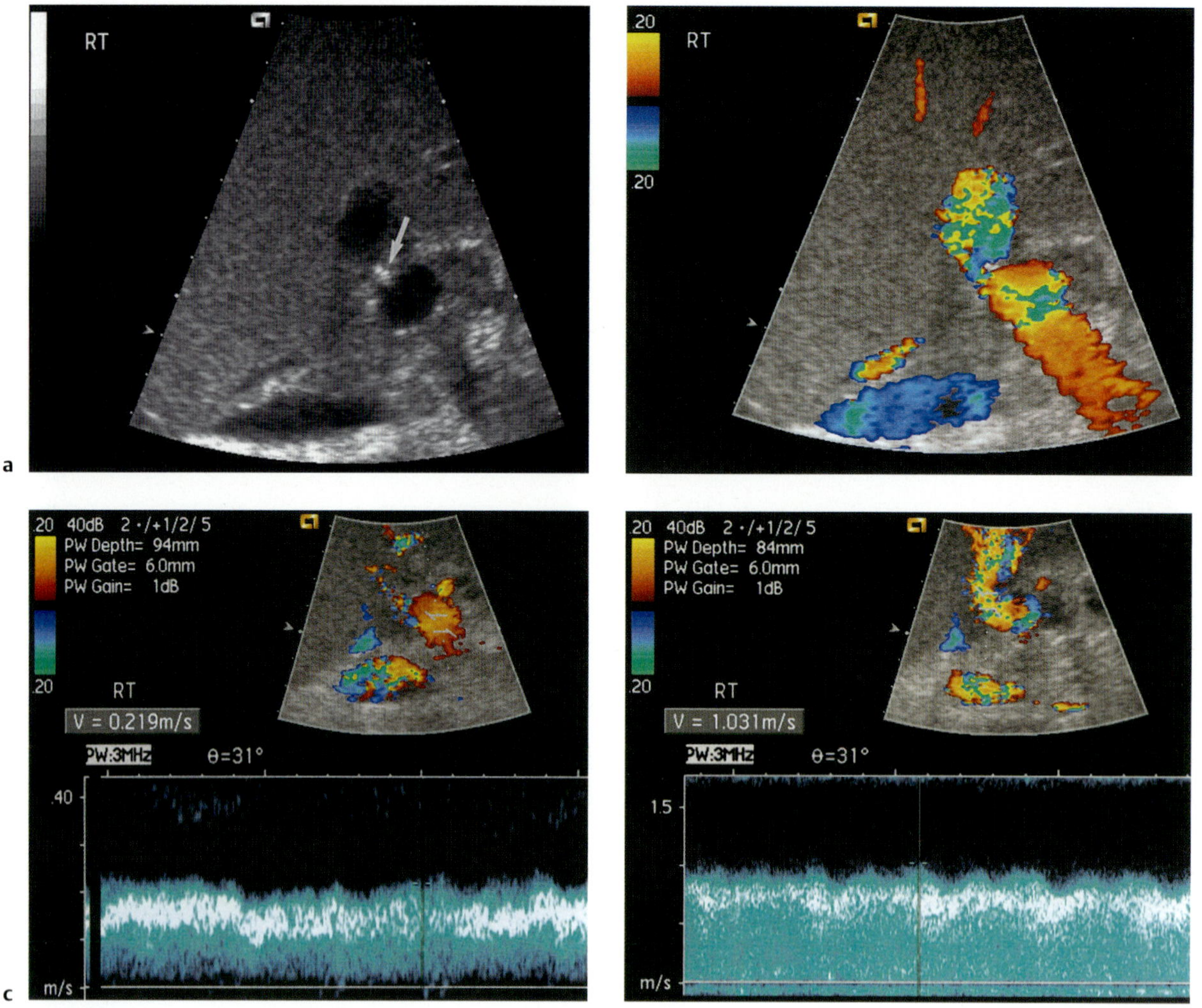

Fig. 10.**15** **a** B mode imaging of echogenic suture material (arrow) at the level of the portal vein anastomoses in a transplant patient. **b** Color Doppler imaging of the portal vein demonstrating marked narrowing and color Doppler disturbance at the site of narrowing in the portal vein. **c** Velocity measurement of 0.22 m/s in the prestenosis region. **d** A velocity of 1.03 m/s in the turbulent region indicates a portal vein stenosis

ring in less than 2% of patients, more often in children.[4,21,22] Portal vein thrombosis is invariably related to technical difficulties; misalignment, and a redundant length of portal vein, leading to kinking and stricturing. Other predisposing factors include previous portal vein shunt surgery, previous portal vein thrombosis and sclerosis, vessel trauma from a portal cannula, and underlying prothrombotic state.[22] Acute rejection with diminished portal venous flow has been proposed as a cause of portal vein thrombosis and may be an important factor in small children with full-size liver grafts.[23] Portal vein thrombus may be demonstrated on ultrasound as internal echoes within the portal vein, expansion of the portal vein, and loss of color Doppler signal. Reduction in the hepatic artery RI accompanies portal vein thrombosis and may be a helpful secondary sign for the determination of portal vein thrombosis. A hepatic artery RI of 0.50 or less, together with an equivocal finding at portal venous CDUS, is reported to have a specificity of 100% and a sensitivity of 44% for portal vein thrombosis.[24]

Assessment of the splenic length in many post-transplant patients shows a small reduction in spleen size; a significant increase suggests portal hypertension.[8] Portal vein stenosis (Fig. 10.**15**) is recognized but is again uncommon.[4] A peak velocity of greater than 1 m/s or a three- to four-fold step-up in velocity across the narrowed portal vein is suggestive of stenosis.[8,21] Transhepatic portal vein cannulation and measurement of venous pressures across the anastomosis may document portal vein stenosis in the absence of any thrombus.[3] Percutaneous transhepatic dilatation of the portal vein stenosis may be successful.[25] However, if this technique fails, patients should be treated by portosystemic shunt or revision of the portal vein anastomosis.[3] If adequate collateralization occurs, both with portal vein stenosis and portal vein thrombosis, graft survival may be unaffected.

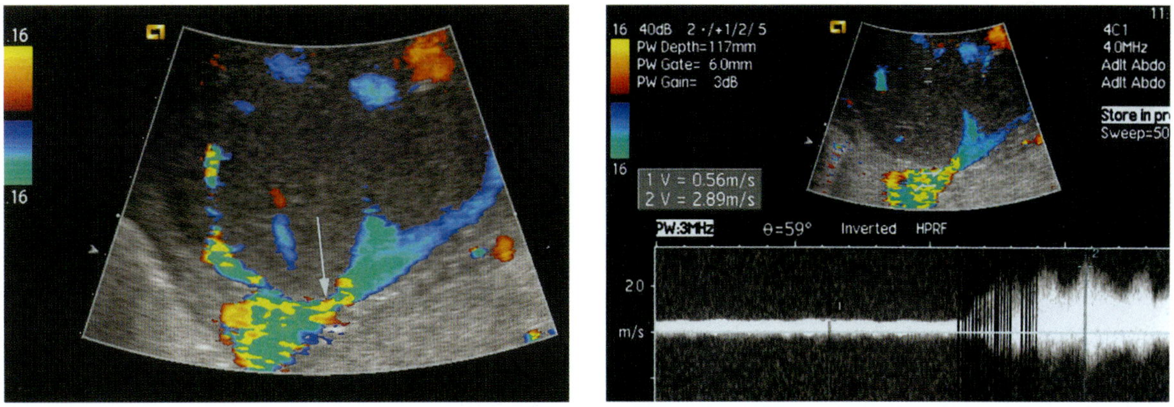

Fig. 10.**16** **a** Color Doppler imaging of a narrowed IVC demonstrating color flow disturbance (arrow). **b** Velocity increases from 0.56 m/s to 2.89 m/s across the narrow segment of transplant IVC

Portal Vein Gas

Intraportal venous gas is occasionally seen as echogenic shadowing within the portal vein, and is a more common finding than previously recognized. While it may be secondary to necrotic bowel or intra-abdominal sepsis, it can also be an incidental finding after liver transplantation, without any sequelae.[26]

Hepatic Veins

Occlusion or stenosis of the IVC anastomosis is rare (Fig. 10.**16**), occurring in less than 1 % of recipients.[4] Suprahepatic stenosis presents with a clinical picture of acute or chronic Budd–Chiari syndrome with ascites, peripheral edema, portal hypertension, and biopsy evidence of hepatic venous congestion.[4] Although CDUS may suggest the diagnosis (Fig. 10.**16**), inferior vena cavography and pressure studies are required for the definitive diagnosis. Hepatic vein thrombosis is rare, as the hepatic veins are not directly involved in a surgical anastomosis. It may be seen when the underlying abnormality recurs in recipients whose transplant was for Budd–Chiari syndrome.[8] Any pathological process that changes liver compliance will alter hepatic vein pulsatility.[27] Perioperative ischemia, vascular catastrophe, rejection, and cholangitis may all cause damping of the spectral Doppler trace.[27]

Summary points:

- The hepatic artery in the post-transplant period is crucial to graft survival as the biliary system is dependent on it, and thrombosis will result in graft loss
- Intrahepatic tardus-parvus spectral Doppler waveform is strongly indicative of a proximal hepatic artery stenosis and should be further investigated with angiography with a view to balloon dilatation

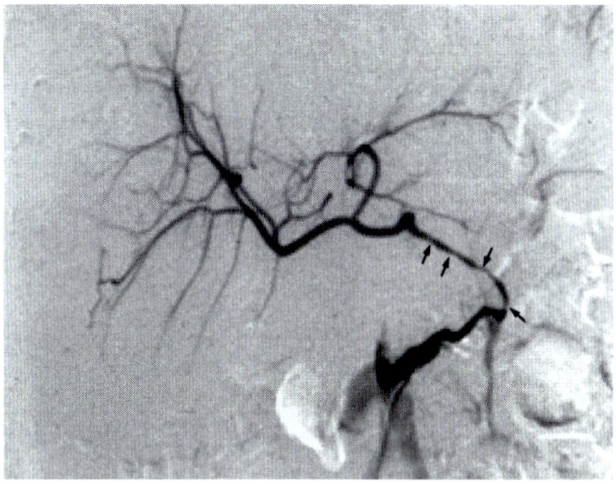

Fig. 10.**17** Multiple nonanastomotic hepatic artery stenosis (arrows) demonstrated in selective “conduit” arteriography in a transplant patient. (Reproduced from *Clinical Radiology*[16] by permission of the Editor)

- Hepatic pseudoaneurysms may be located in an intrahepatic position related to iatrogenic injury or in an extrahepatic position related to sepsis
- Portal vein occlusion following liver transplantation is uncommon but occurs most often in pediatric patients
- A peak velocity greater than 1 m/s or a three- to four-fold step-up in velocity across the narrowed portal vein is suggestive of stenosis

Nonvascular Complications

Rejection

Following hepatic transplantation, acute rejection is the most common serious complication affecting allograft survival, and occurs in more than one third of all liver allografts.[17] Treatment, which is usually successful, involves manipulation of immunosuppressive drug therapy. Nonanastomotic vascular stenosis (Fig. 10.**17**)

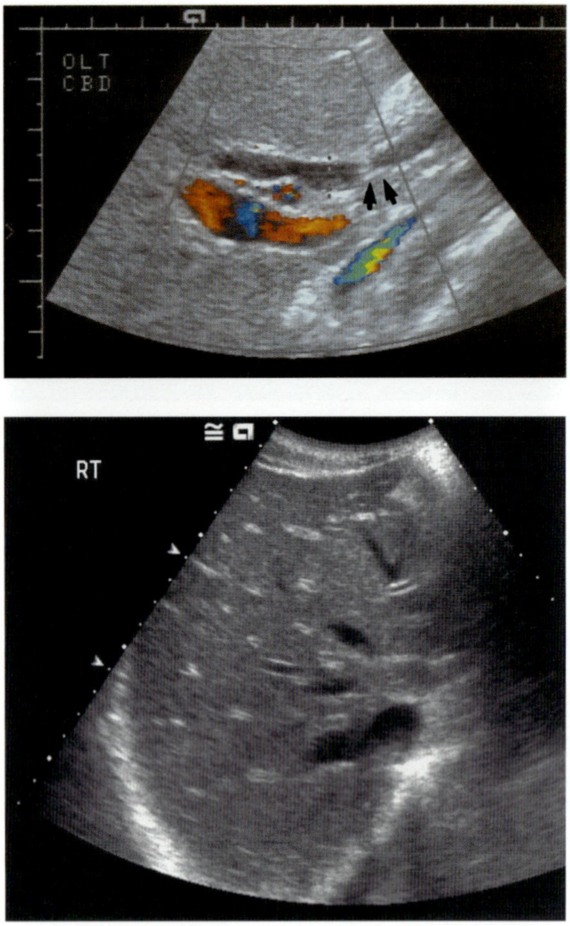

a

b

Fig. 10.**18** **a** Dilated common bile duct after liver transplantation. The surgical sutures at the anastomotic site are visible (arrows). **b** Widespread intrahepatic bile duct dilatation in a post-transplant patient

as well as diffuse intrahepatic arterial narrowing has been seen in patients with transplant rejection. Acute rejection is due to an inflammatory cellular infiltrate and does not significantly affect the peripheral hepatic vasculature.[28] In chronic rejection there is deposition of subintimal foam cells, myointimal foam cells, myointimal hyperplasia, and intimal sclerosis, resulting in progressive arterial narrowing and slow flow with subsequent thrombosis.[29]

CDUS shows a nonspecific profile in acute rejection. Marder et al.[28] found that there was no correlation between the RI and acute rejection, and Longley et al.[30] showed no correlation between loss of hepatic artery diastolic flow and acute rejection. Changes in hepatic arterial and venous velocity profiles reflect alteration in hepatic vascular resistance, which is not specific to rejection, since altered hepatic vascular resistance also occurs with preservation injury, sepsis, and nonthrombotic graft infarction.[6] An area of decreased reflectivity/attenuation on CT and ultrasound respectively has also been described in the periportal region, but this has a low sensitivity and specificity in the diagnosis of rejection.[31] There is no reliable noninvasive diagnostic examination modality to detect liver allograft rejection, the main role of radiology being to exclude other complications prior to a histologic diagnosis with liver biopsy.

Biliary System

Biliary complications are an important cause of postoperative morbidity and mortality in liver transplantation. The three major biliary complications after liver transplantation are biliary obstruction, bile leakage, and generalized bile duct changes (Fig. 10.**18**). The reported incidence of complications has decreased from 50 %, with mortality as high as 30 % in early series,[32–35] to a current complication rate of less than 20 % and a mortality of less than 5 %.[4]

Biliary tract complications are predominantly encountered in the weeks immediately following transplantation, although strictures can be a late manifestation with presentation up to seven years after transplantation.[36] The method of surgical anastomosis, "cold" ischemic time, and associated vascular insufficiency are factors that critically influence the frequency, development, and type of complication. Strictures of the bile duct anastomosis are more common after duct-to-duct reconstruction, occurring in 5–14 % of cases.[32,33] Nonanastomotic strictures (Fig. 10.**19**) carry a worse prognosis, representing a diffuse biliary injury occurring with HAT, prolonged cold ischemia, and ABO-incompatible donors.[3] When nonanastomotic strictures are present, it is important that CDUS be performed to confirm patency of the hepatic artery. In nontransplant patients, ultrasonography is the accepted method for detecting biliary duct dilatation.[37,38] However, the accuracy is lower in liver transplant patients, with a sensitivity of 38–46 % and a specificity of 98 %.[39] Dilatation of the intrahepatic ducts has a higher predictive value for diagnosis of biliary obstruction than does common bile duct diameter.[39] This is explained by the possibility that bile duct dilatation may not have had the opportunity to develop even though obstruction or partial obstruction exists; ultrasound will not identify a bile duct stricture without duct dilatation. If bile duct dilatation is suspected clinically, ultrasound remains the investigation of choice, providing evidence to support the need to proceed to T tube cholangiography, percutaneous transhepatic cholangiography (PTC), or endoscopic retrograde cholangiopancreatography.

Bile leaks are usually secondary to anastomotic complications. Greif et al.[36] surveyed the biliary complications of 1792 patients who had undergone liver transplantation; 50 % of bile leaks were due to anastomotic complications, the remaining leaks were due to HAT (17.2 %), leaks at the T tube site (31 %), and leaks from aberrant ducts.[36] The majority of bile leaks occur early, within the first 30 days of liver transplantation or at the time of removal of the T tube. Diagnosis of a biliary leak is often difficult without cholangiography. Subhepatic collections are common in the early post-transplant period; direct visualization of the biliary tree and site of leak by cholangiography is mandatory.[40] Ultrasound can readily detect intra- and extrahepatic bilomas that occur as a result of post-transplantation bile leaks. However, their appearance may be indistinguishable from that of other collections of fluid in the upper abdomen, such as ascites (Fig. 10.**20**), serum, or hematomas. Ultrasound-guided fine-needle aspiration may confirm the nature of the fluid. Drainage of bile leaks may promote healing of the bile ducts and may save the liver graft.[41]

Fluid Collections

Abscess formation (Fig. 10.**21**) occurs in approximately 10% of liver transplants postoperatively, mostly occurring in subphrenic or subhepatic spaces.[17] Ultrasound guidance will allow drainage of any fluid collection that is found and warrants drainage. Occasionally, fluid collections may be completely obscured by bowel gas on ultrasonography, and CT provides the conclusive imaging modality. Hematoma formation may be seen in the immediate postoperative period and is usually secondary to extensive intraoperative abdominal bleeding from varices. Hematomas may be present at any site, most commonly in the subphrenic and subhepatic space.[17] In the first two weeks following liver transplantation the majority of hematomas are comprised of clotted blood and aspiration is neither necessary nor possible. The development of new collections in the late postoperative period raises the possibility of bile leak as a consequence of HAT, or loculated ascites as a consequence of portal vein or IVC flow abnormalities.[8]

Post-transplantation abdominal bleeding occurs in less than 10% of patients and may be due to hepatic artery pseudoaneurysm, breakdown of a vascular anastomosis, infection, or hemobilia.[42] Radiological investigation may only serve to delay treatment in the unstable patient where surgery is required. However, if the patient is stable, ultrasound-guided aspiration of fluid may help to confirm the presence of free intra-abdominal blood.

Miscellaneous Complications

Infrequently seen complications include pancreatitis and adrenal hemorrhage, both of which may be identified by ultrasound. Enlargement of the pancreas may be seen in uncomplicated pancreatitis, and fluid collections will be detected if a pseudocyst develops. Adrenal infarction, which may be hemorrhagic, occurs on the right side and is caused by inadvertent ligation of the adrenal vein at the time of transplantation.[1] Pleural effusions, which are sympathetic in nature, are

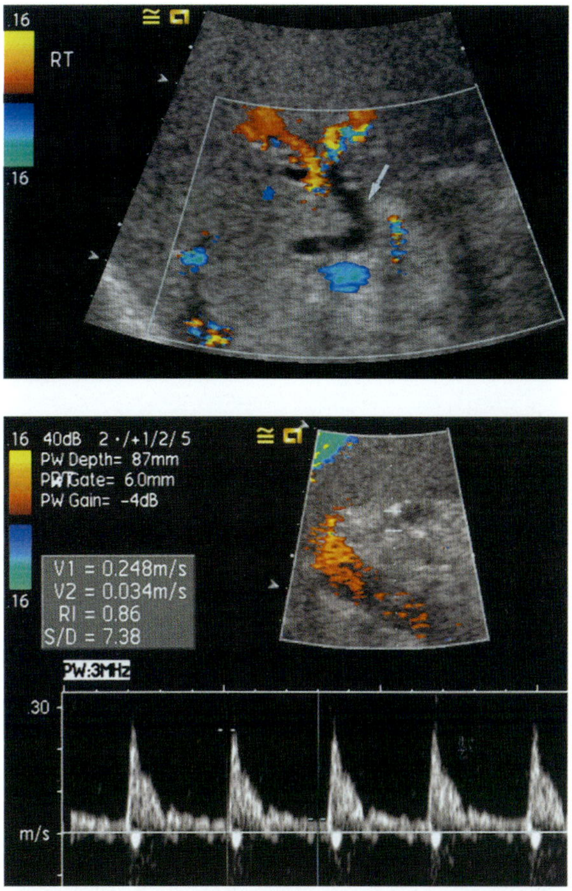

a

b

Fig. 10.**19** **a** Nonanastomotic intrahepatic bile duct dilatation in a post-transplant patient (arrow). **b** High-resistance hepatic artery (RI = 0.86) spectral Doppler waveform in the same patient suggesting an ischemic cause of the biliary abnormality

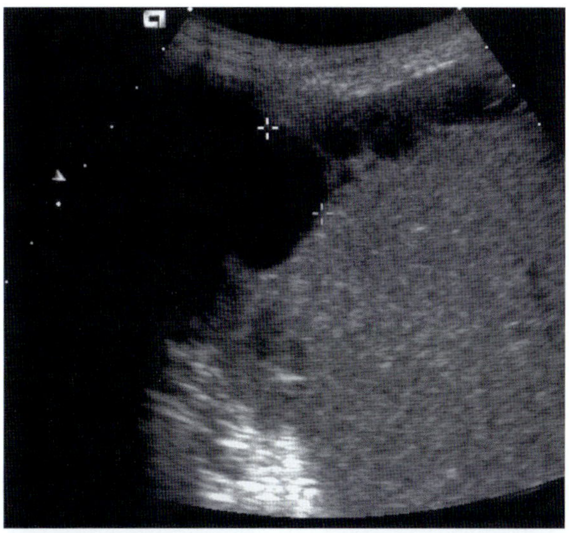

Fig. 10.**20** A fluid collection present at the upper surface of a transplant liver (+–+). On aspiration this was found to be bile and representative of a biloma

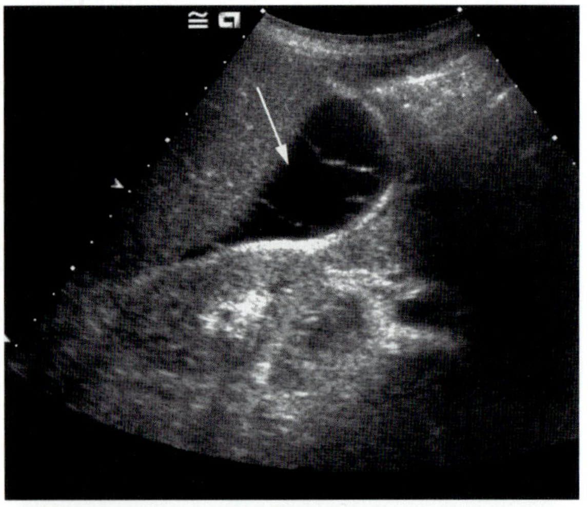

Fig. 10.**21** A septated subhepatic fluid collection representing an infected collection (arrow)

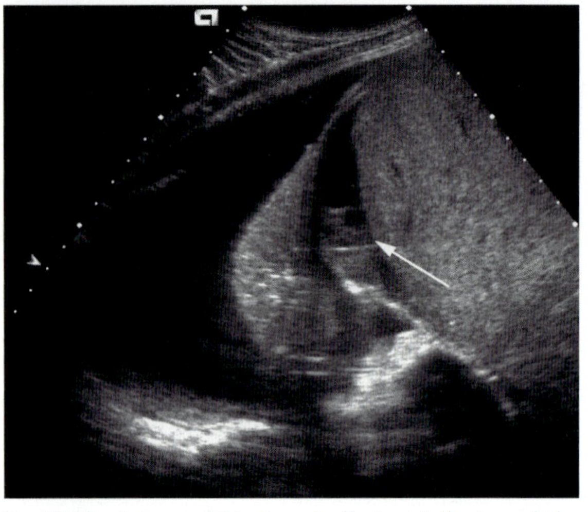

Fig. 10.**22** A large right pleural effusion, tethering of the right lung, and a subphrenic fluid collection (arrow) in a posttransplant patient

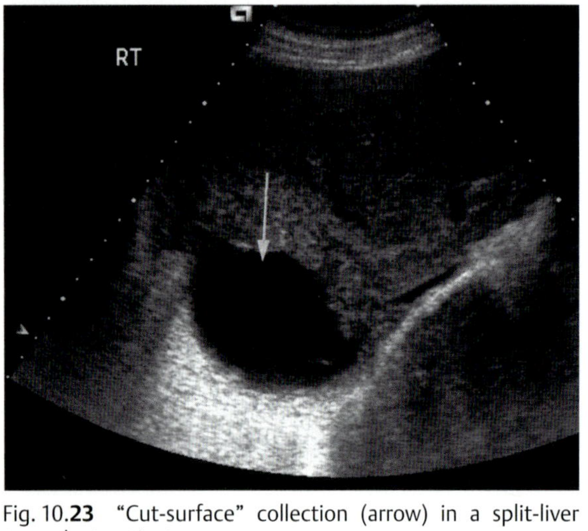

Fig. 10.**23** "Cut-surface" collection (arrow) in a split-liver transplant patient

commonly seen on the right side (Fig. 10.**22**). These can be drained under ultrasound guidance if respiratory compromise is experienced.

Complications of Split Liver Transplantation

While no difference has been noted in the frequency of primary graft nonfunction or arterial thrombosis in split grafts as compared with full-size grafts, the collective European experience suggests an 18.5 % incidence of postoperative hemorrhage, 11 % incidence of HAT, 4 % incidence of PVT, and a 20 % biliary complication rate. Biliary complications include anastomotic and cut-surface leaks and anastomotic and nonanastomotic stricture formation (Fig. 10.**23**).[43]

■ ***Summary points:***

- There are no reliable ultrasound criteria for the diagnosis of rejection; liver biopsy is the definitive investigation, safely guided by ultrasound
- Nonanastomotic bile duct strictures carry a worse prognosis than anastomotic strictures as they are representative of diffuse biliary injury
- There are no distinguishing ultrasound features of fluid collections in the upper abdomen; they may be bilomas, ascites, serum, or hematomas
- Abscess formation occurs in 10 % of liver transplant patients, most often in the subphrenic or subhepatic spaces

Pediatric Liver Transplantation

All vessels are more prone to stenosis and obstruction in children than in adults, presumably due to the small vessel size. The reported incidence of HAT varies from 9 % to 18 % in children.[4] A direct hepatic artery end-to-end anastomosis is used whenever possible; otherwise an iliac artery homograft is used.

In cases of HAT in children, collateral circulation that reestablishes intrahepatic arterial flow occasionally develops, but in most cases the presence of collateral circulation does not appear to protect the liver from eventual ischemic injury.[44] The potential to form collateral circulation may be related to the type of biliary reconstruction performed in the pediatric patient. If there is a pretransplant diagnosis of biliary atresia, a Roux-en-Y choledochojejunostomy with a straight tube or internal stent is used for the biliary anastomosis. This brings the highly vascular jejunal arterial bed close to the transplanted liver; with arterial occlusion, collateral vessels can be recruited from the jejunal vascular arcade.[10] The collateral circulation so formed may result in a decreased sensitivity of CDUS for HAT, because the CDUS examination may detect the network of collaterals around the occluded artery and this may be interpreted as a patent hepatic artery. Confu-

sion with collaterals is reported to occur in 85% of children with HAT.[45,46]
Complications can also be seen secondary to the Roux-en-Y loop, including Roux loop torsion, Roux loop intussusception, Roux loop infarction, and meconium obstruction of the Roux loop.[3,47] In addition, the Roux loop has the disadvantage of impeding access to the biliary tract, so these children require a PTC under general anesthesia for detailed evaluation of the biliary tree.
Finally, diaphragmatic paralysis with consequent respiratory compromise has been identified in a minority of young children following OLT. In these cases ultrasound can provide real-time imaging of the diaphragmatic movement.[8]

Summary point:

- In pediatric liver transplantation, hepatic artery thrombosis in the presence of a Roux-en-Y choledochojejunostomy is less likely to result in graft loss as collaterals are recruited from the highly vascular jejunal arterial bed.

References

1. Zajko AB, Campbell WL, Bron KM, Schade RR, Koneru RR, Van Thiel D. Diagnostic and interventional radiology in liver transplantation. Gastroenterol Clin North Am 1988;17:105–143.
2. Kok T, Slooff MJH, Thijn CJ, et al. Routine Doppler ultrasound for the detection of clinically unsuspected vascular complications in the early post operative phase after orthotopic liver transplantation. Transpl Int 1998;11:272–6.
3. Gimson AES, Karani JB, Heaton ND. Major biliary tract and vascular complications. In: Williams R, Portmann B, Tan KC, editors. The practice of liver transplantation. 1st ed. London: Churchill Livingstone; 1995. p. 199–209.
4. Karani JB, Heaton ND. Imaging in liver transplantation [review]. Clin Radiol 1998;53:317–22.
5. Nolten A, Sproat IA. Hepatic artery thrombosis after transplantation; temporal accuracy of diagnosis with duplex ultrasound and the syndrome of impending thrombosis. Radiology 1996;198:553–9.
6. Sidhu PS, Ryan SM, Richardson HD, Rela M, Heaton ND, Karani JB. The role of Levovist in the assessment of hepatic artery thrombosis following liver transplantation. Radiology 1999;213:210
7. Propeck PA, Scanlan KA. Reversed or absent hepatic arterial diastolic flow in liver transplants shown by duplex sonography: a poor predictor of subsequent hepatic artery thrombosis. AJR Am J Roentgenol 1992;159:1199–1201.
8. Meire H. Transplant liver assessment. In: Meire H, Cosgrove DO, Dewbury K, Farrant P, eds. Abdominal and General Ultrasound. 2nd ed. London: Churchill Livingstone, 2000; 280–294.
9. Tzakis A, Gordon R, Shaw B, Iwatsuki S, Starzl IT. Clinical presentation of hepatic artery thrombosis after liver transplantation in the cyclosporine era. Transplantation 1985;40:667–671.
10. Flint EW, Sumkin JH, Zajko AB, Bowen A. Duplex sonography of hepatic artery thrombosis after liver transplantation in the cyclosporin era. AJR Am J Roentgenol 1988;151:481–3.
11. Katyal S, Oliver JH, Buck DG, Federle MP. Detection of vascular complications after liver transplantation: early experience in multislice CT angiography with volume rendering. AJR Am J Roentgenol 2000;175:1735–9.
12. Kopka L, Rodenwaldt J, Vossherich R, et al. Hepatic blood supply; comparison of optimized dual phase contrast-enhanced 3-D MRA and DSA. Radiology 1999;211:51–8.
13. Stafford-Johnson DB, Hamilton BH, Dong Q, et al. Vascular complications of liver transplantation: evaluation with gadolinium-enhanced MR angiography. Radiology 1998;207:153–60.
14. Glockner JF, Forauer AR, Solomon H, Varma CR, Perman WH. 3-D gadolinium enhanced MRA of vascular complications after orthoptic liver transplantation. AJR Am J Roentgenol 2000;174:1447–53.
15. Abbasoglu O, Levy MF, Vodapally MS, et al. Hepatic artery stenosis after liver transplantation – incidence, presentation, treatment, and long term outcome. Transplantation 1997;27:250–5.
16. Sidhu PS, Ellis SM, Karani JB, Ryan SM. Hepatic artery stenosis following liver transplantation: significance of the tardus parvus waveform and the role of microbubble contrast media in the detection of a focal stenosis. Clin Radiol 2002 [in press].
17. Oliver JH, Federle MP, Campbell WL, Zajko AB. Imaging the hepatic transplant. Radiol Clin North Am 1991;29:1285–98.
18. Dodd GD, Memel DS, Zajko AB, Baron RL, Santaguida LA. Hepatic artery stenosis and thrombosis in transplant recipients: Doppler diagnosis with resistive index and systolic acceleration time. Radiology 1994;192:657–61.
19. Marshall MM, Muiesan P, Kane PA, Rela M, Heaton ND, Karani JB, Sidhu PS. Hepatic pseudoaneurysms following liver transplantation: incidence, presenting figures and management. Clin Radiol 2001;56:579–87.
20. Tobben PJ, Zajko AB, Sumkin JH, et al. Pseudoaneurysms complicating organ transplatation: roles of CT, duplex sonography and angiography. Radiology 1988;169:65–70.
21. Glockner JF, Forauer AR. Vascular or ischemic complications after liver transplantation. AJR Am J Roentgenol 1999;173:1055–9.
22. Lerut J, Tzakis A, Bron KM, et al. Complications of venous reconstruction in human orthotopic liver transplantation. Ann Surg 1987;205:404–14.
23. Samuel D, Gillet D, Reynes M, Bismuth H. Portal and arterial thrombosis in liver transplantation: a frequent event in severe rejection. Transplant Proc 1989;21:2225–7.
24. Platt JF, Rubin JM, Ellis JH. Hepatic artery resistance changes in portal vein thrombosis. Radiology 1995;196:95–8.
25. Raby N, Karani JB, Thomas S, O'Grady JG, Williams R. Stenoses of vascular anastomoses after hepatic transplantation: treatment with ballon angioplasty. AJR Am J Roentgenol 1991;157:167–71.
26. Chezmar JL, Nelson RC, Bernardino ME. Portal venous gas after hepatic transplantation; sonographic detection and clinical significance. AJR Am J Roentgenol 1989;153:1203–5.
27. Coulden RA, Britton PD, Farman P, Noble-Jamieson G, Wright DGD. Preliminary report: hepatic vein Doppler in the early diagnosis of acute liver transplant rejection. Lancet 1990;336:273–5.
28. Marder DM, De Marino GB, Sumkin JH, Sheahan DG. Liver transplant rejection: value of the resistive index in Doppler US of hepatic arteries. Radiology 1989;173:127–9.
29. Demetris JA, Slasky S, Van Thiel DH, Starzl TE, Dekker A. Pathology of hepatic transplantation; a review of 62 adult allograft recipients immunosuppressed with a cyclosporine/steroid regimen. Am J Pathol 1985;118:151–61.
30. Longley DG, Skolnick ML, Sheahan DG. Acute allograft rejection in liver transplant recipients: lack of correlation with loss of hepatic artery diastolic flow. Radiology 1988;169:417–20.
31. Kaplan SB, Sumkin J, Campbell WL, Zajko AB, Demetris AJ. Periportal low attenuation areas on CT; value as evidence of

liver transplant rejection. AJR Am J Roentgenol 1989;152:285–7.
32. Stratta RJ, Wood RP, Langnas AN, et al. Diagnosis and treatment of biliary tract complications after orthoptic liver transplant. Surgery 1989;106:675–84.
33. Lerut J, Gordon RD, Iwatsuki S, et al. Biliary tract complications in human orthoptic liver transplantation. Transplantation 1987;43:47–51.
34. Klein AS, Savador S, Burdick JF, et al. Reduction of morbidity and mortality from biliary complications after liver transplantation. Hepatology 1991;14:818–23.
35. Lopez RR, Bennar KG, Ivanceu K, Keefe EB, Deverney LW, Pinson CW. Management of biliary complications after liver transplantation. Am J Surg 1992;163:519–24.
36. Greif F, Bronsther OL, Van Thiel DH, et al. The incidence, timing and management of biliary tract complications after liver transplantation. Ann Surg 1994;219:40–5.
37. Koenigsberg M, Weiner SN, Walzer A. The accuracy of sonography in the differential diagnosis of obstructive jaundice; a comparison with cholangiography. Radiology 1979;133:157–65.
38. Neimin HL, Mintzer RA. Accuracy of biliary duct ultrasound; conparison with cholangiography. AJR Am J Roentgenol 1977;129:979–82.
39. Kok T, Van der Sluis A, Klein JP, et al. Ultrasound and cholangiography for the diagnosis of biliary complications after orthoptic liver transplantation; a comparative study. J Clin Ultrasound 1996;24:103–15.
40. Evans RA, Raby ND, O'Grady J, et al. Biliary complications following orthoptic liver transplantation. Clin Radiol 1990;41:190–4.
41. Kaplan S, Zajko AB, Koneru B. Hepatic bilomas due to hepatic artery thrombosis in liver transplant recipients:percutaneous drainage and clinical outcome. Radiology 1990;174:1031–5.
42. Woods RP, Shaw BW, Starzl TE. Extrahepatic complications of liver transplantation. Semin Liver Dis 1985;5:377–84.
43. Heaton ND, Corbally MT, Rela M, Tan KC. Surgical techniques of segmental reduction. Split and auxillary liver transplantation. In: Williams R, Portmann B, Tan KC, editors. The practice of liver transplantation. 1st ed. London: Churchill Livingstone; 1995. p. 143–51.
44. Wozney P, Zajko AB, Bron KM, Point S, Starzl TE. Vascular complications after liver transplantation: a five-year experience. AJR Am J Roentgenol 1986;147:657–63.
45. McDiarmid SV. Liver transplantation. The pediatric challenge. Clin Liver Dis 2000;4:879–927.
46. McDiarmid SV. Risk factors and outcomes after pediatric liver transplantation. Liver Transpl Surg 1996;2:44–56.
47. Osorio RW, Freise CE, Stock PG, et al. Non-operative management of biliary leaks after orthotopic liver transplantation. Transplantation 1993;55:1074–7.

Long-Term Ultrasound Follow-Up of Liver Transplantation

R. C. Beese and P. S. Sidhu

Introduction

Ultrasound plays a vital role in the long-term follow-up of liver transplant patients.[1,2] Ultrasound provides a simple first-line noninvasive imaging modality to assess the graft for structural complications; disease recurrence in the graft is an important cause of morbidity and mortality in the transplant patient.[3] Long-term complications of immunosuppression may be assessed with ultrasound. In our institution all post-transplant patients undergo a color Doppler ultrasound examination immediately prior to clinical follow-up, with results available to the consulting hepatologist.

Ultrasound is the imaging modality of choice in patients who develop symptoms or deranged biochemical parameters at any stage following liver transplantation. A detailed knowledge of the surgical anatomy of the transplant graft (including older surgical techniques) is required for accurate assessment of the graft at follow-up. The following chapter reviews the possible long-term structural complications that can occur in the transplanted liver, with disease recurrence dealt with in the context of initial indications for transplantation, and complications of long-term immunosuppression are examined.

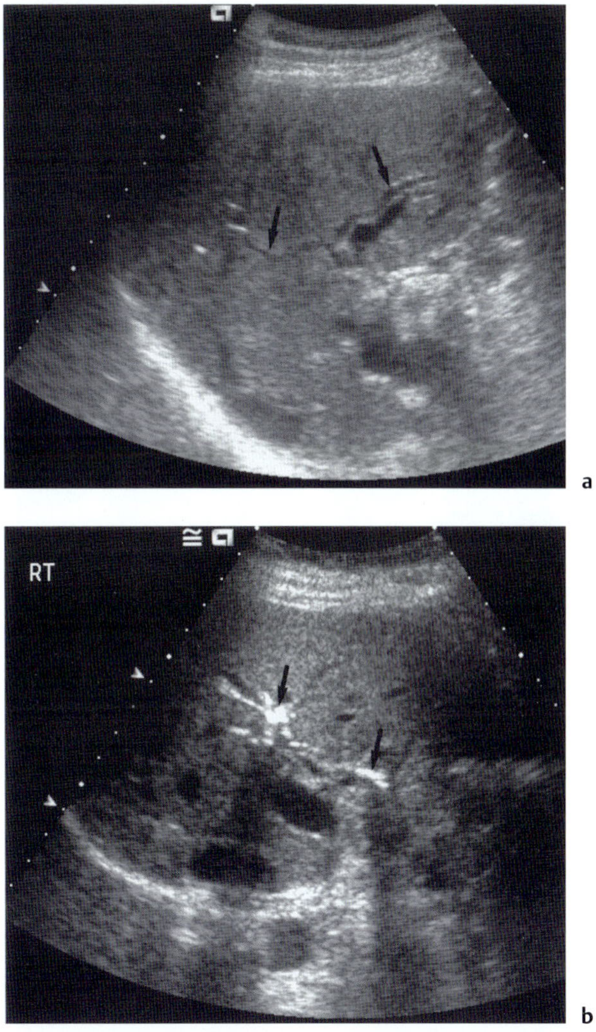

Fig. 11.**1** **a** Roux-en-Y loop in a transplant patient. Narrowing at the anastomosis site has produced intrahepatic bile duct dilatation (arrows). **b** Roux-en-Y loop allows free reflux of air from the jejunal bowel loop, producing "aerobilia" (arrows)

Vascular Complications

All vascular complications discussed in the previous chapter are relevant in the long-term surveillance, with some important differences.

Hepatic Artery

The main hepatic artery "proper" and the left and right branches should be examined with color Doppler ultrasound with a spectral Doppler waveform recorded. Color Doppler studies of the intrahepatic arterial tree become more difficult to interpret with time after the operation. A normal hepatic artery spectral Doppler waveform on serial examinations accurately excludes significant hepatic artery disease.[4] The diagnosis of hepatic artery stenosis may be inferred using color Doppler imaging if serial hepatic arterial spectral Doppler waveform shows a progressive reduction in arterial velocity and the development of the tardus parvus waveform in the absence of parenchymal abnormality.[5–7] Angiography should then be recommended.

Hepatic artery stenosis and occlusion over a long period may have less devastating immediate consequences to the liver graft than acute hepatic artery occlusion in the immediate post-operative period. If the hepatic artery narrows and subsequently becomes occluded, graft function maybe preserved by the formation of a number of collateral arteries. Furthermore, when a Roux-en-Y loop is fashioned in children or adults (Fig. 11.**1**),

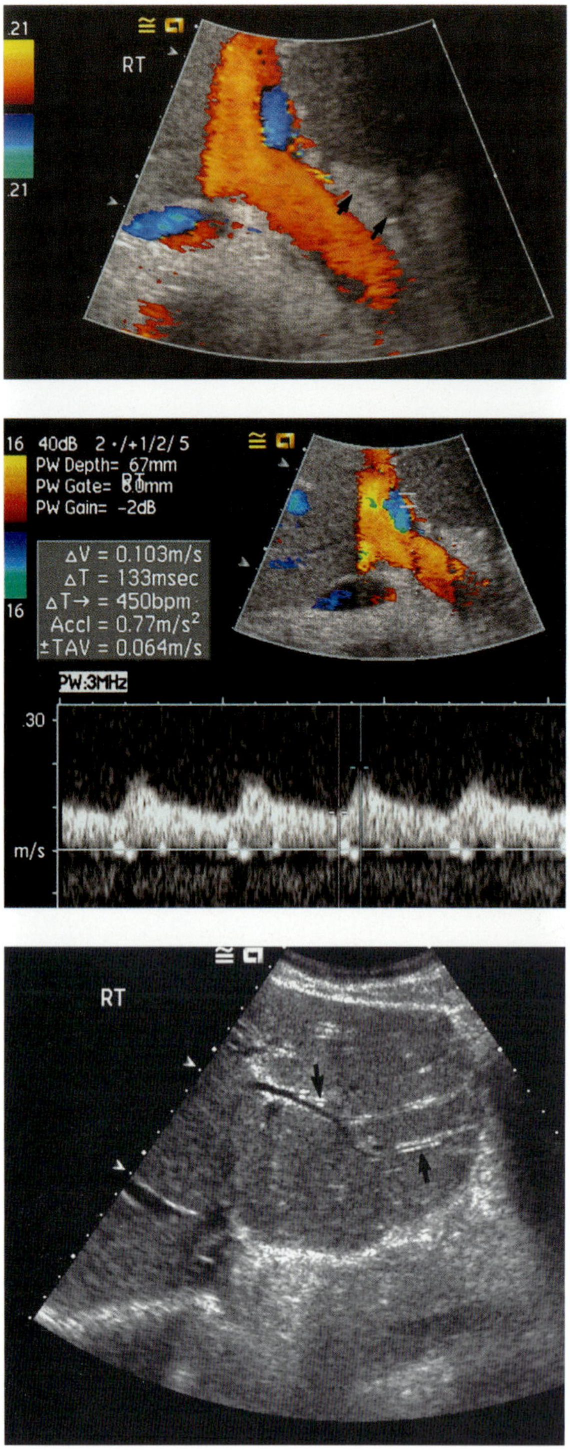

a

b

c

Fig. 11.2 **a** Occluded hepatic artery (arrows) in an adult liver transplant patient, of six months' duration. **b** Intrahepatic hepatic artery spectral Doppler analysis demonstrates the tardus parvus waveform with an acceleration time of 0.13 seconds. **c** Dilated intrahepatic bile ducts (arrows) as a result of ischemic changes secondary to the occlusion of the main hepatic artery

replacing a recipient common bile duct, the highly vascular jejunal bed allows rapid collateralization and protects the graft from acute ischemic complications.[5] In the event of the establishment of a good collateral supply, an entirely normal intrahepatic spectral Doppler waveform may be demonstrated even in the presence of complete main hepatic artery occlusion (Fig. 11.**2**). A more common finding is the damping of the intrahepatic systolic arterial spectral Doppler waveform with the maintenance of high diastolic spectral Doppler waveform.[8] Hence, the presence of hepatic arterial flow within the graft must be taken in the clinical context of graft function.

Although late arterial occlusion may be clinically silent, the majority of patients suffer one or more complications.[9] In the first few weeks after transplantation, arterial occlusion may present as a biliary leak. However, if the biliary tree survives the initial ischemic event, then biliary strictures may develop, particularly at the hilum of the left and right ducts.[10] This in turn may lead to infective complications such as cholangitis and biliary abscess formation. Hepatic abscess formation is also more common with chronic ischemia (Fig. 11.**3**).[9]

Portal Vein

Portal Vein Occlusion

Immediate portal vein complications are rare, with portal vein thrombosis occurring in fewer than 2% of cases of liver transplantation.[11] Long-term portal vein occlusion is a rare late consequence of transplantation (Fig. 11.**4**). It is seen in patients with conditions predisposing to an increased incidence of portal vein thrombosis: coagulopathies, Budd–Chiari syndrome, abnormal portal vein anatomy including cases of cutdown liver or live related donor patients with a portal vein conduit, or patients who have had an operative thrombectomy.[11] Acute portal vein occlusion presents with graft dysfunction and signs and symptoms of portal hypertension. Ultrasound will demonstrate thrombus and features of portal hypertension.

Portal Vein Stenosis

Portal vein stenosis is a rare but important complication, which can lead to portal hypertension and portal vein thrombosis.[12] Turbulent flow is common at the portal vein anastomotic site, and this tends to be the area where a stenosis occurs (Fig. 11.**5**). Patients with portal vein stenosis usually have increasing portal vein velocity measurements and increasing spleen size over time, with a portal vein that demonstrates "waisting," i.e., pre- and poststenotic dilatation.[13]

A portal vein peak systolic velocity of 1.00 m/s indicates significant hemodynamic stenosis that warrants further investigation. In children with a left lobe graft the portal vein may become "stretched" following hypertrophy of the transplanted left lobe. This results in

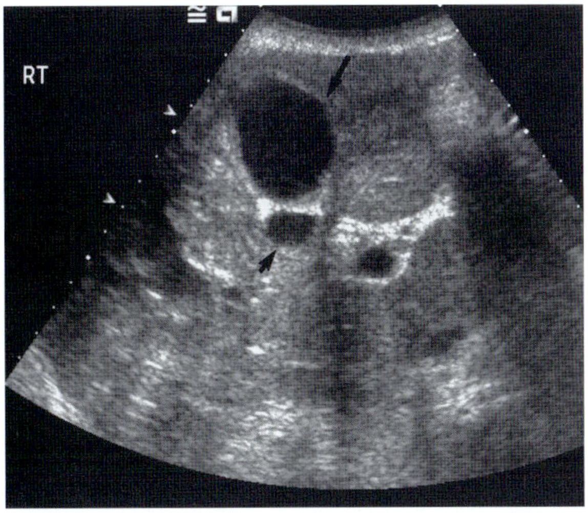

Fig. 11.**3** Multiple biliary abscesses (arrows) in a liver transplant patient with hepatic artery occlusion

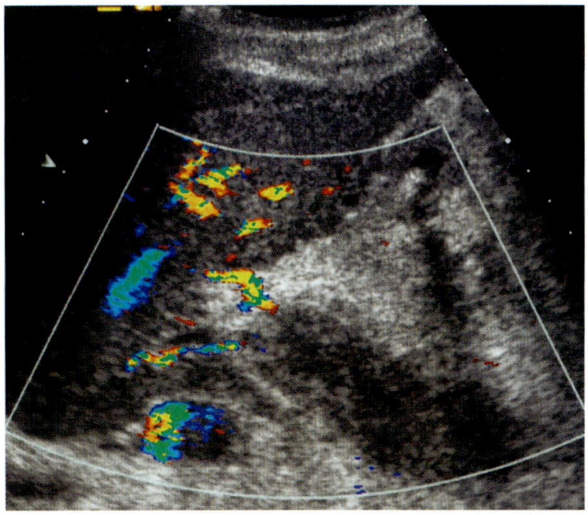

Fig. 11.**4** Portal vein occlusion following liver transplantation

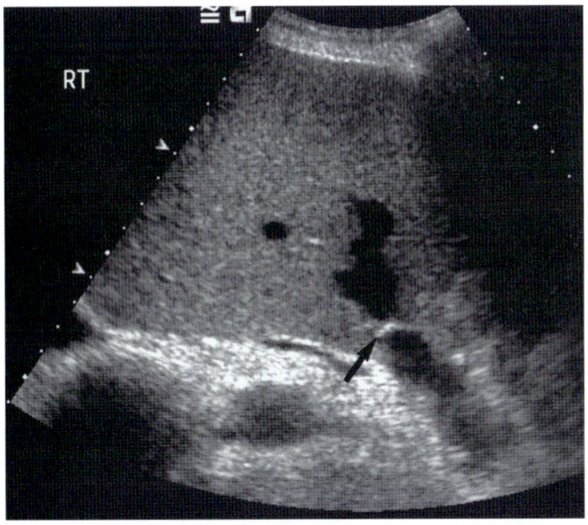

a

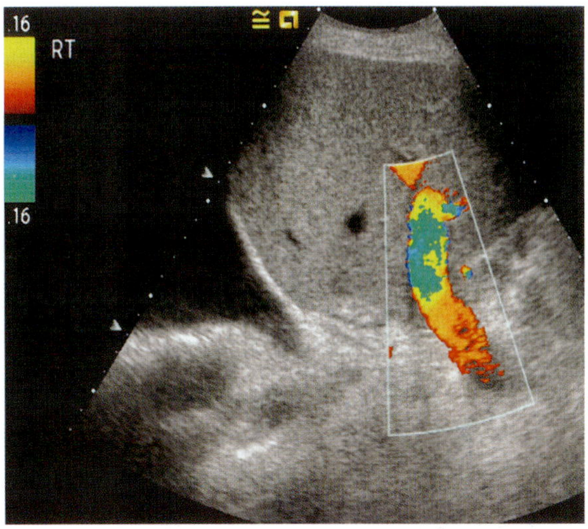

b

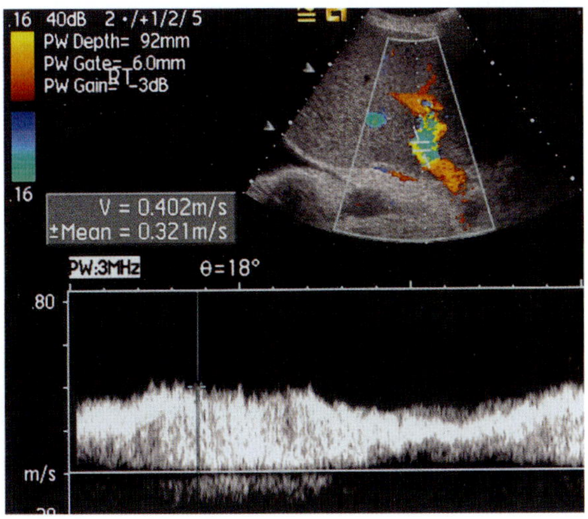

c

Fig. 11.**5** **a** Suture material is seen as an echogenic area (arrow) in the portal vein. **b** Minor narrowing with turbulence on color Doppler imaging is present at the anastomotic site in the portal vein. **c** Spectral Doppler analysis demonstrates a velocity of 0.40 m/s, not suggestive of a stenosis of the portal vein

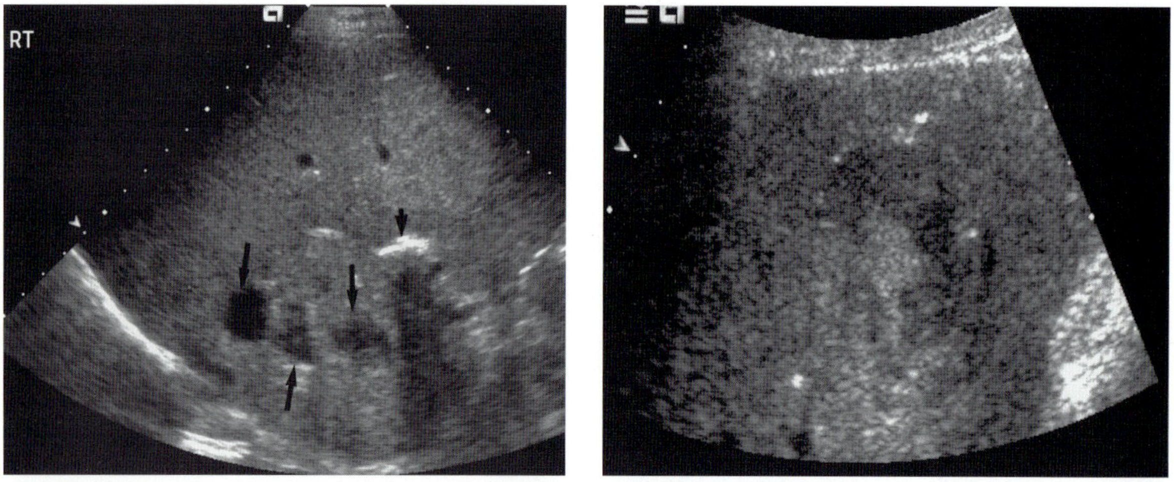

a b

Fig. 11.**6** **a** Abscess in the right lobe of a transplant liver. Pockets of low reflectivity (arrows) and high reflectivity (short arrow) indicate the pressure of fluid and air. **b** Abscess in the left lobe of a transplant liver. A more echogenic collection than the previous example

portal vein occlusion, which may be treated using a jump graft. Serial measurements of the spleen should be made at all ultrasound examinations, as an increase in spleen size may be an indicator of portal hypertension.

Inferior Vena Cava

Thrombosis or stenosis of inferior vena cava (IVC) anastomoses are rare, occurring in less than 1–4% of patients, and are usually due to technical surgical problems or a consequence of compression by a fluid collection.[14] Infrahepatic stenosis may cause only lower extremity swelling. Suprahepatic stenosis presents with a Budd–Chiari-like picture of ascites, liver enlargement, and pleural effusion. Color Doppler studies will demonstrate these changes and demonstrate absence or dampening of the normal hepatic vein spectral Doppler waveform. There may also be distension of the hepatic veins and IVC.[15]

■ ***Summary points:***

- A normal hepatic artery spectral Doppler waveform on serial ultrasound examinations accurately excludes significant hepatic artery disease
- Hepatic artery occlusion and stenosis over a long period may have less devastating consequences for liver graft function than acute hepatic artery occlusion in the immediate postoperative period; hepatic abscess formation is more common

Nonvascular Complications

Renal Complications

Renal insufficiency due to nephrotoxic effects of the immunosuppressive therapy is a common complication and has been reported in up to 25% of pediatric recipients.[16] Ultrasound may be used to exclude obstruction in patients with deteriorating renal function and give information about the size and reflectivity of the kidneys.

Graft-Versus-Host Disease

Graft-versus-host disease is a common complication following bone marrow transplantation and is becoming increasingly recognized following solid organ transplantation.[17] It has serious consequences and may be fatal. Imaging has no role in the assessment of graft versus host disease other than to exclude structural abnormalities of the graft.

Rejection

Rejection is common in liver transplant recipients but imaging is neither sensitive nor specific for detecting rejection.[18] Ultrasound is used to exclude structural abnormalities in the graft that may have a similar clinical presentation to rejection. The diagnosis of rejection is made on histological study following liver biopsy.

Infection

Infection is the most common complication of liver transplantation, with immunosuppressive therapy the major risk factor.[19] In the presence of a structural abnormality of the graft, such as hepatic artery thrombosis or a biliary stricture, infection may be localized to

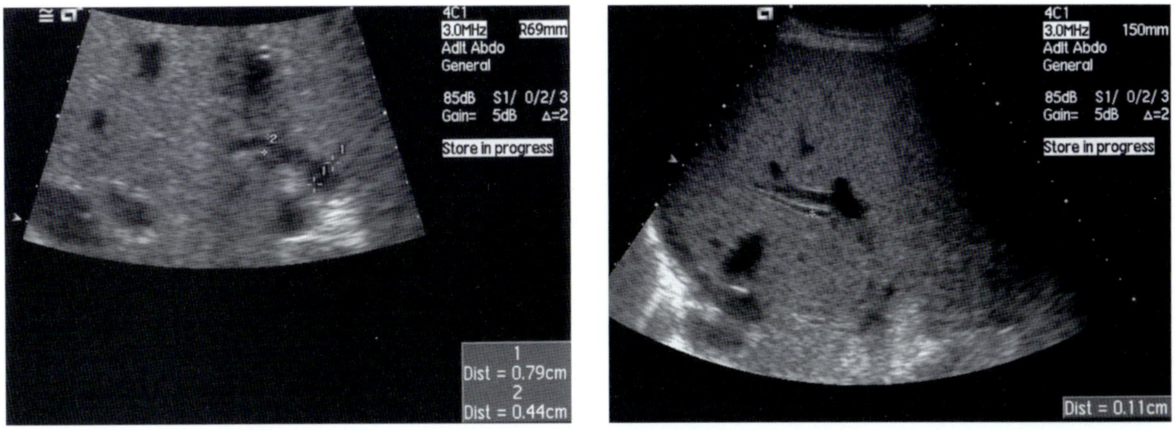

a b

Fig. 11.7 Nonanastomotic biliary strictures. **a** Irregular dilatation of the more central bile ducts in a liver transplant patient. **b** Peripheral isolated bile duct dilatation in the same patient

the graft. Hepatic abscess formation may be readily visualized with ultrasound and treated by ultrasound-guided drainage. Abscesses may be visualized as either increased echogenicity or decreased echogenicity (Fig. 11.**6**). A retrospective review of adult liver transplantation over a nine-year period demonstrated an incidence of hepatic abscess of 3.9%.[9] Eighty-five percent of abscesses were bacterial in origin, 15% fungal and contributed to eventual graft failure.

Biliary Complications

The current surgical practice for biliary reconstruction is end-to-end anastomoses, where the recipient bile duct may be used. However, if the recipient has an underlying biliary abnormality with an insufficient length of common bile duct, such as in biliary atresia or sclerosing cholangitis, or when a cut-down graft is transplanted, it will be necessary to construct a Roux-en-Y-loop.

Bile duct dilatation is unusual in the early postoperative period.[6] On ultrasound, in the early postoperative period it is practice to measure the common, left, and right bile ducts to confirm nondilatation and record the baseline measurement. This is particularly important in cut-down grafts in children, where intrahepatic bile duct dimensions are of adult proportions and early measurement will avoid an erroneous call of bile duct dilatation. The presence of a normal biliary system on ultrasound makes the presence of a structural biliary complication unlikely.[2] If the bile duct size increases are accompanied by biochemical changes or persist for more than three months after transplantation, a biliary system abnormality is invariably present and cholangiography is then required (Fig. 11.**7**).[2]

Nonanastomotic biliary strictures at the hilum of the liver are most commonly associated with ischemia as a consequence of hepatic artery stenosis or thrombosis.[10,20] Other established causes of nonanastomotic strictures include chronic rejection and infection, particularly with cytomegalovirus.[2] Anastomotic strictures arise secondary to operative difficulties and respond to transhepatic balloon dilatation.[21] A small group of patients with postoperative biliary system obstruction have extensive epithelial casts forming within the biliary tree (Fig. 11.**8**). These patients usually have a patent hepatic artery, suggesting that the lesions are unlikely to be vascular in origin. It is possible that this is a late manifestation of preservation injury affecting the harvested liver, leading to epithelial sloughing within the biliary system. Most patients with this condition require retransplantation.[22]

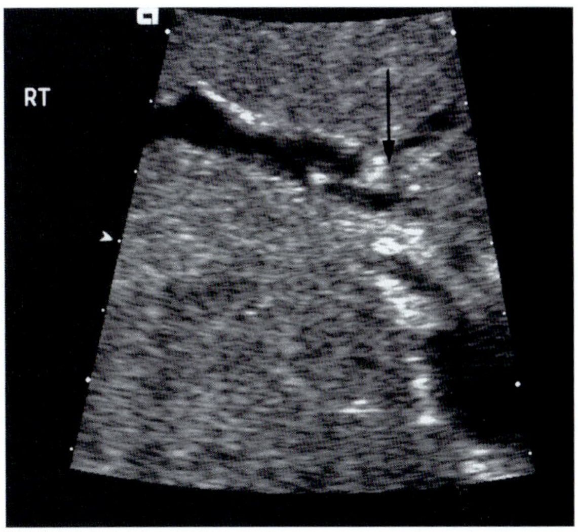

Fig. 11.**8** Intrahepatic bile duct dilatation, with echogenic material (arrow) within the bile ducts, in a liver transplant patient

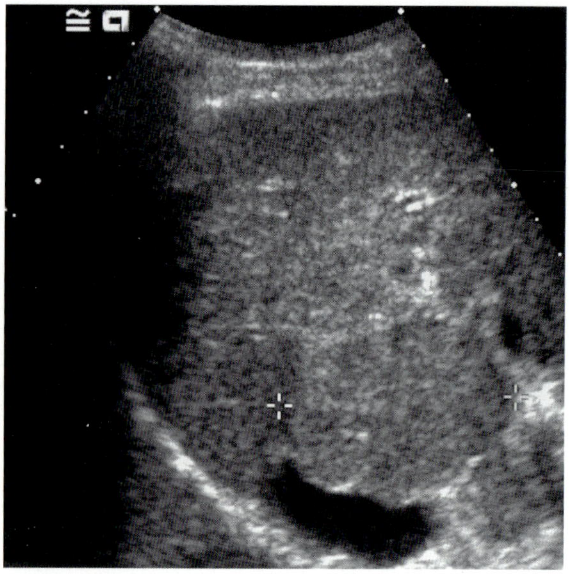

Fig. 11.**9** Recurrent HCC (cursors) in a liver transplant patient with underlying HCV infection

■ ***Summary points:***

- Renal insufficiency due to nephrotoxic effect of immunosuppressive therapy is a common complication, occurring in 25 % of pediatric liver transplant patients
- Imaging is not specific for rejection
- Immunosuppressive therapy is a risk factor for infection
- Nonanastomotic biliary strictures are associated with ischaemia.

Disease Recurrence

The initial indication for liver transplantation should be taken into account (although not often offered by the referring physician) when surveillance ultrasound is performed in the post-transplant phase, to allow for the possibility of disease recurrence.

Viral Infection

Viral infection does recur in the transplant liver. Biopsy evidence of recurrence of hepatitis C is seen in 87 % of transplants and tends to occur within two years of transplantation.[23] Early recurrence is associated with a higher incidence of rejection and cirrhosis leading to eventual graft loss. The role of ultrasound is limited to the exclusion of other complications when the biochemical parameters become abnormal. Ultrasound is useful to monitor complications of recurrent infection such as cirrhosis and portal hypertension, and for surveillance for the development of focal liver lesions.

The recurrence rate for hepatitis B (HBV) is also high at 90 %.[24] This reinfection leads to early graft loss, estimated at 41 % at 14 months. Recurrent HBV infection in a transplant patient is more aggressive than in the pretransplant patient; furthermore, patients who have undergone transplantation for chronic HBV may develop end-stage liver disease within a number of months.[3] This poor outcome of chronic HBV infection was initially considered a contraindication to transplantation; however, now the aim of treatment in the post-transplant period is to prevent reinfection with immunoprophylaxis and antiviral therapy.

Hepatocellular Carcinoma

Ultrasound has a low sensitivity to the presence of hepatocellular carcinoma (HCC) in the pretransplant liver, so other imaging modalities must be relied upon. It is difficult to identify focal lesions on ultrasound in the presence of the abnormal architecture of advanced cirrhosis. Liver transplantation is indicated in patients with cirrhosis and an unresectable HCC.[25-27]

The histological pattern and degree of differentiation of HCC give no indication of the subsequent course of disease, as it is the preoperative staging of the tumor that indicates the recurrence rate. The lowest recurrence rates occur in small tumors measuring less than 5 cm without evidence of disease spread[28]: a recurrence rate of 7 % is seen with tumors less than 5 cm as against 62 % for tumors greater than 5 cm in size.[29] Furthermore, infiltration of regional lymph nodes or the presence of gross or microscopic vascular invasion of the tumor at the time of transplantation significantly influences the prognosis.[30] A combination of ultrasound, computed tomography (CT), and magnetic resonance imaging (MRI) is accurate in detecting HCC recurrences in the liver transplant (Fig. 11.**9**).[31]

Overall, children who have received a liver transplant for primary hepatic malignancy have a better prognosis than adults; the quoted 10-year survival rate is 21 % in adults and 50 % in children. The recurrence of HCC in a noncirrhotic liver transplant should be readily detected on ultrasonography, but there are no available published data to confirm this.[32]

Fibrolamellar HCC

Fibrolamellar hepatocellular carcinoma, a rare variant of HCC, is a slow-growing, usually unicentric neoplasm occurring in the absence of cirrhosis, with a peak incidence in adolescence and young adulthood.[33]

The recurrence rate for fibrolamellar HCC following transplantation is unexpectedly high for a tumor that is slower-growing and has a higher resectability rate than the classic HCC.[34,35] This may in part be due to the late presentation of these tumors, generally with a large bulk of tumor. The survival rate at five years following transplantation is 50 %.[28]

Cholangiocarcinoma

The rate for recurrence of cholangiocarcinoma is higher than that of HCC.[36,37] Although bloodstream spread is rare, both central and peripheral cholangiocarcinomas invade the lymphatic system at an early stage. Involvement of the lymphatic system is invariably associated with tumor recurrence such that liver transplantation is precluded; if lymphatic involvement is discovered at surgery, transplantation must be abandoned.[36]

Epithelioid Hemangioendothelioma

Epithelioid hemangioendothelioma is an unusual tumor of endothelial origin affecting young adults with a normal noncirrhotic liver, rarely presenting as a liver tumor with or without associated soft tissue and lung involvement.[38] If liver involvement is present, the tumor may manifest clinically as liver failure for which the only treatment is liver transplantation. Liver transplantation has been successful even in the presence of metastatic disease at the time of surgery.[39] However, the tumor does recur, depending on the stage at presentation.

Primary Biliary Cirrhosis

The assessment of recurrence of primary biliary cirrhosis (PBC) in the transplanted graft is a subject of controversy.[40,41] The most accurate method of determining the possibility of recurrence is based on histology. The presence of pruritus, antimitochondrial antibodies, and elevated IgM in the post-transplant patient are nonspecific findings.

The rejection process complicates the histology as this too is centered on the bile ducts. Normally the presence of granulomas is required for the diagnosis of recurrent PBC, but studies indicate that histological features of PBC such as granulomatous bile duct damage, ductopenia, and biliary fibrosis may also be seen in the allograft. These histological features of PBC are variable and do not reflect the level of abnormality of liver function indices. The rate of recurrence increases with time, so that by 10 years recurrence may be seen in up to 30–50% of liver biopsy specimens.[41] In the medium term recurrence of PBC has little clinical impact, and ultrasound has no role in the detection of recurrence except to exclude structural abnormalities that may present a similar fashion.

Primary Sclerosing Cholangitis

Ultrasound has limited use in the assessment of primary sclerosing cholangitis (PSC) recurrence; as in the pretransplant condition, the ultrasound findings may be entirely normal.[42,43] However, the presence of bile duct dilatation in the transplant graft invariably indicates a newly developed biliary abnormality,[2] for which recurrence of PSC must be considered in the differential diagnosis. Most patients undergoing transplantation for PSC will have a Roux-en-Y loop as a consequence of abnormal recipient extrahepatic ducts, and this is prone to a higher incidence of cholangitis and biliary strictures leading to a cholangiopathy similar to PSC. This presents difficulty for both cholangiographic and histological methods of determining absolute PSC recurrence. Furthermore, patients transplanted for PSC are known to have a higher incidence of biliary complications, again reflecting the use of a Roux-en-Y reconstruction.[43] Again, recurrence of the disease has little clinical impact on graft survival in the medium term.

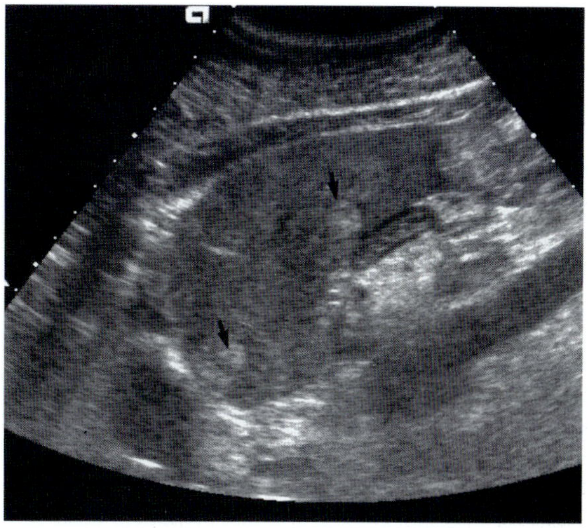

Fig. 11.**10** Multiple echogenic lesions in the liver due to metastatic lesions of carcinoid tumor (arrows)

Autoimmune Chronic Active Hepatitis

Autoimmune hepatitis does recur in the graft of patients transplanted for chronic active hepatitis, has little impact in the medium term, and, as in PBC, ultrasound is insensitive in diagnosing recurrence.[44–46]

Metastatic Disease

Recurrence rates in the transplant liver when transplantation is performed for primary bowel and pancreatic malignancies have been so high as not to justify liver transplantation.[47]

Neuroendocrine Tumors

These rare tumors, which include gastrinomas, glucagonomas, VIPomas, carcinoids, and insulinomas, metastasize to the liver, resulting in the development of associated syndromic symptoms (Fig. 11.**10**). When conventional therapy fails, liver transplantation may be curative, but normally mere removal of tumor bulk results in a reduction of symptomatic ectopic hormonal secretion. To date, 10 patients at our institution have undergone transplantation for such an indication,

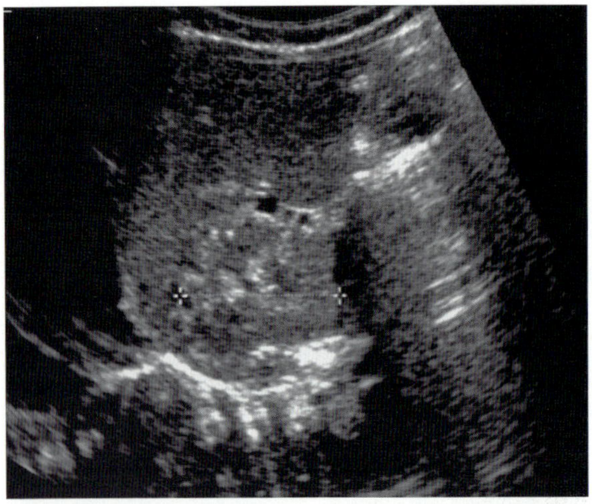

Fig. 11.**11** Hepatoblastoma in a four-month-old male child prior to surgery (cursors)

with a 50% survival rate at two years.[48] Ultrasound is useful to monitor disease recurrence or progression.

Alcoholic Liver Disease

Patients who have undergone a liver transplantation for cirrhosis due to alcoholic liver disease tend to resume alcohol consumption after transplantation. However, only a small percentage resume heavy consumption. Generally, patients with alcohol-related liver disease will not consume more alcohol than their counterparts who have received a liver transplant for liver disease of other causes. Survival after transplantation for alcoholic liver disease is similar to that after transplantation for other forms of chronic liver disease.[49,50]
Unwillingness to offer a liver transplant to individuals with alcoholic liver disease because of failure to demonstrate complete long-term alcohol abstinence appears difficult to justify in the face of good survival with social rehabilitation.[50]

Sarcoidosis

Recurrent sarcoidosis in human lung, renal, and cardiac allografts is well recognized. Liver transplant allograft recurrence, however, has only been reported on one occasion.[51] Five-year survival of patients who receive transplants for sarcoidosis is marginally better than that of patients undergoing transplantation for viral hepatitis or alcoholic liver disease.[52] It is thought that the use of prednisolone and cyclosporine to prevent rejection also prevents recurrence of sarcoidosis and halts the progression of extrahepatic disease.

Budd–Chiari Syndrome

Liver transplantation in Budd–Chiari syndrome represents a viable treatment option with a favorable long-term survival.[53] However, depending on the initial cause of the Budd–Chiari thromboembolic phenomena, the syndrome may recur not only in the hepatic veins but also in the portal vein and hepatic artery.[54] This contributes significantly to postoperative morbidity and mortality.[55] Patients are placed on long-term full anticoagulation to prevent recurrent thrombosis. A full color Doppler ultrasound examination of all hepatic vessels at follow-up is mandatory to exclude recurrent disease.

Summary points:

- Biopsy evidence of recurrence of hepatitis C is seen in 87% and hepatitis B in 90% of liver transplants
- The lowest recurrence rate of HCC occurs with tumors smaller than 5 cm without evidence of disease spread
- A combination of ultrasound, CT, and MRI is accurate at detecting HCC recurrences in the liver transplant
- The recurrence rate for fibrolamellar HCC following transplantation is unexpectedly high for a tumor that is slow-growing
- The most accurate method of determining recurrence of primary biliary cirrhosis and primary sclerosing cholangitis is histological analysis

Recurrent Disease in Children

Hepatoblastoma

Hepatoblastoma is the commonest primary liver tumor in children under five years of age for which transplantation is a recognized treatment (Fig. 11.**11**).[56] Factors associated with a poor prognosis and disease recurrence include previous resection, portal vein invasion by tumor, multifocal disease, other vascular invasion, and the presence of extrahepatic disease. Unifocal disease, irrespective of tumor size, with fetal epithelium on histology is associated with a better outcome, whilst the presence of anaplastic cells has been associated with a poor prognosis.[56]

Hepatocellular Carcinoma

The common age range for HCC is between 5 and 15 years, but it remains less common than hepatoblastoma. As in adults, any preexisting conditions that lead to cirrhosis will predispose to HCC development. These include biliary atresia, Fanconi syndrome, and metabolic diseases such as tyrosinemia. HCC in children has a worse prognosis than hepatoblastoma as it often presents late with evidence of metastatic disease. Children undergoing transplantation for a benign disease, where HCC was incidentally detected, have equivalent survival rates to those without neoplasia. The children with the worst survival were those transplanted for

HCC with preexisting underlying liver disease.[57] Children with tyrosinemia undergo transplantation to prevent the development of HCC; the incidence of HCC increases with age in these patients.

Post-Transplant Lymphoproliferative Disease

Post-transplant lymphoproliferative disease (PTLD) is a B cell proliferation in lymph nodes and solid organs associated with the Epstein–Barr virus, typically developing within the first year after solid organ transplantation.[58] The reported incidence of PTLD increases with decreasing age of liver transplant patient and is associated with potent immunosuppression agents.[59] The incidence of PTLD ranges from 2% to 10% in adults[60] and from 2.9% to 18.9% in children.[58] Children are more at risk for the development of PTLD primarily because they are likely to be seronegative for Epstein–Barr virus before transplantation and acquire primary infection after transplantation.[58,59] PTLD has a broad clinical spectrum, ranging from an infectious mononucleosis-like syndrome to manifestations of frank lymphoma.[61]

The clinical, histopathological, and imaging features of PTLD in liver transplant patients differ from those of lymphoma in immunocompetent patients, but bear some resemblance to the lymphomas that arise in other immunocompromised patients, most notably with AIDS and congenital T cell immunodeficiencies.[62] Recognized characteristics of PTLD include a tendency toward extranodal involvement and a variable response to treatment. For example, localized disease such as presentation with head and neck lymphadenopathy or single organ involvement tends to regress with reduction of immunosuppression and has a good prognosis. However, multiorgan or disseminated disease has a poor prognosis with up to 50% mortality.[58,63] Systemic chemotherapy in advanced disease results in long-term remission, but this is achieved at the expense of considerable patient morbidity.[58]

The aim of imaging is initial detection, then staging, and finally treatment follow-up of the disease. The earlier PTLD is detected, the better the response to treatment, and ultrasound surveillance is usually responsible for the initial discovery of the disease. Once an abnormality is demonstrated, imaging may be used to guide biopsy for histological confirmation. CT is the imaging modality of choice for staging and assessing the bulk of disease and follow-up of treatment response.

The abdomen is the commonest site of involvement with PTLD, and up to 50% of patients present with isolated abdominal disease.[64] Extranodal abdominal disease is three to four times more frequent than nodal disease; 88% of liver transplant recipients assessed with CT had extranodal abdominal PTLD.[65]

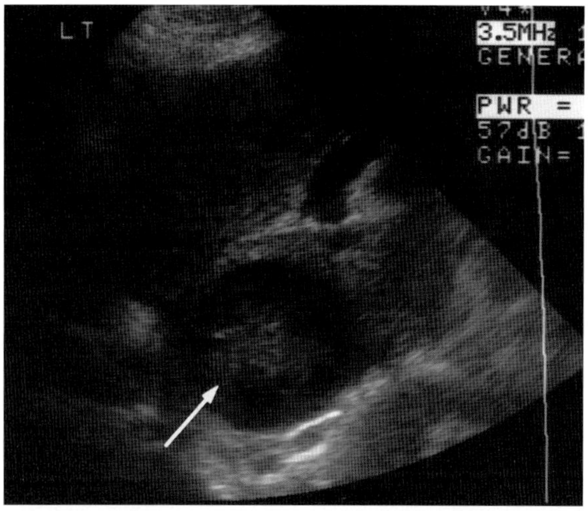

Fig. 11.**12** Focal tumor in a liver transplant recipient (arrow). This proved on biopsy to be an example of intrahepatic post-transplant lymphoma

Three distinct patterns of hepatic PTLD may be seen at ultrasound. The most common is focal areas of low echogenicity measuring between 1 and 4 cm, followed by a diffuse parenchymal involvement with no discrete lesions resulting in hepatomegaly and progressing to liver failure (Fig. 11.**12**).[64] The third pattern involves the porta hepatis, which may result in biliary obstruction and is postulated to originate within the biliary tree (Fig. 11.**13**).[66] Rarely, fulminant disease may present as a consequence of PTLD, causing extensive graft necrosis.[67]

Other extranodal manifestations of abdominal PTLD include involvement of the gastrointestinal tract (approximately 30%), with the small bowel most frequently involved, splenic involvement (28% of cases, manifests as focal low-echogenic lesions), splenomegaly, or both, and renal involvement (less than 20% of patients).[65] Unlike renal lymphoma in the nontransplant patient, PTLD kidney involvement tends to be unilateral and unifocal. A solitary, round, low-echogenic lesion without renal enlargement is the most common manifestation; diffuse renal enlargement, which may extend beyond the capsule, occurs less commonly.[65]

Abdominal lymph node involvement, seen in about 20% of patients, appears as nonspecific nodal enlargement. These involved nodes are typically 2–3 cm in diameter but may coalesce to form larger masses, with central low-reflective areas of necrosis being an uncommon finding.[64,65] Any combination of peritoneal, retroperitoneal, and extraperitoneal lymph nodes may be enlarged. Omental and mesenteric involvement by PTLD is less common, seen in about 10% of patients with abdominal disease, and manifests an "extranodal mass." Such masses may be well circumscribed or infiltrative, representing either primary tumor involvement or direct extension from an abdominal organ.

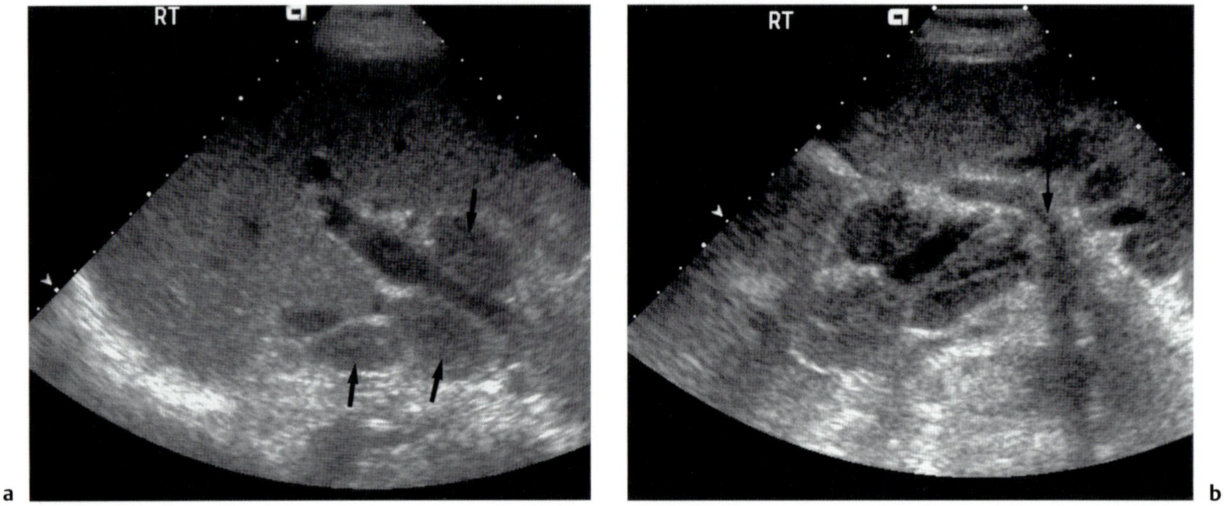

Fig. 11.**13** **a** PTLD in a liver transplant patient demonstrating multiple portal hilar lymph nodes (arrows). **b** Same patient with multiple lymph nodes surrounding the celiac axis (arrow)

Uncommon sites for disease occurrences in the abdomen include the gallbladder, abdominal wall musculature, and subcutaneous fat.

Summary points:

- Post-transplant lymphoproliferative disease (PTLD) is a B cell proliferation in lymph nodes and solid organs associated with the Epstein–Barr virus that develops after solid organ transplantation
- Children are more at risk than adults of developing PTLD
- Three patterns of PTLD are seen in the transplant liver on ultrasound: focal lesion, diffuse parenchymal abnormality: and involvement of the porta hepatis causing biliary obstruction

References

1. Morton MJ, James EM, Wiesner RH, Krom RA. Applications of duplex ultrasonography in the liver transplant patient. Mayo Clin Proc 1990;65:360–72.
2. Raby N, Meire HB, Forbes A, Williams R. The role of ultrasound scanning in the management after liver transplantation. Clin Radiol 1988;39:507–10.
3. Davern TJ, Lake JR. Recurrent disease after liver transplantation. Semin Gastrointest Dis 1998;9:86–109.
4. Maceneaney PM, Malone DE, Skehan SJ, et al. The role of hepatic arterial Doppler ultrasound after liver transplantation: an ‚audit cycle' evaluation. Clin Radiol 2000;55:517–24.
5. Wozney P, Zajko AB, Bron KM, Point S, Starzl TE. Vascular complications after liver transplantation: a five-year experience. AJR Am J Roentgenol 1986;147:657–63.
6. Meire HB, Farrant P. Liver Transplants. In: Meire H, Cosgrove DO, Dewbury K, Farrant P, editors. Clinical ultrasound. 2nd ed. London: Churchill Livingstone; 2000. p. 273–95.
7. Dodd GD, Memel DS, Zajko AB, Baron RL, Santaguida LA. Hepatic artery stenosis and thrombosis in transplant recipients: Doppler diagnosis with resistive index and systolic acceleration time. Radiology 1994;192:657–61.
8. Hall TR, Diarmid SV, Grant EG, Boechat MI, Busuttil RW. False-negative duplex Doppler studies in children with hepatic artery thrombosis after liver transplatation. AJR Am J Roentgenol 1990;154:573–75.
9. Desai SR, Beese RC, Karani JB. Intrahepatic abscess formation following adult orthoptic liver transplantation. Br J Radiol 1996;96:200
10. Zajko AB, Campbell WL, Logsdon G. Cholangiographic findings in hepatic artery occlusion after liver transplantation. AJR Am J Roentgenol 1987;149:485–89.
11. Lerut J, Tzakis A, Bron KM, et al. Complications of venous reconstruction in human orthotopic liver transplantation. Ann Surg 1987;205:404–14.
12. Malassangne B, Suobrane O, Dousset B, Legmann P, Houssin D. Extrahepatic portal hypertension following liver transplantation: a rare but challenging problem. HPB Surg 1998;10:357–63.
13. Lee J, Ben-Ami T, Yousefzadeh D, et al. Extrahepatic portal vein stenosis in recipients of living-donor allografts: Doppler sonography. AJR Am J Roentgenol 1996;167:90
14. Brouwers MAM, deLong KP, Peeters PMJG, Bijleveld CMA, Klompmaker IJ, Slouff MJ. Inferior vena cava obstruction after orthoptic liver transplantation. Clin Transplant 1994;8:19–22.
15. Rossi AR, Pozniak MA, Zarvan NP. Upper inferior vena caval anastomotic stenosis in liver transplant recipients: Doppler US diagnosis. Radiology 1993;187:387–9.
16. McDiarmid SV, Busuttil RW, Ascher NL, et al. FK506 (tacrolimus) compared with cyclosporine for primary immunosuppression after paediatric liver transplantation: results from the US multicenter trial. Transplantation 1995;59:530–6.
17. Cattral MS, Langas AN, Wisecarver JL, et al. Survival of graft versus host disease in a liver transplant recipient. Transplantation 1994;57:1271–4.

18. Holbert BL, Campbell WL, Skolnick ML. Evaluation of the transplanted liver and postoperative complications. Radiol Clin North Am 1998;33:521–40.
19. Nicholson V, Johnson PC. Infectious complications in solid organ transplant recipients. Surg Clin North Am 1994;74:1223–45.
20. Sankary HN, McChesney L, Hart M, Foster P, Williams J. Identification of donor and recipient risk factors associated with non anastomatic biliary strictures in human hepatic allografts. Transplantation Proc 1993;25:1964–7.
21. Lopez RR, Bennar KG, Ivanceu K, Keefe EB, Deverney LW, Pinson CW. Management of biliary complications after liver transplantation. Am J Surg 1992;163:519–24.
22. Gimson AES, Karani JB, Heaton ND. Major biliary tract and vascular complications. In: Williams R, Portmann B, Tan KC, editors. The practice of liver transplantation. 1st ed. London: Churchill Livingstone; 1995. p. 199–209.
23. Testa G, Crippin JS, Netto GJ, et al. Liver transplantation for hepatitis C: recurrence and disease progression in 300 patients. Liver Transpl 2000;6:553–61.
24. O'Grady JG, Smith HM, Davies SE, et al. Hepatitis B reinfection after orthoptic liver transplantation. Serological and clinical implications. J Hepatol 1992;14:104–11.
25. Mazzaferro V, Regalia E, Doci R, et al. Liver transplantation for the treatment of small hepatocellular carcinomas in patients with cirrhosis. N Engl J Med 1996;334:693–9.
26. Neuhaus P, Jonas S, Bechstein WO. Hepatoma of the liver—resection or transplantation? Langenbecks Arch Surg 2000;385:171–8.
27. Yokoyama I, Takagi H. Liver transplantation and hepatocellular carcinoma. Semin Surg Oncol 1996;12:212–6.
28. McPeake JR, O'Grady J, Zaman S, et al. Liver transplantation for primary hepatocellular carcinoma: tumor size and number determine outcome. J Hepatol 1993;18: 226–34.
29. Imatsuki S, Gordon RD, Shaw BJ, Starzl TE. Role of liver transplantation in cancer therapy. Ann Surg 1985;202:401–7.
30. Ismail T, Angrisani L, Gunson BK, et al. Primary hepatic malignancy: the role of liver transplantation. Br J Surg 1990;77:983–7.
31. Rizzi PM, Kane PA, Ryder SD, et al. Accuracy of radiology in detection of hepatocellular carcinoma before liver transplantation. Gastroenterology 1994;107:1425–9.
32. Migliazza L, Lopez Santamaria M, Murcia J, et al. Long-term survival expectancy after liver transplantation in children. J Pediatric Surg 2000;35:5–7.
33. Craig JR, Peters RL, Edmondson HA, Omata M. Fibrolamellar carcinoma of the liver: a tumour of adolescents and young adults with distinctive clinicopathological features. Cancer 1980;46:372–9.
34. El-Gazzaz G, Wong W, El-Hadary MK, et al. Outcome of liver resection and transplantation for fibrolamellar hepatocellular carcinoma. Transpl Int 2000;13:S406–9
35. Schlitt HJ, Neipp M, Weimann A, et al. Recurrence patterns of hepatocellular and fibrolamellar carcinoma after liver transplantation. J Clin Oncol 1999;17:324–31.
36. O'Grady JG, Polson RJ, Rolles K, Calne RY, Williams R. Liver transplantation for malignant disease. Results in 93 consecutive patients. Ann Surg 1988;207:373–9.
37. Penn T. Hepatic transplantation for primary and metastatic cancers of the liver. Surg 1991;110:726–34.
38. Weiss JW, Enzinger FM. Epitheloid haemangioendothelioma: a vascular tumour often mistaken for a carcinoma. Cancer 1982;50:970–81.
39. Scoazec JY, Lamy P, Degott C, et al. Epithelioid haemangioendothelioma of the liver. Diagnostic features and the role of liver transplantation. Gastroenterology 1988;94:1447–53.
40. Garcia RF, Garcia CE, McMaster P, Neuberger J. Transplantation for primary biliary cirrhosis: retrospective analysis of 400 patients in a single center. Hepatology 2001;33:22–7.
41. Neuberger J. Recurrent primary biliary cirrhosis. Baillières Clin Gastroenterol 2000;14:669–80.
42. Gow PJ, Chapman RW. Liver transplantation for primary sclerosing cholangitis. Liver 2000;20:97–103.
43. Letourneau JG, Day JL, Hunter DW, et al. Biliary complications after liver transplantation in patients with pre-existing sclerosing cholangitis. Radiology 1988;167:349–51.
44. Neuberger J. Recurrence of primary biliary cirrhosis, primary sclerosing cholangitis and autoimmune hepatitis. Liver Transpl Surg 1995;5:109–15.
45. Tillmann HL, Jackel E, Manns MP. Liver transplantation in autoimmune liver disease-selection of patients. Hepatogastroenterology 1999;46:3053–9.
46. Balan V, Abu-Elmagd K, Demetris AJ. Autoimmune liver diseases. Recurrence after liver transplantation. Surg Clin North Am 1999;79:147–52.
47. Iwatsuki S, Busuttil RW, Klintmalm GBG. Liver transplantation for metastatic hepatic malignancy. In: Busuttil R, Klintmalm GBG, editors. Transplantation of the liver. 1st ed. Philadelphia: WB Saunders; 1996. p. 130–3.
48. Arnold JC, O'Grady JG, Bird GL, Calne RY, Williams R. Liver transplantation for primary and secondary apudomas. Br J Surg 1989;76:248–9.
49. Mackie J, Groves K, Hoyle A, et al. Orthoptic liver transplantation for alcholoic liver disease: a retrospective analysis of survival and risk factors predisposing to recidivism. Liver Transpl 2001;7:418–27.
50. Berlakovich GA, Stenniger R, Herbst F, Barlan M, Mittlbock M, Muhlbacher M. Transplantation for alcoholic cirrhosis: how does recurrence of disease harm the graft? Transpl Int 1994;7:S123–7
51. Fidler HM, Hadgiyannis SJ, Dhillon AP, Sherlock S, Burroughs AK. Recurrent hepatic sarcoidosis following liver transplantation. Transplant Proc 1997;29:2509–10.
52. Casavilla AF, Gordon R, Wright HI, Garater JS, Starzl TE, VanThiel DH. Clinical course after liver transplantation in patients with sarcoidosis. Ann Intern Med 1993;118:865–6.
53. Jamieson NV, Williams R, Calne RY. Liver transplantation for Budd Chiari syndrome 1976–1990. Ann Chir 1991;45:362–5.
54. Ruckert JC, Ruckert RI, Rudolph B, Muller JM. Recurrence of the Budd–Chiari syndrome after orthotopic liver transplantation. Hepatogastroenterology 1999;46:867–71.
55. Hulff G, Todo S, Tzakis AG, Gordon RD, Starzl TE. Liver transplantation for Budd Chiari syndrome. Ann Surg 1990;211:43–9.
56. Koneru B, Flye MW, Busuttil RW, et al. Liver transplantation for hepatoblastoma. The American experience. Ann Surg 1991;213:118–21.
57. Ryckman FC, Alonso MH, Busuttil RW, Klintmalm GBG. Transplantation for primary hepatic malignancy in children. In: Busuttil RW, Klintmalm GB, editors. Transplantation of the liver. 1st ed. Philadelphia: WB Saunders; 1996. p. 216–26.
58. Cox KL, Lawerence-Miyasaki LS, Garcia-Kennedy R, et al. An increased incidence of Epstein–Barr virus infection and lymphoproliferative disorders in young children on FK506 after liver transplantation. Transplantation 1995;59:524–9.
59. Younes BS, McDiarmid MG, Martin JH, et al. The effect of immunosuppression on post-transplant lymphoproliferative disease in pediatric liver transplant patients. Transplantation 2000;70:94–7.
60. McCarthy M, Ramage JK, McNair A, et al. The clinical diversity and role of chemotherapy in lymphoproliferative disorder in liver transplantation recipients. J Hepatol 1997;27:1015–21.
61. Morrison VA, Dunn DL, Manivel JC, Galjl-Peczalska KJ, Peterson BA. Clinical characteristics of post-transplant lymphoproliferative disorders. Am J Med 1994;97:14–24.
62. List AF, Grelo FA, Vogler LB. Lymphoproliferative disease in immunocompromised hosts: the role of Epstein–Barr virus. J Clin Oncol 1987;5:1673–89.

63. Reyes J, Tzakis A, Green M, et al. Post-transplant lymphoproliferative disorders occurring under primary FK506 immunosuppression. Transplant Proc 1991;23:3044–6.
64. Pickhardt PJ, Siegel MJ. Abdominal manifestations of post transplantation lymphoproliferative disorder. AJR Am J Roentgenol 1998;171:1007–13.
65. Pickhardt PJ, Siegel MJ. Post transplantation lymphoproliferative disorder of the abdomen: CT evaluation in 51 patients. Radiology 1999;213:73–8.
66. Navarro F, Pyda P, Pageaux GP, et al. Lymphoproliferative disease after liver transplantation: primary biliary location. Transplant Proc 1998;30:1486–8.
67. Bowen A, Hungate RG, Kaye RD, Reyes J, Towbin RB. Imaging in liver transplantation. Radiol Clin North Am 1996;34:757–78.

Interventional Radiology in Liver Transplantation

S. Babar and J. Tibballs

Introduction

Orthotopic liver transplantation (OLT) has become a well-established technique since the first reported human transplant performed in 1963, with survival rates of over 80% at 1 year in both adults and children.[1,2] OLT is now the treatment of choice for irreversible liver cell failure and selected cases of hepatocellular carcinoma (HCC). Nonetheless it remains a technically challenging procedure and its success is highly dependent upon the correct selection of patients before transplantation and the accurate diagnosis and treatment of complications after the transplantation procedure. Radiology plays an essential role in both of these areas.

The commonest liver transplantation procedure is whole-organ OLT. The shortage of available donor organs has led to innovative techniques of reduced-size "split" and living related donor liver transplantation, which were driven largely by the need to provide donor livers for pediatric recipients; However, living related transplantation is now being used in the adult population as well.

The role of interventional radiology (IR) in pre-OLT assessment has decreased as noninvasive imaging modalities have improved, but the introduction of the transjugular intrahepatic portosystemic shunt (TIPS) procedure has had a notable impact in selected patients awaiting OLT. The role of IR in the assessment and treatment of post-OLT complications remains vital. In its simplest form, successful OLT requires effective anastomosis of the donor and recipient inferior vena cava (IVC), portal vein, hepatic artery, and bile duct, and the correct level of immunosuppression to prevent rejection but avoid infection or malignancy.

Interventional Radiology Before Transplantation

The aims of pre-OLT imaging are to evaluate technical feasibility by determining hepatic vascular anatomy, and to determine the suitability of OLT in cases of HCC by assessing the presence and extent of hepatic malignancy. Whilst noninvasive imaging with ultrasound, multiphase contrast-enhanced spiral computed tomography (SCT), and gadolinium-enhanced magnetic resonance imaging (MRI) are the mainstays of this evaluation, IR techniques are still of use in specific instances.

Hepatic Artery

A detailed knowledge of hepatic arterial anatomy is not required for OLT, and extrahepatic arterial anatomy is readily appreciated on noninvasive imaging. Detailed segmental hepatic arterial anatomy is, however, required in the setting of living related OLT in order to plan the segmental splitting of the donor liver and avoid devascularization of individual segments. Formal angiography currently has superior resolution to both SCT and MR angiography and is indicated in this setting. Ultrasonography is inaccurate for assessing hepatic arterial anatomy.

Portal Vein

An adequate portal vein inflow is essential to graft survival. Portal vein thrombosis is present to some degree in 5–10% of patients with end-stage cirrhosis, notably those with HCC. Portal vein thrombosis does not necessarily preclude OLT, but it may necessitate modification of surgical technique. Patency of the portal vein is usually demonstrable on noninvasive imaging, but occasionally angiographic delineation is required to confirm the exact extent of portal vein thrombosis and anatomy of venous collaterals. The portal vein thrombosis is usually demonstrated by means of indirect hepatic arterioportography, unless there is hepatofugal flow, in which case it can be demonstrated by wedged hepatic venography using either iodinated contrast medium or carbon dioxide.

Transjugular Intrahepatic Portosystemic Shunt

TIPS has become an important pre-OLT interventional technique in selected patients. It is very effective at reducing portal hypertension and is used to "buy time" for end-stage cirrhotic patients suffering the complications of portal hypertension, notably variceal hemorrhage and ascites, and is described in both the adult[3–6] and pediatric[7] populations. Although TIPS can, rarely, precipitate a rapid decline in liver function necessitating emergency transplantation, in most patients there is an improvement in liver and renal function, allowing optimization of the patient's condition prior to transplantation. In this situation TIPS acts as a "bridge to transplantation."

Comparison of OLT in patients with and without TIPS show no difference in terms of perioperative transfu-

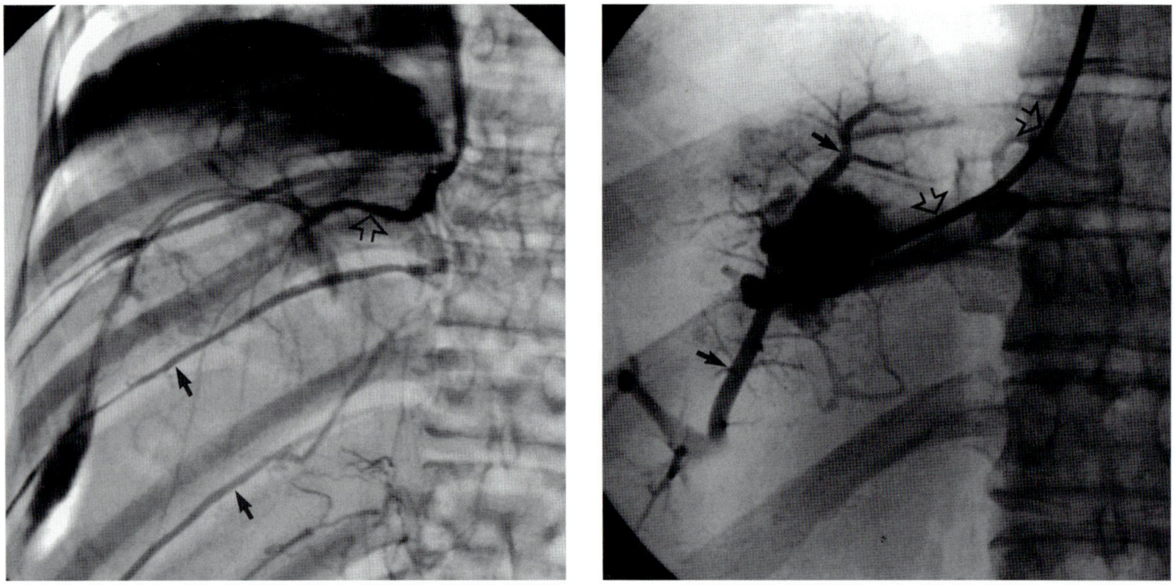

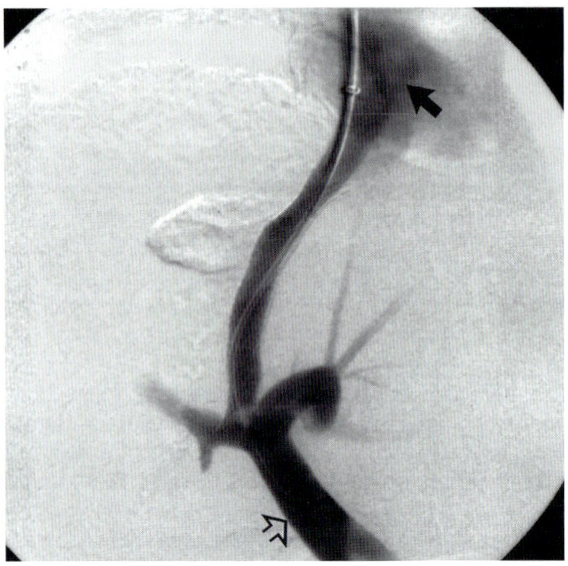

Fig. 12.1 **a** Hepatic venogram showing a small-caliber, irregular right hepatic vein (open arrow) and venous collaterals in established Budd–Chiari syndrome. Intercostal veins (solid arrows) are also filling. **b** The TIPS needle assembly (open arrows) has been advanced into the liver parenchyma and contrast injected demonstrating right portal vein branches (solid arrows). **c** Digital subtraction angiogram following TIPSS stent deployment showing flow of contrast from the portal vein (open arrow) to the right atrium (solid arrow)

sion requirements, operative time, length of hospital stay, and outcome. Therefore, TIPS is not indicated simply to reduce portal venous pressure prior to transplantation.[3–6]

Although these studies show that TIPS has no direct bearing on the outcome of surgery, they do report modification of surgical technique being required in 22–35 % of patients.[3,6] In most cases this is due to migration or misplacement of the stent. If the upper end of the stent extends too far proximally into the IVC or right atrium or the lower end too far into the portal vein, it can interfere with cross-clamping at surgery, making it difficult to control these vessels and perform the necessary anastomoses. Fortunately, transplantation surgeons have developed various techniques for dealing with poorly positioned stents[8] so these rarely jeopardize the procedure. Nevertheless, extreme care should be taken when deploying the TIPS stent in patients who are candidates for OLT.

It is worth noting that comparisons of OLT in patients who have previously undergone surgical portosystemic shunting to patients with TIPS[9,10] do show a higher mean operative time and similar or increased blood-product transfusion requirements and duration of hospital stay in the surgical group. No difference in long-term survival was seen; nonetheless TIPS remains the preferred method of portal decompression prior to OLT.

A particularly interestingly indication for TIPS as a “bridge to transplantation” is Budd–Chiari syndrome.[11,12] Although technically challenging in this syndrome because of the variable degree of obliteration of the hepatic veins, TIPS has been successfully performed in both acute and chronic cases (Fig. 12.**1**).

Occasionally TIPS allows recovery of liver function to such a degree that transplantation is no longer required.

TIPS has also been used to treat portal vein thrombosis prior to OLT,[13] thereby eliminating the need for surgical thrombectomy or bypass grafts.

Hepatocellular Carcinoma

Long-term success following OLT for HCC depends mainly upon avoiding recurrent disease. The risk of recurrent disease is related to the size and number of tumors, the presence of vascular invasion, and the presence of extrahepatic spread. Stages I and II of HCC have five-year survival rates of 60–75%, compared to only 15–20% for stages III and IV of the disease.[14]

The presence and extent of HCC is usually determined with noninvasive imaging, but IR retains a role as a problem-solving tool in equivocal cases and in the temporary control of HCC in patients awaiting OLT.

Lipiodol Angiography

Lipiodol is known to be retained by HCC. An emulsion of Lipiodol and iodinated contrast medium is injected selectively into the hepatic artery and unenhanced CT performed 10–14 days later. Dense focal retention of Lipiodol is highly suggestive of HCC, with a positive predictive value of 90%,[15] and therefore may help in characterizing indeterminate focal lesions. This technique, however, has low sensitivity in screening for occult foci of HCC before OLT.[16]

Temporary Control of Disease

Having diagnosed HCC amenable to OLT, there is frequently a wait of weeks or even months for a suitable donor organ to become available. The question then arises as to whether treatment should be instituted to delay tumor growth but which could jeopardize the success of future OLT. As HCC is resistant to systemic chemotherapy and radiotherapy, targeted local treatments are required. These fall into two groups: (1) transarterial and (2) percutaneous.

Transarterial Therapy

Targeted chemotherapy or radiotherapy using chemotherapeutic agents or iodine-131 emulsified with Lipiodol can be delivered to the tumor by selective catheterization of its feeding hepatic artery. The effect of these agents can be enhanced by additional embolization of the feeding artery with either Gelfoam or polyvinyl alcohol (PVA) particles. There is some evidence that Lipiodol–iodine-131 therapy following resection of HCC reduces tumor recurrence and increases disease-free survival,[17] but such adjuvant treatment has not been assessed in patients undergoing transplantation for HCC.

Percutaneous Therapy

Numerous techniques for percutaneous ablation of HCC now exist. Percutaneous ethanol injection (PEI) and radiofrequency thermal ablation are most commonly used for HCC, but percutaneous acetic acid injection, interstitial laser hyperthermia, microwave coagulation, and cryotherapy are also described. Percutaneous and transarterial techniques may be combined. No controlled trials of pre-OLT use of these techniques exist, but PEI has been reported to produce survival rates comparable to those for HCC resection.[18] A potential concern with these procedures is the risk of percutaneous seeding of tumor, reported at 2.3% for PEI,[19] which could compromise long-term survival after OLT. It is worth noting that percutaneous needle biopsy of HCC is associated with a needle-tract implantation rate of 3.4–5.1%[21] and should therefore be avoided in potential OLT candidates.

■ *Summary points:*

- Detailed knowledge of segmental hepatic artery anatomy is required in the setting of living related donor liver transplantation in order to plan the segmental splitting of the donor liver and avoid devascularization of individual segments.
- Patency of the portal vein is usually demonstrable on ultrasound, but angiographic delineation is required to confirm the exact extent of portal vein thrombosis and anatomy of venous collaterals.
- TIPS is very effective at reducing portal hypertension and is used to "buy time" for end-stage cirrhotic patients suffering the complications of portal hypertension, notably variceal hemorrhage and ascites.
- TIPS may performed in the setting of both acute and chronic Budd–Chiari syndrome and occasionally allows recovery of liver function to such a degree that transplantation is no longer required.
- Dense focal retention of Lipiodol is highly suggestive of HCC, with a positive predictive value of 90%.

Interventional Radiology After Liver Transplantation

The role of radiology after OLT is to assess the integrity of the vascular and biliary anastomoses and associated complications, and to assess and treat complications related to immunosuppression, namely rejection, infection, and malignancy.

Post-transplantation complications may be divided into the early and the late. There are four main causes of poor or deteriorating graft function immediately after OLT: acute rejection, primary graft nonfunction,

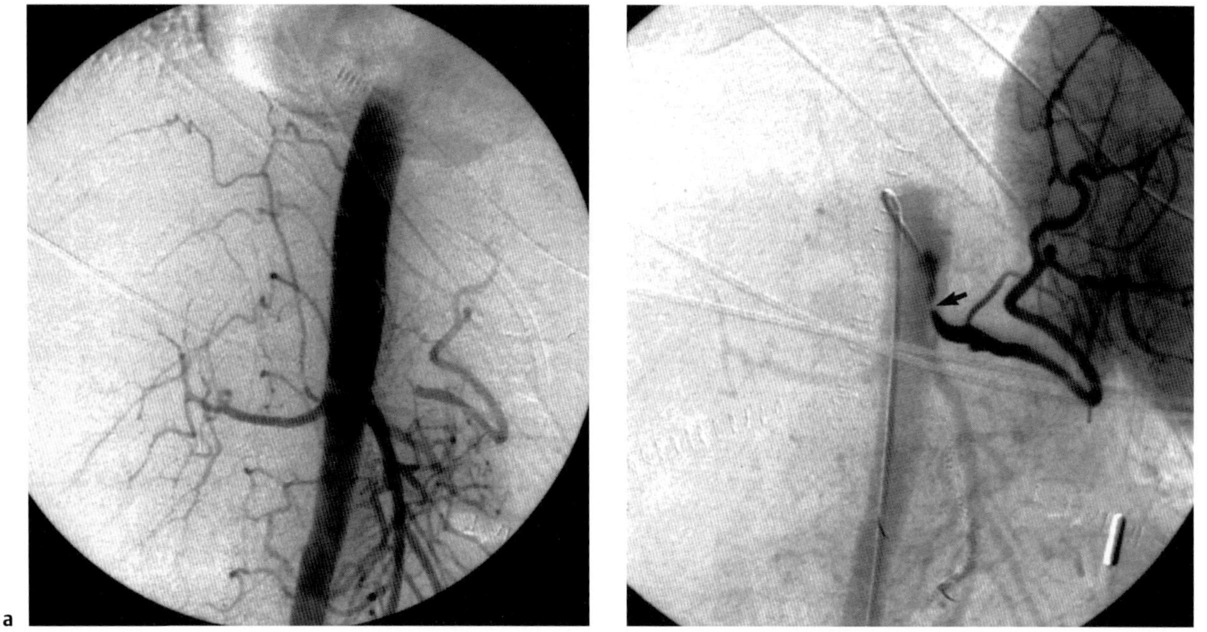

Fig. 12.**2** **a** Flush aortogram in a patient with clinical signs of HAT seven days after orthotopic liver transplantation (OLT). No hepatic artery filling is seen. **b** Selective celiac injection in the same patient confirms complete occlusion of the hepatic artery with stenosis of the splenic artery origin (arrow)

infection, and technical problems (vascular or biliary). It is in the last category that IR plays an important and an ever-increasing role. The main late complications are chronic rejection and malignancies—non-Hodgkin lymphoma, post-transplant lymphoproliferative disease, and skin malignancies.

Acute Rejection

There are well-recognized clinical and histological criteria for acute rejection. Noninvasive imaging is generally unhelpful and the role of IR is limited to liver biopsy. This is usually performed percutaneously using a 'Tru-Cut' needle and has a major complication rate of less than 0.2%.[22] If there is coagulopathy (International normalized ratio 1.5, platelets $< 50 \times 10^9$/l) or ascites, a transjugular approach is used which is safe and effective in these high-risk patients.[23]

Infection

Sepsis is the commonest cause of morbidity and mortality after OLT. However, the role of IR is generally limited to diagnostic fine-needle aspiration (FNA) or drainage of potentially infected perihepatic fluid collections. Post-transplantation pleural effusions and ascites are common and without a specific cause, and most resolve spontaneously. Larger collections or focal collections in the context of clinical sepsis require FNA or drainage. In a series of pediatric patients, intervention for fluid collections was required in 16% of cases.[24] Percutaneous FNA or drainage is usually performed under ultrasound guidance using a Seldinger technique and flexible polyurethane locking-pigtail catheters. Bile collections typically present with pain and sepsis and require drainage, as discussed below.

Vascular Complications

Conventional OLT involves four vascular anastomoses:

- Suprahepatic IVC anastomosis
- Infrahepatic IVC anastomosis
- Hepatic artery anastomosis
- Portal vein anastomosis

Complications are usually related to stenosis or occlusion at these sites, but aneurysm formation, sepsis, and vessel rupture are occasionally seen.

Hepatic Artery

Hepatic artery thrombosis (HAT) is the commonest vascular complication of OLT, occurring in 4–12% of adults and 9–42% of children.[25,26] Portal vein inflow remains the major source of blood supply to the transplanted liver, and is in fact increased in the postoperative period. Unlike the native liver, however, the transplanted organ is uniquely dependent upon hepatic artery inflow as the biliary tree is supplied solely by this artery. Early HAT is associated with hepatic infarction, biliary tract necrosis, bile leak, and graft failure. Biochemically it manifests as persistently elevated or rising transaminase levels and prothrombin time. Doppler ultrasonography usually demonstrates absent hepatic arterial inflow, and urgent hepatic angiography is required to confirm the diagnosis (Fig. 12.**2**). Complete

HAT requires urgent re-transplantation. Hepatic artery stenosis typically occurs close to the arterial anastomosis and should be treated, as there is a risk of progression from stenosis to thrombosis. Successful balloon angioplasty has been reported in small numbers of patients,[27,28] but definitive surgical revascularization may be needed. Late-onset HAT (6 months) may be asymptomatic, but biliary necrosis has been reported.[29]

Arterial vascularization of the graft may be achieved by means of a conduit fashioned from donor iliac artery anastomosed from the infrarenal aorta to the donor hepatic artery. This is typically used in cases of revascularization following HAT, and in reduced-size grafts. The complication rate is similar to that of conventional donor–recipient hepatic artery anastomoses.

Portal Vein

Portal vein stenosis or thrombosis is much less common than stenosis or thrombosis of the hepatic artery, with a reported incidence of 2%.[25] Acute PVT may cause graft failure, mimicking HAT. Portal vein stenosis causes portal hypertension and therefore presents with ascites and variceal bleeding. The diagnosis can be made on noninvasive imaging and confirmed with indirect arterioportography. PVT requires urgent surgical portal vein thrombectomy or retransplantation. Portal vein stenosis may be treated by balloon angioplasty via a transhepatic approach,[30] with success in over 90% of cases. Stent insertion may be performed if angioplasty fails.

Portal vein stenosis is more common in reduced-sized grafts, due to tension related to short donor portal vein length or as a result of graft growth, and consequently is more frequent in children. Treatment is by angioplasty or stenting as described above.[31]

Hepatic Venous Outflow

Stenoses of the hepatic veins or IVC are rare complications of OLT, with a reported incidence of less than 1%.[32] Hepatic vein stenosis is commoner in living related donor transplantation in which the donor hepatic vein is anastomosed to the intact recipient IVC.[33] Hepatic vein and suprahepatic IVC stenosis may result in Budd–Chiari syndrome, whereas infrahepatic IVC stenosis leads to the development of lower limb edema.

Doppler ultrasonography is the initial mode of investigation of suspected hepatic vein outflow obstruction. Venography via either the femoral, internal jugular, or transhepatic route is then performed to delineate any stenoses and assess their hemodynamic significance by measuring the pressure gradient across them. A pressure gradient of more than 7–10 mmHg is significant. Hepatic vein and IVC stenoses may be treated by balloon angioplasty, with stent insertion reserved for recurrent stenoses or lesions that fail to respond to initial angioplasty.[34,35]

Uncommon Vascular Complications

Intrahepatic hepatic artery pseudoaneurysms and arterioportal fistulas have been reported as complications of post-OLT liver biopsy.[36] Pseudoaneurysms may rupture, resulting in intrahepatic and intraperitoneal hemorrhage (Fig. 12.**3**). The diagnosis is usually made with Doppler imaging or SCT and confirmed angiographically. Pseudoaneurysms may be excluded by placing microcoils immediately distal and proximal to the aneurysm neck, or they may be packed using detachable coils. Bleeding arterial branches may also be embolized. Larger pseudoaneurysms may be punctured percutaneously and directly packed with coils or injected with thrombin. Pseudoaneurysms of the main hepatic artery can result from sepsis, anastomotic breakdown, or following percutaneous transluminal angioplasty of stenosis,[37] and may be amenable to endovascular treatment, although definitive surgical repair is often needed.

Biliary Complications

Biliary tract complications occur in 10–20% of adult OLT patients[38] and up to 38% of children.[39] The usual biliary anastomosis is an end-to-end choledochocholedochostomy with or without T tube insertion. In cases of unfavorable anatomy, biliary reconstruction, or reduced-size grafts, a choledochojejunostomy with a Roux-en-Y loop is fashioned.

The main complications seen are bile leaks and duct strictures. Bile leaks may result from surgical complications or from ischemia due to stenosis or thrombosis of the hepatic artery (Fig. 12.**4**). Resulting bilomas require percutaneous drainage and antibiotic therapy.[40] Bilomas may resemble simple fluid collections on ultrasound and SCT imaging, and therefore the decision to perform drainage must be based upon a clinical picture of bile leak, usually manifested as abdominal pain with evidence of sepsis.

Biliary strictures are an important cause of morbidity in transplant patients. They are more frequently seen in patients with a choledochocholedochostomy and can cause bile stasis and secondary infection. Strictures may be anastomotic, nonanastomotic or intrahepatic and again are usually due to ischemia, although intrahepatic strictures are also associated with chronic rejection, infection, long cold-ischemic time, and ABO incompatibility.[41] Severe ischemia may result in bile duct necrosis.

Ultrasound is insensitive in detecting biliary obstruction after OLT, so cholangiography is indicated if biliary complications are suspected. Endoscopic retrograde cholangiopancreatography is the initial method of choice but is precluded if a choledochojejunostomy is present; in which case percutaneous transhepatic cholangiography is necessary. If a bile leak is shown, nasobiliary or percutaneous drainage or endoscopic stent insertion is performed. This may be definitive

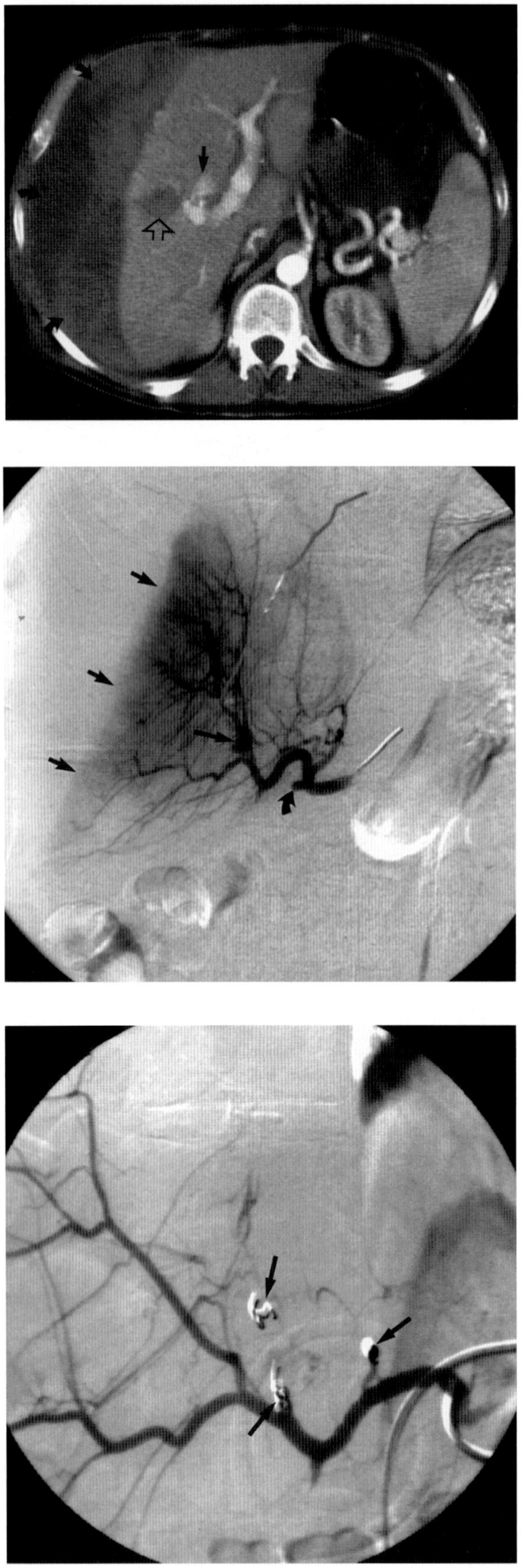

a

b

c

treatment for small leaks from the T tube exit site or anastomosis, but is usually only a temporizing measure in larger anastomotic leaks or in the setting of duct necrosis, which require surgical reconstruction or retransplantation.

Focal strictures may be treated by percutaneous balloon dilatation. Nonanastomotic strictures respond better than anastomotic strictures, which may require repeat dilatations to achieve a sustained improvement. Ultimately all strictures tend to recur, and therefore surgical reconstruction is the best hope of long-term improvement. Metal stents have been used with reasonable medium-term results, but these will also ultimately occlude. Metal stents preclude further attempts at surgical reconstruction and can cause erosion of the bile ducts and adjacent arteries, and for this reason their use is not recommended.[42] Multiple duct strictures may necessitate retransplantation.

Stones, sludge, and casts can produce bile duct filling defects on cholangiography. There are several causal factors for bile duct filling defects. Most cases of necrotic debris are caused by ischemia due to hepatic artery occlusion. It is difficult to differentiate between stones and sludge on imaging, and there may be underlying biliary strictures. Percutaneous transhepatic biliary drainage is not only useful for removal or irrigation of these bile duct filling defects, but also allows balloon dilatation of underlying strictures.[43]

Post-OLT Malignancy

Non-Hodgkin lymphomas and post-transplant lymphoproliferative disorder uncommonly occur as a result of immunosuppression. The role of IR is limited to percutaneous biopsy to establish the diagnosis.

◁ Fig. 12.**3** **a** Late arterial phase spiral computed tomography (SCT) performed 24 hours following a percutaneous liver biopsy on day 5 after OLT. A low-density area (open arrow) is seen corresponding to the path of the biopsy needle. There is a large hemoperitoneum (curved arrows). A small vascular blush is seen anterior to the right hepatic artery, consistent with a pseudoaneurysm (solid arrow). **b** Selective common hepatic angiogram showing compression of the liver by the large hemoperitoneum (short arrows) and confirming the small pseudoaneurysm (long arrow). Note the stump of the tied-off donor gastroduodenal artery (curved arrow). **c** Selective common hepatic angiogram following coil embolization of three feeding arteries (arrows), confirming exclusion of the pseudoaneurysm

■ ***Summary points:***

- Pseudoaneurysms may be excluded by placing microcoils immediately distal and proximal to the aneurysm neck, or they may be packed using detachable coils.
- Biliary tract complications occur in 10–20% of adult liver transplant patients and up to 38% of children.
- Ultrasound is insensitive in detecting biliary obstruction after liver transplantation, and cholangiography is indicated if biliary complications are suspected.
- Nonanastomotic biliary strictures respond better than anastomotic strictures, which may require repeat dilatations to achieve a sustained improvement.

Conclusion

Radiology plays a vital role in a successful liver transplantation program. Advances in noninvasive imaging have diminished the role of IR in pre-OLT imaging, although TIPS has emerged as an important technique in selected patients. After OLT, IR retains a pivotal role in the assessment and management of postoperative complications, and its role is likely to increase further as technological advances expand the scope for minimally invasive therapies.

References

1. Neuberger J, Lucey MR. Survival after transplantation. In: Neuberger J, Lucey MR editors. Liver transplantation: practice and management. London: BMJ Publishing Group; 1994. p. 169–75.
2. Kelly DA. Specific indications: paediatric liver transplantation. In: Neuberger J, Lucey MR editors. Liver transplantation: practice and management. London: BMJ Publishing Group; 1994. p. 85–104.
3. Millis JM, Martin P, Gomes A, et al. Transjugular intrahepatic portosystemic shunts: impact on liver transplantation. Liver Transpl Surg 1995;1:229–33.

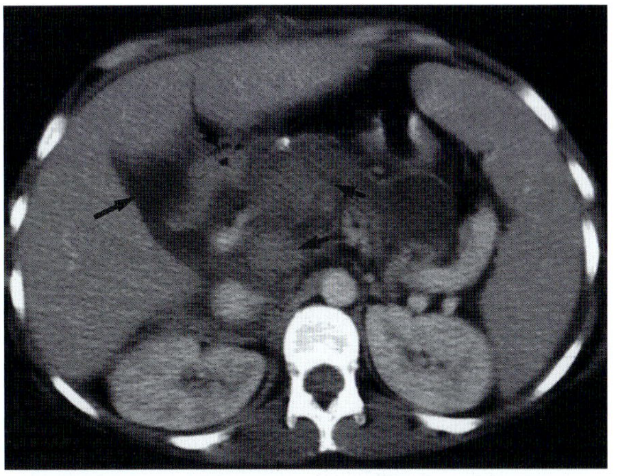

a

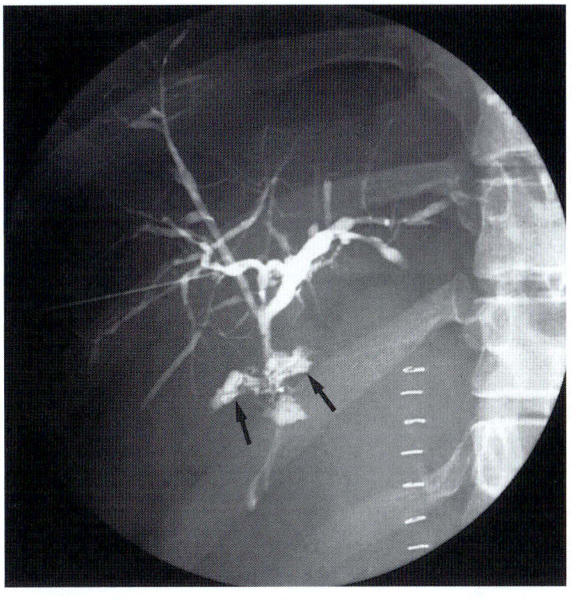

b

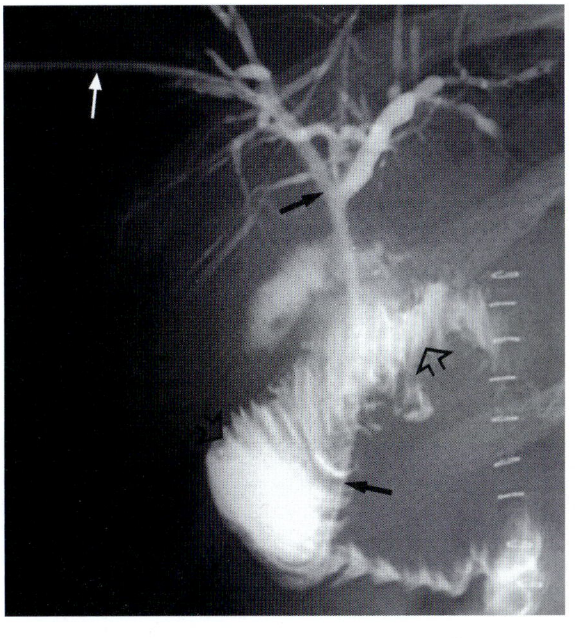

c

Fig. 12.**4** **a** Portal venous phase enhanced SCT day 5 after ▷ OLT. A low-density collection (long arrow) is seen in the gallbladder fossa, consistent with simple fluid or bile. The intermediate density collection adjacent to the portal vein is consistent with hematoma (short arrows). Air is noted within the Roux loop of a choledochojejunostomy (curved arrow). **b** Percutaneous transhepatic cholangiogram demonstrating diffuse irregularity of the intrahepatic ducts consistent with ischemia. There is contrast extravasation (arrows) at the choledochojejunostomy anastomosis indicating bile leak. **c** An internal–external biliary drain (solid arrows) has been inserted through into the Roux loop (open arrows). Further investigations confirmed hepatic artery occlusion and the patient underwent retransplantation

4. Somberg KA, Lombardero MS, Lawlor SM, et al. A controlled analysis of the transjugular intrahepatic portosystemic shunt in liver transplant recipients. The National Institute of Diabetes and Digestive and Kidney Diseases (NIDDK) Liver Transplantation Database. Transplantation 1997;63: 1074–9.
5. John TG, Jalan R, Stanley AJ, et al. Transjugular intrahepatic portosystemic stent-shunt (TIPSS) insertion as a prelude to orthotopic liver transplantation in patients with severe portal hypertension. Eur J Gastroenterol Hepatol 1996;12:1145–9.
6. Lerut JP, Laterre PF, Goffette P, et al. Transjugular intrahepatic portosystemic shunt and liver transplantation. Transpl Int 1996;9:370–5.
7. Johnson SP, Leyendecker JR, Joseph FB, et al. Transjugular portosystemic shunts in pediatric patients awaiting liver transplantation. Transplantation 1996;62:1178–81.
8. Hutchins RR, Patch D, Tibballs J, et al. Liver transplantation complicated by embedded transjugular intrahepatic portosystemic shunt: a new method for portal anastomosis—a surgical salvage procedure. Liver Transpl 2000;6:237–8.
9. Abouljoud MS, Levy MF, Rees CR, et al. A comparison of treatment with transjugular intrahepatic portosystemic shunt or distal splenorenal shunt in the management of variceal bleeding prior to liver transplantation. Transplantation 1995;59:226–9.
10. Menegaux F, Keeffe EB, Baker E, et al. Comparison of transjugular and surgical portosystemic shunts on the outcome of liver transplantation. Arch Surg 1994;129:1018–23.
11. Ryu RK, Durham JD, Krysl J, et al. Role of TIPS as a bridge to hepatic transplantation in Budd-Chiari syndrome. J Vasc Interv Radiol 1999;10:799–805.
12. Shrestha R, Durham JD, Wachs M, et al. Use of transjugular intrahepatic portosystemic shunt as a bridge to transplantation in fulminant hepatic failure due to Budd-Chiari syndrome. Am J Gastroenterol 1997;92:2304–6.
13. Liatsos C, Vlachigiannakos, Patch D, et al. Successful recanalization of portal vein thrombosis before liver transplantation using transjugular intrahepatic portosystemic shunt (TIPS). Liver Transpl 2001 (in press).
14. Iwatsuki S, Starzl TE, Sheahan DG, et al. Hepatic resection versus transplantation for hepatocellular carcinoma. Ann Surg 1991;214:221–9.
15. Lencioni R, Pinto F, Armillotta N, et al. Intrahepatic metastatic nodules of hepatocellular carcinoma detected at lipiodol-CT: imaging-pathologic correlation. Abdom Imaging 1997;22:253–8.
16. Saada J, Bhattacharya S, Dhillon AP, et al. Detection of small hepatocellular carcinoma in cirrhotic livers using iodised oil computed tomography. Gut 1997;41:404–7.
17. Lau WY, Leung TW, Ho SK, et al. Adjuvant intra-arterial iodine-131-labelled lipiodol for resectable hepatocellular carcinoma: a prospective randomised trial. Lancet 1999;353:797–801.
18. Livraghi T, Giorgio A, Marin G, et al. Hepatocellular carcinoma in cirrhosis in 746 patients: long term results of percutaneous ethanol injection. Radiology 1995;197:101–8.
19. Ishii H, Okada S, Okusaka T, et al. Needle tract implantation of hepatocellular carcinoma after percutaneous ethanol injection. Cancer 1998;82:1638–42.
20. Kim SH, Lim HK, Lee WJ, et al. Needle-tract implantation in hepatocellular carcinoma: frequency and CT findings after biopsy with a 19.5-gauge automated biopsy gun. Abdom Imaging 2000;25:246–50.
21. Takamori R, Wong LL, Dang C, et al. Needle-tract implantation from hepatocellular cancer: is needle biopsy of the liver always necessary? Liver Transpl 2000;6:67–72.
22. Van Thiel DH, Gavaler JS, Wright H, et al. Liver biopsy. Its safety and complications as seen at a liver transplant center. Transplantation 1993;55:1087–90.
23. Papatheodoridis GV, Patch D, Watkinson A, et al. Transjugular liver biopsy in the 1990s: a 2-year audit. Aliment Pharmacol Ther 1999;13:603–8.
24. Adetiloye VA, John PR. Intervention for pleural effusions and ascites following liver transplantation. Paediatr Radiol 1998;28:539–43.
25. Langnas A, Marujo W, Stratta R, et al. Vascular complications after liver transplantation. Am J. Surg 1991 23:76–9.
26. Wozney P, Zajko AB, Bron KM, et al. Vascular complications after liver transplantation: a 5-year experience. AJR Am J Roentgenol 1986;147:657–63.
27. Raby N, Karani J, Thomas S, et al. Stenoses of vascular anastomoses after hepatic transplantation: treatment with balloon angioplasty. AJR Am J Roentgenol 1991;157:167–71.
28. Mondragon RS, Karani JB, Heaton ND, et al. The use of percutaneous transluminal angioplasty in hepatic artery stenosis after transplantation. Transplantation 1994;57:228–31.
29. Valente JF. Alonso MH, Weber FL, et al. Late hepatic artery thrombosis in liver allograft recipients is associated with intrahepatic biliary necrosis. Transplantation 1996;61:61–5.
30. Zajko AB, Sheng R, Bron K, et al. Percutaneous transluminal angioplasty of venous anastomotic stenosis complicating liver transplantation: intermediate-term results. J Vasc Interv Radiol 1994;5:121–6.
31. Funaki B, Rosenblum JD, Leef JA, et al. Angioplasty treatment of portal vein stenosis in children with segmental liver transplants: mid-term results. AJR Am J Roentgenol 1997;169:551–4.
32. Lerut J, Tzakis A, Born K, et al. Complications of venous reconstruction in human orthotopic liver transplantation. Ann Surg 1987;205:404–14.
33. Egawa H, Inomata Y, Uemoto S, et al. Hepatic vein reconstruction in 152 living-related donor liver transplantation patients. Surgery 1997;121:250–7.
34. Rossi AR, Pozniak MA, Zarvan NP. Upper inferior vena caval anastomotic stenosis in liver transplant recipients: Doppler US diagnosis. Radiology 1993;187:387–9.
35. Zajko AB, Claus D, Clapuyt P, et al. Obstruction to hepatic venous drainage after liver transplantation: treatment with balloon angioplasty. Radiology 1989;170:763–5.
36. Otobe Y, Hashimoto T, Shimizu Y, et al. Formation of fatal arterioportal fistula following needle liver biopsy in a child with living related transplant: report of a case. Surg Today 1995;25:916–19.
37. Sheng R, Orons PD, Ramos HC, et al. Dissecting pseudoaneurysm of the hepatic artery: a delayed complication of angioplasty in a liver transplant. Cardiovasc Intervent Radiol 1995;18:112–14.
38. Lerut J, Gordon R, Iwatsuki S, et al. Biliary tract complications in human orthotopic liver transplantation. Transplantation 1987;43:47–51.
39. Heffron TG, Edmond JC, Whitington PF, et al. Biliary complications in pediatric liver transplantation. Transplantation 1992;53:391–5.
40. Hoffer FA, Teek RL, Lillehei CW, et al. Infected bilomas and hepatic artery thrombosis in infant recipients of liver transplants. Interventional radiology and medical therapy as an alternative to retransplantation. Radiology 1988;169:435–8.
41. Campbell WL, Sheng R, Zajko AB, et al. Intrahepatic biliary strictures after liver transplantation. Radiology 1994;191:735–40.
42. Culp WC, McCowan TC, Lieberman RP, et al. Biliary strictures in liver transplant recipients: treatment with metal stents. Radiology 1996;199:339–46.
43. Sheng R, Ramirez CB, Zajko AB, et al. Biliary stones and sludge in liver transplant patients: a 13 year experience. Radiology 1996;198:243–7.

Pancreas Transplantation

A. Khanna, N. H. Patel, Z. Song, and R. M. Jindal

Introduction

Diabetes mellitus (DM) is a very common disease, which affects approximately 2–6% of the general population; the overall incidence is increasing worldwide. It is currently the third most common disease and the fourth leading cause of death by disease in the USA. It is estimated that, by 2010, the number of people with DM will exceed 350 million. About 10% of DM patients have insulin-dependent diabetes mellitus (IDDM). The syndrome of IDDM includes abnormal glucose metabolism and specific microvascular complications that include retinopathy, nephropathy, and neuropathy. Intensive insulin therapy will improve glucose control; nevertheless, most patients will eventually develop some or all of these secondary complications.

DM is currently the leading cause of kidney failure and blindness in adults, the commonest cause of amputations and impotence, and one of the leading chronic diseases of childhood. Apart from the latest report on a small number of patients by the Edmonton group on consecutive successful allogenic islet cell transplantations,[1] vascularized pancreas transplantation is the only available treatment of IDDM that can establish insulin independence, with normoglycemia and normal glycosylated hemoglobin levels for as long as the graft functions.

Unlike other organ transplantation, pancreatic transplantation is not considered a life-saving operation, and the recipients are subject to life-long immunosuppression. The Diabetes Control and Complications Trial (DCCT), showed the importance of euglycemia in preventing and controlling the progression of complications.[2–4] Nevertheless, completely normal glycosylated hemoglobin can only be obtained by a pancreas transplant.

The first pancreatic transplant was performed by Kelly and Lillihei at the University of Minnesota in 1966. In the 1980s, developments in immunosuppression therapy and surgical management of pancreatic exocrine secretions combined with careful candidate selection resulted in dramatic improvements in both patient and graft survival. In the 1990s, the incorporation of additional new antirejection agents into the immunosuppression protocols resulted in a further decrease in the incidence of acute rejection.

Patient Selection

Patient selection for pancreatic transplantation involves a comprehensive multidisciplinary pretransplant evaluation with additional work-up tailored to the individual patient. Overall, the evaluation confirms the diagnosis of IDDM, determines the patient's ability to withstand a major operation, establishes the absence of any exclusion criteria, and documents end-organ complications to study the effect of pancreas transplantation on the secondary complications of diabetes.

■ *Summary points:*

Patient selection for pancreas transplants should include the following:

- Objective measures to exclude irreversible cardiac ischemia
- Exclusion of irreversible severe peripheral vascular disease
- Consideration that previous stroke and transient ischemic attacks increase postoperative risk
- As routine, ECG, stress thallium scan, coronary angiograms, Doppler examination of limbs
- Exclusion of chronic sepsis

Technical Aspects of Pancreas Transplantation

Advances in organ retrieval and preservation technology have played an important role in the improving results of pancreas transplantation. Most North American transplant centers have chosen vascularized pancreas transplantation with the duodenal segment method of bladder drainage as the procedure of choice, but an increasing number of centers have switched to exocrine drainage into the bowel to avoid the metabolic and urological complications of bladder drainage. The majority of pancreas transplants are performed in conjunction with a simultaneous renal transplant from the same donor through a midline intraperitoneal approach. The operation usually lasts from three to five hours, depending on whether the patient is having a pancreas alone or combined simultaneous kidney and pancreatic transplant (SKPT). Most pancreas transplants have been performed using the standard technique of endocrine drainage into the systemic venous

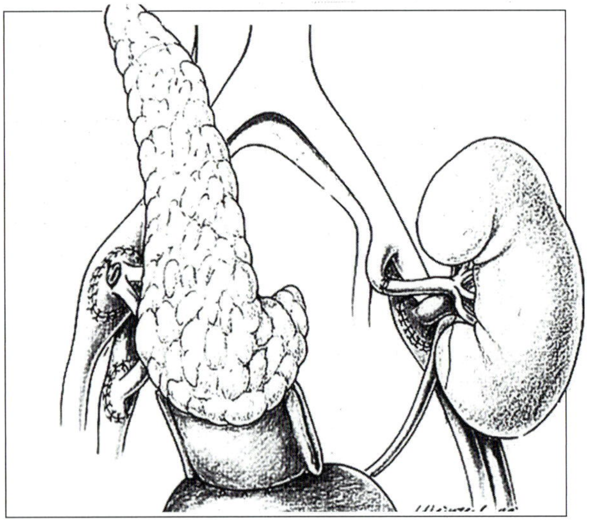

Fig. 13.**1** Standard surgical technique of simultaneous kidney and pancreatic transplant

circulation (iliac vein) and exocrine drainage into the urinary bladder (Fig. 13.**1**). A new technique of draining the endocrine secretion into the portal venous system in combination with enteric drainage of the exocrine secretions is gradually replacing the standard technique. The recipient's native pancreas and kidneys are not removed.

Following operation, the patient usually spends two to three days in the intensive care unit and two to three weeks in the hospital. SKPT is associated with a greater morbidity than a kidney transplant alone, mainly due to reoperation, pancreas-specific morbidity, increased rejection episodes, and infections.[5,6]

Long-Term Outcome After Pancreas Transplantation

With newer immunosuppressive regimens and an optimized safe, standardized surgical procedure that has minimized technical complications related to exocrine secretions and graft thrombosis, the results of vascularized pancreas transplantation have improved significantly in the past decade. The one-year patient survival rate for all categories—SKPT, PAKT (pancreas after kidney transplant), and PTA (pancreas transplant alone)—is 95 %, with an 85 % one-year survival rate of pancreas graft after SKPT, 74 % after PAKT, and 69 % after PTA. The one-year kidney graft survival rate after SKPT is 91 %. Rejection accounts for 18 % of graft failures in the first year following pancreatic transplantation. The overall average pancreas graft survival rates for combined kidney–pancreas transplants at one, three, and five years are 83.6 %, 72.9 %, and 65.5 % respectively. Results of pancreatic transplants are frequently updated and can be found on www.insulin-free.org./article/inp.htm.

Complications

Early Complications

Complications can arise shortly following pancreas transplantation, they include surgical complications such as vascular thrombosis, urinary leak, graft rejection, allograft pancreatitis, and intra-abdominal infection. Kidney allograft rejection can be used to guide treatment in SKPT patients as kidney graft rejection is believed to precede or parallel pancreatic rejection. The bladder drainage technique has allowed direct monitoring of pancreatic exocrine function, and urine amylase and cytology have both been used as noninvasive markers of early rejection.

Vascular thrombosis is the most common complication associated with pancreatic transplantation, with an overall rate of approximately 12 %, of which 5 % are arterial and 7 % venous in origin (Fig. 13.**2**). Several donor risk factors for thrombosis have been identified, including old age and cardio-cerebrovascular diseases. Surgical related risk factors are left-sided implantation, arterial reconstruction, and portal vein extension. Surgical complications related to exocrine pancreatic drainage and allograft pancreatitis are usually due to technical errors (leak or fistula) or infection leading to fluid collections, pseudocysts, or abscesses surrounding the pancreatic graft. Reflux graft pancreatitis, hematuria, and bleeding are also quite common complications. Perioperative antibacterial prophylaxis with imipenem–cilastatin alone or in combination with vancomycin, or with antibiotics chosen according to the results of duodenal culture, and antifungal and antiviral prophylaxis with fluconazole, nystatin, or clotrimazole, and aciclovir or ganciclovir, are recommended and have been shown to reduce the incidence of infective complications. The repeat laparotomy rate following pancreatic transplantation is 24–32 % in the USA. This is commonly for intra-abdominal infections, vascular thrombosis, and anastomotic leaks. Uncommon complications after pancreas transplantation have been reported, such as mesenteric arteriovenous fistula, iliac artery–bladder fistula, arterial mycotic aneurysm and rupture, urethral diverticula, and cytomegalovirus pancreatitis.

In addition to these surgical complications, pancreas transplant recipients may also develop urological or metabolic complications due to the unusual physiology of the transplanted pancreas and bladder drainage of the exocrine secretions. Urinary tract infections and chemical cystitis or urethritis due to pancreatic enzyme activation are commonly seen. Some patients may develop a urethral stricture, hematuria, or perforation of the bladder or duodenal segment. Pancreas transplant recipients are uniquely susceptible to metabolic acidosis and dehydration because of the loss of pancreatic secretions rich in sodium and bicarbonate into the urinary tract. Recent reports from several centers have shown that enteric drainage can avoid these complications.

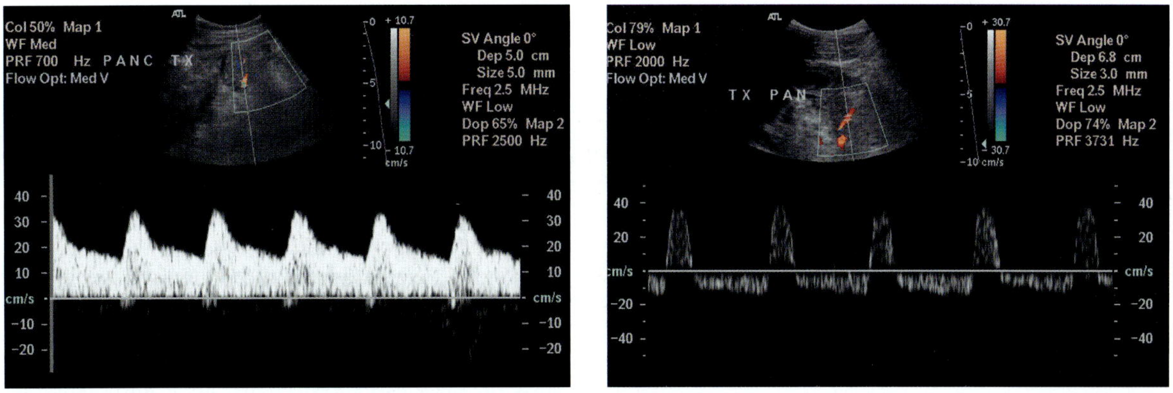

a b

Fig. 13.**2** **a** Normal color Doppler image of a pancreatic transplant showing multiple small vessels within it. Spectral Doppler examination of one of those vessels shows a normal low-resistance arterial waveform. **b** Color Doppler image showing absent small vessel flow within the pancreas itself. Only the main supplying artery can be seen. Spectral Doppler shows reverse diastolic flow within this vessel in keeping with a venous thrombosis. This was confirmed at surgery

■ *Summary points:*

Postoperative complications after pancreas transplantation can include:

Immunological:

- Recurrence of autoimmune process in the transplanted pancreas
- Rejection

Nonimmunological:

- Thrombosis
- Bleeding
- Pancreatitis
- Anastomotic leak
- Sepsis
- Pancreatic ascites
- Pancreatic fistula
- Primary nonfunction
- Intestinal obstruction, perforation
- Metabolic acidosis
- Urethretis, balanitis, cystitis

Late Complications

Long-term complications of pancreas transplantation include the side effects of chronic immunosuppression, hyperinsulinemia, and progression of diabetic complications. Chronic immunosuppression is associated with an increased risk of infection, malignancy such as lymphoma, and specific drug toxicity. Corticosteroids and calcineurin inhibitors such as cyclosporine and tacrolimus are associated with insulin resistance, hypertension, and detrimental changes in lipid metabolism that can lead to accelerated atherosclerosis.

Pancreas transplantation can establish a euglycemic insulin-independent state immediately following operation; however, diabetic retinopathy may not improve even after glucose control has been achieved. DCCT data has demonstrated that nephropathy is also preventable and neuropathy can be reversed by improved glucose control. Atherosclerotic vascular disease is the most common cause of morbidity and mortality following solid organ transplantation. For most pancreas transplant recipients, the quality of life is improved. This include opportunities for social interaction, ability to return to work, an increased energy level, and psychological well-being.

Specific Immunosuppression for Pancreas Transplantation

Traditionally, it was believed that the additional load of the pancreas would result in a greater susceptibility to rejection, and therefore a heavier immunosuppression regime would be required than for kidney transplantation alone. There is also a unique susceptibility of the pancreas allograft to the diabetogenicity of some immunosuppressants, whilst the transplanted pancreas continues to remain susceptible to recurrence of autoimmune disease. Most pancreas transplant centers have traditionally employed quadruple drug immunosuppression with anti-T-lymphocyte induction using either a monoclonal (OKT3) or a polyclonal (antithymic globulin or anti-lymphocytic globulin) antibody agent. Maintenance immunosuppression involves triple therapy consisting of a calcineurin inhibitor (cyclosporine or tacrolimus), an antimetabolite (azathioprine or mycophenolate mofetil) (MMF, CellCept), and corticosteroids. This traditional view of immunosuppressive therapy for pancreatic transplants is now being reevaluated. Furthermore, the advent of newer immunosuppressants has given the clinician a greater choice of antirejection therapy.

Maintenance therapy in pancreatic transplantation entails the use of triple drug therapy consisting of either

Table 13.**1** Immunosuppressive agents used in pancreas transplantation

Tacrolimus	Daclizumab/ basiliximab	OKT3 or ATG
Prednisone	Cyclosporine/ tacrolimus	Cyclosporine/ tacrolimus
MMF	Prednisone MMF	Prednisone MMF

Each column represents an immunosuppressive regimen. The trend is to avoid the use of antibody for induction. Daclizumab (Zenapax) and basiliximab (Simulect) are the recently introduced anti-IL-2 antibodies. MMF, mycophenolate mofetil

cyclosporine or tacrolimus, corticosteroids, and an antimetabolite, such as azathioprine or MMF. From the 1980s to the middle of the 1990s, cyclosporine (Sandimmune) was used for almost all pancreas transplant patients. For the last few years, a new microemulsion formulation of cyclosporine (Neoral) has replaced the original formulation. The new formulation has clearly shown an improved pharmacokinetic profile and has a pharmacoeconomic and immunological advantage; however, there is no evidence that it improves pancreas graft survival.

Tacrolimus is a calcineurin inhibitor, similar to cyclosporine, which provides a highly specific and reversible blockade of calcineurin in T lymphocytes, thus resulting in the inhibition of IL-2 transcription in the nucleus and the prevention of T helper cell activation. Tacrolimus has been widely accepted in solid organ transplantation as both a primary and rescue agent since the late 1980s and became available for use in pancreatic transplantation immunosuppression protocols in 1994. An additional advantage of this drug is its steroid-sparing effects, with complete steroid withdrawal possible in up to 60% of renal allograft recipients. The use of tacrolimus for all categories of transplantation (SKPT, PAKT, PTA) has been increased in recent years. Comparing tacrolimus with cyclosporine, the one-year graft survival rates were similar for SKP and PTA transplant recipients. For PAKT recipients, the one-year graft survival rates was better with tacrolimus than with cyclosporine (84% versus 65%). Bruce et al.[7] reported their experience with cyclosporine/MMF/prednisone and tacrolimus/MMF/prednisone in 51 consecutive SPK transplantations and found that cyclosporine/MMF/prednisone was only marginally more effective than cyclosporine/azathioprine/prednisone, whereas the tacrolimus regimen showed excellent results with one-year patient, pancreas, and kidney survival rates of 97%, 94%, and 97% respectively.

The introduction of tacrolimus has also revived interest in solitary pancreas transplantation as an option in patients with unstable diabetes and a functioning kidney. In contrast to the results of SKPT (graft survival about 75–90% at 1 year), the results of pancreas transplantation alone have remained poor (about 50% at 1 year). Bartlett et al.[8] in a landmark study showed that using tacrolimus and percutaneous biopsy of the pancreas to diagnose rejection at an early stage, they could increase graft survival to 90.1% as compared with 53.4% in the cyclosporine group.

The majority of pancreas transplants are still performed using antilymphocyte induction with either the monoclonal antibody OKT3 or polyclonal preparations such as anti-thymic globulin. In recent years, there has been an overall decrease in the use of antibody induction therapy from 90% during the period 1987–1993 to 82% of pancreas transplants performed during 1994–1998. In the last decade, the use of polyclonal agents declined from 61% to 33%, while the use of OKT3 increased from 27% to 49%. Antibodies are usually given intravenously during the transplantation procedure or immediately after the operation to provide an immunosuppressive umbrella, allowing the administration of potentially nephrotoxic compounds to be delayed.

Patients usually receive a 5- to 14-day course of induction therapy. OKT3 is by far the most extensively studied of these. This first dose effect frequently causes fever, chills, tachycardia, gastrointestinal disturbances, bronchospasm, and elevation or depression of blood pressure; dosage adjustments may be required. Although the addition of an antilymphocyte agent provides enhanced immunosuppression in the early posttransplantation period, it is associated with added costs and side effects.

Investigators have recently reported that potent new immunosuppressive compounds—tacrolimus combined with either MMF or azathioprine—and steroid without antibody induction can achieve similar results to the traditional antibody preparations in recipients of SPKT. The one-year pancreas graft survival rate for SKPT without anti-T-lymphocyte induction is 85%, which is similar to treatment regimens employing polyclonal or monoclonal antibody induction. However, anti-T-cell induction is still associated with superior pancreatic graft survival in the PAKT and PTA categories (Table 13.**1**).

Pancreatic Islet Cell Transplantation

Pancreatic islet cell transplantation is arguably the most logical approach to restoring homeostasis in patients with diabetes. However, there are a number of problems to be overcome, including the limited supply of human islet tissue, the adverse effects of current immunosuppressive protocols, the problems of primary nonfunction, rejection, and recurrence of disease. There have been numerous clinical trials of human islet cell allografts at various centers worldwide. According to data compiled by the International Islet Transplant Registry, up to December 1998 a total of 407 adult islet allografts had been performed world-wide. A detailed analysis (one-year follow up) performed on 200 pretransplant C-peptide-negative patients with

type 1 DM undergoing transplantation between 1990 and 1997 showed one-year patient and allograft survival rates of 96% and 35% respectively. The definition of graft survival was de novo production of C-peptide; however, only 8% of recipients were insulin-independent at one year. The longest duration of function of an islet allograft as defined by C-peptide production is now over eight years, with insulin independence maintained for over 5 years. The latest results of pancreatic islet transplantation can be found at www.med.uni-giessen.de/itr.
Analysis of the results and the data presented to the registry have shown the following variables to be critical to the overall success of islet transplantation:

- Preservation time of the organ should be less than eight hours.
- A minimum number of 6000 IE/kg (IE=islet equivalents, a notional expression of the islet tissue volume).
- Anti-lymphocyte antibodies (anti-thymic or anti-lymphocyte globulin) given at the time of induction.
- Intrahepatic transplantation site (portal vein) for implantation of islets.

A group at the University of Giessen have achieved significantly better results which were attributed to the following additional factors: total parenteral nutrition and insulin administration to rest the islets metabolically, and administration of nicotinamide and pentoxifylline to prevent primary nonfunction. At one year, 30% of their patients had achieved insulin independence. Although the overall results are not encouraging, with few patients achieving insulin independence, two points need to be stressed. First, in many patients in whom C-peptide production is demonstrated but insulin independence is not achieved, HbA_{1c} can be normalized with better metabolic control than can be obtained with the use of exogenous insulin alone. The results obtained are significantly better than those achieved with intensive insulin treatment as defined by the DCCT Research group. Moreover, despite the improved control, unlike in the DCCT trial, hypoglycemia has not been observed. This is despite the gradual decline in allograft function as monitored by a decline in C-peptide response during Sustacal (a standardized oral glucose challenge) tests over the six-year period. More recently, the Edmonton group has shown that using a steroid-free immunosuppressive protocol, they were able to achieve 100% success in seven diabetic patients up to a year.[1] Other centers are attempting to reproduce these results.

Future Directions

Fine-needle aspiration biopsy of the transplanted pancreas to diagnose rejection has resulted in an improvement in graft survival, and surgeons are increasingly using the more physiological portal and enteric drainage procedure in pancreas transplantation. Immunosuppressive strategies will evolve to achieve control of rejection while minimizing injury to the allograft and risk to the patient. In addition, new regimens must not only address the issue of specific drug toxicities but also the long-term economic, metabolic, and quality-of-life outcomes. Pancreatic transplantation will remain an important alternative in the treatment of diabetic patients until other strategies are developed that can provide equal glycemic control with less immunosuppression and overall morbidity (see summary points below). Novel strategies to produce tolerance such as the use of donor bone marrow together with pancreas transplantation are being attempted.

Summary points:

The effects of pancreas transplantation on metabolism and secondary complications of diabetes include the following:

- Blood sugar levels are consistently normal
- Early transplantation may prevent the occurrence of secondary complications of diabetes. The effect on established lesions is not clear.
- Neuropathy clearly improves in most patients
- After renal transplantation, recurrence of diabetic nephropathy is prevented in the new kidney

References

1. Shapiro AMJ, Lakey JRT, Ryan EA, et al. Islet transplantation in seven patients with type 1 diabetes mellitus using a glucocorticoid-free immunosuppressive regimen. N Engl J Med 2000;343:230–8.
2. The Diabetes Control and Complications Trial Research Group. Hypoglycemia in the Diabetes Control and Complications Trial. Diabetes 1997;46:271–86.
3. Diabetes Control and Complications Trial (DCCT) Research Group. The effect of intensive treatment on the development and progression of long-term complications in insulin-dependent diabetes mellitus. N Engl J Med 1993;329: 976–86.
4. American Diabetes Association. Position statement: implications of the Diabetes Control and Complications Trial. Clin Diabetes 1993;11:91.
5. Gaber AO, Shokouh-Amiri H, Grewal HP, et al. A technique for portal pancreas transplantation with enteric drainage. Surg Gynecol Obstet 1993;177:417–9.
6. Reddy KS, Stratta RJ, Shokouh-Amiri MH, Alloway R, Egidi MF, Gaber AO. Surgical complications after pancreas transplantation with portal-enteric drainage. J Am Coll Surg 1999;189:305–13.
7. Bruce DS, Woodle ES, Newell KA, et al. Tacrolimus/mycophenolate provides superior immunosuppression relative to Neoral/mycophenolate in synchronous pancreas-kidney transplantation. Transplant Proc 1998;30:1538–40.
8. Bartlett ST, Schweitzer EJ, Johnson LB, et al. Equivalent success of simultaneous pancreas kidney and solitary pancreas transplantation: a prospective trial of tacrolimus immunosuppression with percutaneous biopsy. Ann Surg 1996;224:440–52.

Suggested Further Reading

Jindal RM, Sidner RA. Milgrom ML. Post-transplant diabetes mellitus: the role of immunosuppression. Drug Safety 1997;16:242–57.

Becker BN, Brazy PC, Becker YT, et al. Simultaneous pancreas–kidney transplantation reduces excess mortality in type 1 diabetic patients with end-stage renal disease. Kidney Int 2000;57:2129–35.

McAlister VC, Gao Z, Peltekian K, Domingues K, Mahalati K, MacDonald AS. Sirolimus-tacrolimus combination immunosuppression. Lancet 2000;355:376–7.

Jordan NL, Shapiro R, Gritsch HA, et al. Long-term results of pancreas transplantation under tacrolimus immunosuppression. Transplantation 1999;67:266–72.

Gruessner RWG, Sutherland DER, Drangstveit MB, Wrenshall L, Humar A, Gruessner AC. Mycophenolate mofetil in pancreas transplantation. Transplantation 1998;66:318–23.

Jindal RM, Dubernard J-M. Towards a specific immunosuppression for pancreas and islet grafts. Clin Transplant 2000;14:242–5.

Humar A, Parr E, Drangstveit MB, Kandaswamy R, Gruessner AC, Sutherland DER. Steroid withdrawal in pancreas transplant recipients Clin Transplant 2000;14:75–8.

Corry RJ, Chakrabarti PK, Shapiro R, et al. Simultaneous administration of adjuvant donor bone marrow in pancreas transplant recipients. Ann Surg 1999;230:372–9.

Small Bowel and Multivisceral Transplantation

A. Khanna and R.M. Jindal

Introduction

Small bowel transplantation is indicated for intestinal failure resulting from surgical loss of most of the small bowel (resulting in short gut syndrome) or absence of functional bowel (e.g., motility disorders). Experimental intestinal transplantation was first performed by Lillehei et al. 1959 in dogs.[1] Starzl and Kaupp later reported multivisceral transplantation in dogs.[2] The first report of a clinically successful multivisceral transplantation was in 1987 by Starzl et al.[3] The limited success was due to unrelenting rejection of the allografts, related mainly to the absence of specific and more potent immunosuppressive agents.

With rapid advances in transplant immunology and the introduction of newer immunosuppressants, physicians are now better equipped to prevent and treat allograft rejection. Moreover, the techniques of organ allograft procurement, preservation, and transplantation have been standardized over the course of the last ten years. This has led to better graft outcomes and has rapidly transformed the field of small bowel and multivisceral transplantation for patients with intestinal and/or liver failure.

Indications

Isolated Small Bowel Transplantation

The indications for transplantation of small bowel alone may be divided into the surgical and the nonsurgical. Surgical causes of small bowel loss are:

- Acute loss of intestinal function (surgical resection) due to necrotizing enterocolitis, volvulus, or mesenteric thrombosis
- Chronic loss of intestinal function due to Crohn disease or radiation enteritis
- Absence of vascular access in the presence of short gut syndrome

Nonsurgical causes are:

- Motility disorders: intestinal pseudo-obstruction, Hirschsprung disease
- Absorptive defects: microvillous inclusion disease, polyposis, desmoid tumors

Liver–Small Bowel Transplantation

The main indication for combined liver and small bowel transplant is end-stage liver disease due to prolonged hyperalimentation for short gut syndrome. The liver is transplanted with the small bowel especially if there is biopsy-proven cirrhosis, portal hypertension, and evidence of synthetic and biochemical dysfunction.

Multivisceral Transplantation

Multivisceral transplantation may include[4,5] stomach, duodenum, pancreas, liver, and small bowel with or without colon. The main indications are pseudo-obstruction/aganglionosis syndrome with hepatic failure, diffuse splanchnic venous thrombosis, and hepatic failure.

Patient Selection

Due to the complex nature of problems associated with patients who are candidates for small bowel and multivisceral transplantation, the work-up is best done at a transplant center where there is expertise in short gut problems and small bowel transplantation. Not all patients referred for small bowel transplantation necessarily need one. One of the most important aspects when evaluating these patients is to ensure that all attempts have been made to maximize the use of the remaining gut. This requires a dedicated team of gastroenterologists, nutritionists, social workers, and surgeons to evaluate the patient and, very often, make changes in the feeding formula and the duration of feeding. This has resulted in some patients with short gut syndrome being weaned off hyperalimentation successfully.

Once the need for small bowel transplantation is established, however, the need for other organs (e.g., liver) to be transplanted at the same time is assessed. The patient is evaluated by gastroenterologists, hepatologists, social workers, nutritionists, transplant coordinator, and a transplant surgeon. A complete work-up consists of sending blood for typing, biochemical analysis, liver panel tests, protein S and C deficiency testing, and serological testing for hepatitis and human immunodeficiency virus (HIV). Radiological studies are performed to confirm the absence of

functional small bowel and the patency of the portal venous system. The diagnosis of motility disorders is established by motility studies and bowel biopsy. The social worker looks into the family structure and support system.
Recipients of small bowel transplants require very close monitoring and are a "high-maintenance" group especially during the first few months following transplantation. Hence it is mandatory that they have excellent family support. Once the candidate work-up is completed, the patient is presented to the transplant selection committee and listed for the appropriate transplant.

Technical Aspects

Donor Operation

Careful donor selection is extremely important. The donor should be of the same blood type as the recipient and should not weigh more than 20% more than the recipient. It is important that the cold ischemic time is kept as short as possible. Occasionally, small bowel grafts with up to 17 or 18 hours of cold ischemia time have been used with good results. Donor hypernatremia, dependency on vasopressors, and the presence of infection are contraindications to procurement.
Donor surgery consists of mobilizing the small bowel and liver and isolating the infrarenal aorta. A mixture of amphotericin B, gentamicin, and polymyxin is administered to the small bowel via nasogastric tube to decontaminate the gut. The donor is heparinized, the aorta cross-clamped, and the organs perfused with cold University of Wisconsin solution administered via a catheter in the infrarenal aorta. The small bowel is procured en bloc with the liver. If the recipient needs isolated small bowel transplantation, the two organs are separated on the back table.

Recipient Operation

Figure 14.**1** shows isolated small bowel; liver and small bowel, and multivisceral grafts. The recipient operation consists of an exploratory laparotomy and the taking down of adhesions, as some of these patients have had several explorations. In isolated small bowel transplantation the arterial inflow to the graft is most commonly provided by anastomosing the donor superior mesenteric artery to the infrarenal aorta. Venous outflow is provided by anastomosing the superior mesenteric vein of the donor to the side of the recipient portal vein or into the inferior vena cava.
In liver and small bowel transplantation the arterial inflow is provided by a common Carrel patch made out of the donor celiac axis and superior mesenteric artery which is anastomosed to the infrarenal aorta.[6–8] The suprahepatic cava of the donor is anastomosed to the suprahepatic cava of the recipient. Once the vascular anastomosis is carried out the clamps are released and the graft is perfused. Solumedrol (methylprednisolone; 10 mg/kg in children, 1 g/kg in adults) is administered intravenously by the anesthesiologist to circumvent any immunological response by the recipient. Intestinal continuity is restored by performing donor-to-recipient bowel anastomosis proximally and distally. The terminal end of the small bowel is brought out as an ileostomy that is used for surveillance endoscopy to monitor rejection.

Immunosuppression

A commonly practiced regimen includes the use of an antibody (basiliximab or daclizumab), a calcineurin inhibitor (tacrolimus), an inhibitor of T cell proliferation (mycophenolate), and steroids.
Induction[9] is usually with basilixumab (Simulect) 20 mg i. v. preoperatively and postoperative day 4 or daclizumab[10] (Zenapax) 1 mg/kg intravenously, first dose within 24 hours before transplantation, with subsequent doses given two, four, six, and eight weeks after transplantation.
Tacrolimus (0.15 mg/kg p.o. or i. v. per day) is given to achieve a target trough level of 15–20 ng/ml (microparticle enzyme immunoassay). Mycophenolate mofetil is administered at a dosage of 15–30 mg/kg per day p.o. or i. v.
Methylprednisolone taper starts at a dose of 5 mg/kg per day for children or 200 mg/day for adults and is reduced over a period of five days to 1 mg/kg per day for children or 20 mg/day for adults.
Episodes of acute rejection are treated with steroid boluses, optimization of tacrolimus levels, and, in cases of severe rejection, with OKT3. Recently, sirolimus (previously known as rapamycin) has been used in some patients with limited success.[11]

Postoperative Care

Patients are nursed in an intensive care setting. The majority of the patients can be extubated within a day or two following surgery. Occasionally, due to discrepancies in donor–recipient organ size, extubation may not be possible in the early postoperative period. Careful attention must be paid to extubation parameters and a good trial on continuous positive airway pressure is recommended before extubation is attempted.
Close attention is given to the fluid status of small bowel or multivisceral transplant patients, who can lose a lot of fluid through the stoma. Strict intake/output recording is mandatory, and any unexpected change in stomal output should be immediately brought to attention. Care must be taken to ensure that the patient maintains a good urine output in the postoperative period.

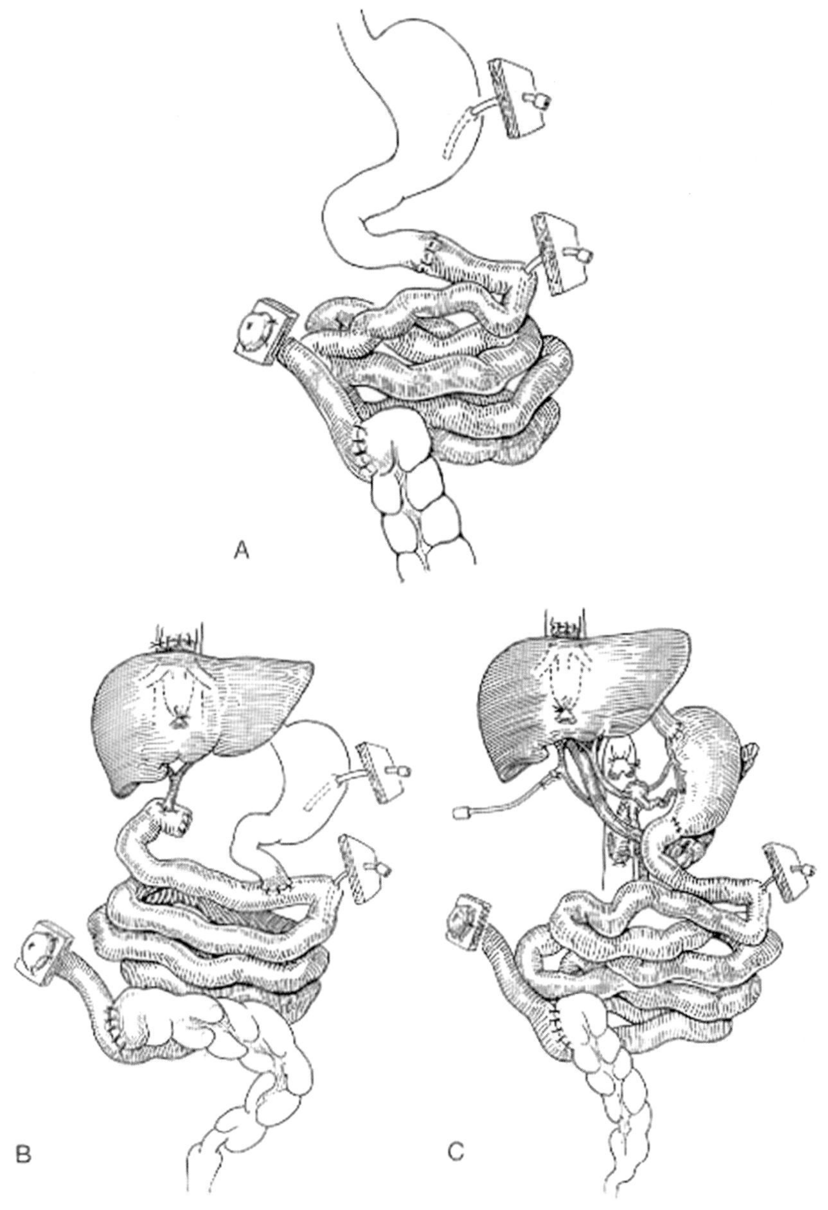

Fig. 14.**1** Intestinal transplantation can be performed as an isolated intestine graft (**a**), as a component of composite grafts such as liver/small bowel (**b**), and as multivisceral grafts (**c**). (Reproduced from Reyes et al. 1998,[6] with permission)

Infection prophylaxis is ensured by intravenous administration of broad-spectrum antibiotics in the postoperative period. All patients are given an antibiotic "cocktail" consisting of amphotericin B, gentamicin, and polymyxin E orally every six hours for the first two to four weeks. This is to decontaminate the gut and prevent bacterial translocation from the allograft. Stool samples are cultured weekly. A positive stool culture in the presence of signs of systemic sepsis indicates allograft rejection causing translocation due to breakdown of the mucosal barrier.[12]

Antiviral prophylaxis in the form of ganciclovir (5 mg/kg i. v. b.d.) is given for the first two weeks following transplantation. Lifetime oral trimethoprim–sulfamethoxazole is used as prophylaxis for *Pneumocystis carinii* pneumonia.

Monitoring of Small Bowel Grafts

During the postoperative period, the stoma is observed for any change in color or bleeding. An accurate record of stomal output is kept. With the introduction and use of zoom videoendoscopy, subtle changes in the small bowel mucosal pattern and loss of microvillous architecture can be appreciated, leading to rapid diagnosis

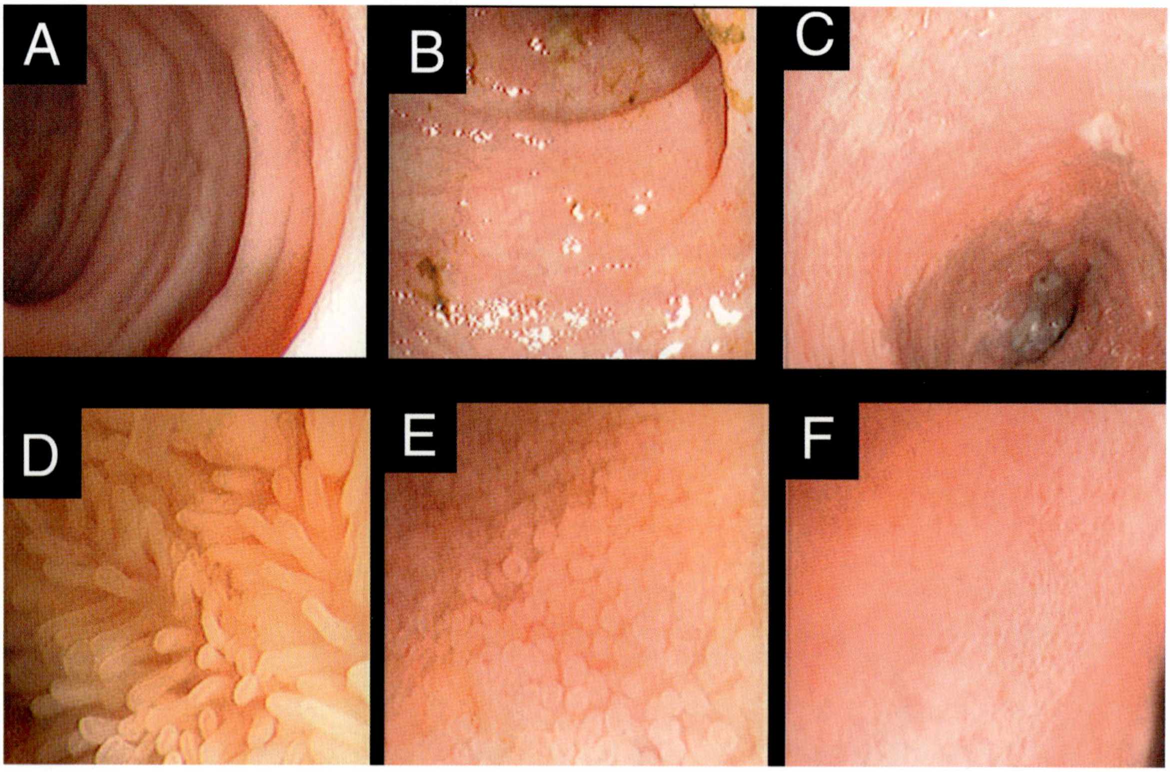

Fig. 14.2 Zoom videoendoscopic view of small bowel graft mucosa. **a**, **d** Normal mucosa. Villi appear tall and thin. No significant erythema is seen on the background of mucosa. **b**, **e** Moderate rejection of the small bowel graft. Villi appear shortened and irregular. Increased erythema is seen on the background. **c**, **f** Severe rejection of the small bowel graft. Villus architecture is completely destroyed and the surface epithelium is lost. (Reprinted from XX, with permission)

and treatment of acute cellular rejection (Fig. 14.**2**).[13,14] Biopsy is confirmatory.

Patients are fed crystalloids via a feeding tube from the third or fourth postoperative day. If tolerated, enteral feeding is started, followed by switching to oral intake. Surveillance endoscopy is performed twice a week for the first four weeks and then weekly thereafter. In pediatric patients, weight gain on enteral feeds is a sign of a satisfactorily functioning graft, an event that is usually catastrophic.

Early Complications

Graft Thrombosis

Vascular thrombosis presents as a dusky looking stoma and absence of peristalsis. An immediate ultrasound scan is obtained to confirm vascular patency. Reexploration is necessary if there is thrombosis of the major vessel supplying the graft.

Graft Rejection

In acute rejection the stoma can undergo changes in color, and this is often associated with a reduction or a sudden increase in stomal output or bleeding. Rejection also causes the stoma to become friable, erythematous, and edematous. Rejection is often associated with abdominal pain, distension, nausea, and vomiting. Immediate enteroscopy through the stoma can establish a diagnosis of rejection based on the gross appearance[13–15] (Fig. 14.**2**).

Gastrointestinal Bleeding

Gastrointestinal bleeding occurs in cases of severe uncontrollable rejection leading to sloughing and ulceration of the mucosa. Translocation may lead to septic shock or respiratory distress syndrome. Gastrointestinal bleeding may also result from coagulopathy as a result of liver dysfunction and fibrinolysis, especially in patients receiving combined liver and small bowel grafts. Treatment consists of infusion of blood products. Occasionally primary nonfunction of the liver may develop, requiring retransplantation.

Enteric Leak

This can occur at the proximal or distal anastomosis. Treatment consists of reexploration and repair of dehiscence. Early diagnosis is essential.

Biliary Leak

In standard liver–small bowel grafts the biliary enteric anastomosis can break down, resulting in biliary peritonitis. The presence of bile in the abdominal drains confirms the diagnosis. Immediate reexploration and revision of the anastomosis is mandatory.

Infections

Complications resulting from infections are high in small bowel transplant patients, owing to the degree of immunosuppression to which patients are subjected and which predisposes them to both bacterial and fungal infections. The first sign of infection should prompt for a thorough search for an intra-abdominal abscess or phlegmon. Reexploration and drainage can be lifesaving. Cytomegalovirus infections are common in small bowel transplant patients. Treatment is with intravenous ganciclovir together with cytomegalovirus-specific immune globulin (Cytogam).

■ ***Summary points:***

- Small bowel transplantation is indicated for intestinal failure due to short gut syndrome and certain motility disorders.
- The liver is also transplanted if there is biopsy-proven cirrhosis, portal hypertension, or biochemical dysfunction.
- The donor should not weigh more than 20% more than the recipient.
- Strict postoperative fluid monitoring is mandatory.
- Observation of the stoma, videoendoscopy, and biopsy are used to diagnose rejection.
- Expected survival is 72% at one year and 48% at five years.

Late Complications

Post-transplant Lymphoproliferative Disease

Post-transplant lymphoproliferative disease (PTLD) can occur in these patients.[16] Presenting features include lymphadenopathy, nonspecific systemic symptoms, and gastrointestinal bleeding, depending upon the organ involved. Treatment includes a reduction or withdrawal of immunosuppression and the administration of antiviral ganciclovir. High-grade PTLD requires immunotherapy with anti-CD20 antibody and chemotherapy. Serial monitoring of Epstein–Barr virus titers in serum by polymerase chain reaction is helpful in monitoring progress of PTLD.[17]

Graft-Versus-Host Disease

Graft-versus-host disease is a manifestation of passenger leukocytes leaving the graft, colonizing the recipient, and generating an immune response. It can present as skin rash, diarrhea, and fever. Skin biopsy confirms the diagnosis. Treatment consists of optimizing tacrolimus levels and maintaining immunosuppression.

Chronic Rejection

Chronic rejection can present several months to years after small bowel transplantation. Presenting features include diarrhea, gut failure, and weight loss. Barium studies show a diffuse tubular gut with strictures and loss of the absorptive surface (Fig. 14.**3**). Biopsy shows fibrosis and chronic arteriolar changes.

Future Directions

The field of small bowel transplantation is evolving continuously. To circumvent organ shortage, living related donor small bowel transplantation is being practiced at a few centers. Strategies to reduce the number of lymphocytes transplanted with the graft (and hence the incidence of GVHD) are being developed. These include OKT3 administration to the donor or in vitro irradiation of the graft following procurement and before implantation. Attempts at increasing chimerism and hence tolerance are being made by the transfusion of donor bone marrow during the peritransplant period in clinical trials.

Newer immunosuppressive agents such as IL-2R antibodies and rapamycin are being introduced. The overall survival rates in the largest series of patients have been 72% and 48% at one and five years respectively, with full nutritional support having been achieved in 91% of the survivors. Small bowel transplantation has now become the standard of care and an established therapeutic modality for patients with short gut syndrome. It requires a dedicated team and the highest degree of cooperation from patients and their families in order for it to be successful.

References

1. Lillehei RC, Goott B, Miller FA. The physiologic response of the small bowel of the dog to ischemia including prolonged in vitro preservation of the bowel with successful replacement and survival. Ann Surg 1959;150:543–60.
2. Starzl TE, Kaupp HA Jr. Mass homotransplantations of abdominal organs in dogs. Surg Forum 1960;11:28–30.
3. Starzl TE, Rowe M, Todo S, et al. Transplantation of multiple abdominal viscera. JAMA 1989;261:1449–57
4. Kato T, Romero R, Verzaro R, Misiakos E, Khan FA, Pinna AD, et al. Inclusion of entire pancreas in the composite liver and intestinal graft in pediatric intestinal transplantation. Pediatr Transpl 1999;3:210–4.

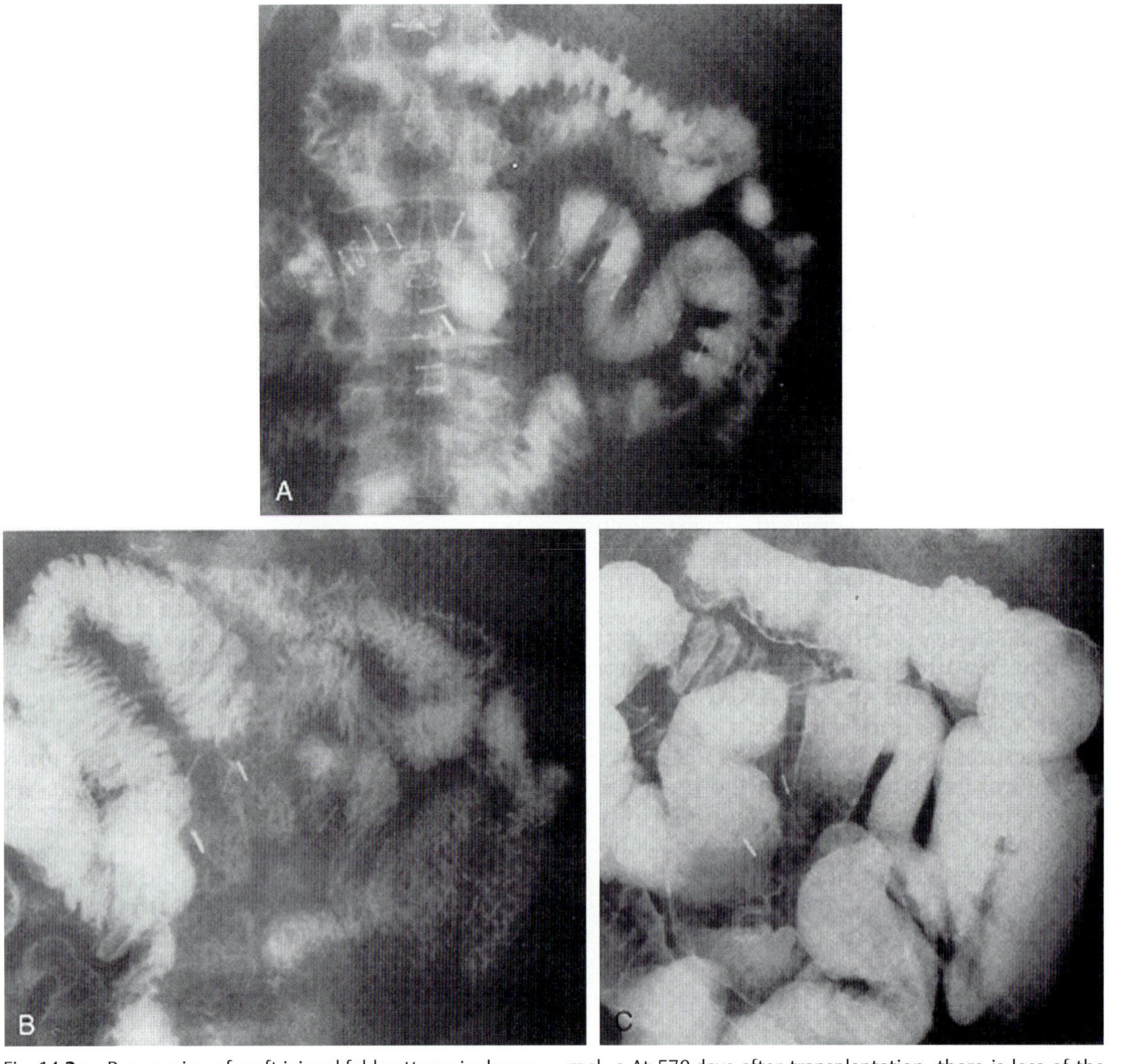

Fig. 14.**3a** Progression of graft jejunal fold patterns is shown on three small bowel series in a 31-year-old man who underwent intestinal transplantation for short gut syndrome. **a** Thick jejunal mucosal folds consistent with preservation injury are seen 22 days after transplantation. **b** At 29 days after transplantation, the mucosal fold pattern has reverted to normal. **c** At 570 days after transplantation, there is loss of the mucosal fold pattern caused by chronic and acute rejection and infection. The graft was eventually removed at 667 days after transplantation because of marked chronic rejection and irreversible graft failure. (From Campbell et al.,[18] with permission)

5. Masetti M, Rodriguez MM, Thompson JF, Pinna AD, Kato T, Romaguera RL, et al. Multivisceral transplantation for megacystis microcolon intestinal hypoperistalsis syndrome. Transplantation 1999;68:228–32.
6. Reyes J, Bueno J, Kocoshis S, Green M, Abu-Elmagd K, Furukawa H, et al. Current status of intestinal transplantation in children. J Pediatr Surg 1998;33:243–54.
7. Bueno J, Abu-Elmagd K, Mazariegos G, Madariaga J, Fung J, Reyes J. Composite liver–small bowel allografts with preservation of donor duodenum and hepatic biliary system in children. J Pediatr Surg 2000;35:291–5; discussion 295–6.
8. Abu-Elmagd KM, Reyes J, Fung JJ, Mazariegos G, Bueno J, Martin D, et al. Clinical intestinal transplantation in 1998: Pittsburgh experience. Acta Gastroenterol Belg 1999;62: 244–7.
9. Pinna AD, Weppler D, Nery JR, Khan F, Ruiz P, Kato T, et al. Induction therapy for clinical intestinal transplantation: comparison of four different regimens. Transplant Proc 2000;32:1193–4.
10. Abu-Elmagd K, Fung J, McGhee W, Martin D, Mazariegos G, Schaefer N, et al. The efficacy of daclizumab for intestinal transplantation: preliminary report. Transplant Proc 2000;32:1195–6.
11. Pappas PA, Weppler D, Pinna AD, Rusconi P, Thompson JF, Jaffe JS, Tzakis AG. Sirolimus in pediatric gastrointestinal transplantation: the use of sirolimus for pediatric transplant patients with tacrolimus-related cardiomyopathy. Pediatr Transplant 2000;4:45–9.
12. Sigurdsson L, Reyes J, Kocoshis SA, Mazariegos G, Abu-Elmagd K, Green M. Bacteremia after intestinal transplanta-

tion in children correlates temporally with rejection or gastrointestinal lymphoproliferative disease. Transplantation 2000;70:302–5.

13. Kato T, O'Brien CB, Berho M, Nishida S, Levi D, Khan FA, et al. Improved rejection surveillance in intestinal transplant recipients with frequent use of zoom video endoscopy. Transplant Proc 2000;32:1200.
14. Kato T, O'Brien CB, Nishida S, Hoppe H, Gasser M, Berho M, et al. The first case report of the use of a zoom videoendoscope for the evaluation of small bowel graft mucosa in a human after intestinal transplantation. Gastrointest Endosc 1999;50:257–61.
15. Sigurdsson L, Reyes J, Putnam PE, del Rosario JF, Di Lorenzo C, Orenstein SR, et al. Endoscopies in pediatric small intestinal transplant recipients: five years experience. Am J Gastroenterol 1998;93:207–11.
16. Nalesnik M, Jaffe R, Reyes J, Mazariegos G, Fung JJ, Starzl TE, Abu-Elmagd K. Posttransplant lymphoproliferative disorders in small bowel allograft recipients. Transplant Proc 2000;32:1213.
17. Green M, Cacciarelli TV, Mazariegos GV, Sigurdsson L, Qu L, Rowe DT, Reyes J. Serial measurement of Epstein–Barr viral load in peripheral blood in pediatric liver transplant recipients during treatment for posttransplant lymphoproliferative disease. Transplantation 1998;66:1641–4.
18. Campbell WL, Abu-Elmagd K, Federle MP, Thaete FL, Furukawa H, Tzakis AG, Todo S. Contrast examination of the small bowel in patients with small-bowel transplants: findings in 16 patients. AJR Am J Roentgenol 1993;161:969–74.

Index

Note: Since the major subjects of this book are ‚abdominal transplantation' and ‚ultrasound,' entries under these terms have been kept to a minimum. Readers are advised to seek more specific entries.

K

L

M

N

O

P

R